Interdisciplinary Advances in Endocrinology

Hossein Gharib • Bagher Larijani
Mandana Hasanzad
Editors

Interdisciplinary Advances in Endocrinology

Springer

Editors
Hossein Ghárib
Division of Endocrinology
Mayo Clinic College of Medicine
Rochester, MN, USA

Mandana Hasanzad
Personalized Medicine Research Center,
Endocrinology and Metabolism Clinical
Sciences Institute
Tehran University of Medical Sciences
Tehran, Iran

Bagher Larijani
Endocrinology and Metabolism Research
Center, Endocrinology and Metabolism
Clinical Sciences Institute
Tehran University of Medical Sciences
Tehran, Iran

ISBN 978-981-95-2285-9 ISBN 978-981-95-2286-6 (eBook)
https://doi.org/10.1007/978-981-95-2286-6

This Springer imprint is published by the registered company Springer Nature Singapore Pte Ltd.
The registered company address is: 152 Beach Road, #21-01/04 Gateway East, Singapore 189721, Singapore

Acknowledgments

The successful compilation of *Interdisciplinary Advances in Endocrinology* has been made possible through the dedication, expertise, and collaborative spirit of many individuals and institutions. First and foremost, we extend our sincere appreciation to all the contributing authors whose scholarly work and commitment to excellence form the foundation of this volume. Their interdisciplinary perspectives have greatly enriched the discourse in the field of endocrinology. We would also like to acknowledge the editorial and production teams whose professionalism and attention to detail ensured the smooth preparation and publication of this work. Finally, we thank our colleagues for their continued encouragement and patience throughout the editorial process. It is our hope that this book will serve as a valuable resource for researchers, clinicians, and students, and contribute meaningfully to the ongoing evolution of endocrinology as an integrative and dynamic field.

Contents

About the Editors

Hossein Gharib a graduate of University of Michigan Medical School, has been a Professor of medicine at the Mayo Clinic College of Medicine, in Rochester, Minnesota, for the last four decades. He is widely recognized as an international authority on thyroid disorders and has published more than 200 peer-reviewed papers, lectured at more than 350 national and international endocrine events, served on the editorial boards of major endocrine journals, and has published four endocrine textbooks, including "The Thyroid Nodule," in 2017. He has received numerous awards and honors, including the Master of the American College of Physicians (MACP) and the Master of the American College of Endocrinology (MACE). He is a past president of the American Association of Clinical Endocrinology, the American College of Endocrinology, and the American Thyroid Association.

Bagher Larijani MD, FACE, has authored numerous textbooks and journal articles; with h-index of 91, he is considered one of the most renowned Iranian academics in the field of endocrinology and related clinical and basic sciences. Through the foundation of Endocrinology and Metabolism Research Institute of the Tehran University of Medical Sciences, the highest-ranking medical research center in Iran, he laid the foundation of the interdisciplinary approach to clinical medicine for the first time in the country. His main field of interest has always been developing a comprehensive and holistic approach to medicine through forging collaboration among scientists and scholars from different fields whose achievements may promote the prevention, diagnosis, and treatment of endocrine diseases. He has also contributed to many global-scale scientific projects, such as the Lancet Commission on Obesity and Climate Change.

Mandana Hasanzad is a Professor of Genetics at Tehran University of Medical Sciences whose research focuses on precision medicine, pharmacogenomics, and the integration of big data and artificial intelligence in human genomics. Her scientific work is particularly centered on noncommunicable diseases, with an emphasis on internal medicine and cardiometabolic disorders. She is the author of several peer-reviewed scientific articles and multiple academic books that contribute to the cutting edge of knowledge in genetics and personalized medicine. She leads two major research initiatives in the field of precision medicine and pharmacogenomics approach. She is a member of the International Consortium for Personalised Medicine (ICPerMed) and an active member of the Clinical Pharmacogenetics Implementation Consortium (CPIC).

Chapter 1
Historical Aspects of Endocrinology and Hormones

Bagher Larijani and Nafiseh Tavasoli

Endocrinology is the branch of medicine that studies the endocrine system, the glands and hormones that regulate various functions of the body. The history of endocrinology spans from ancient times to the present day, revealing the discoveries and developments that have shaped our understanding of this fascinating field. In this chapter, we will explore the origins and evolution of endocrinology, from the first description of Goiter and Diabetes, to the identification and synthesis of the first hormones, to the current advances and challenges in the diagnosis and treatment of endocrine disorders.

1.1 Endocrinology in Ancient Times

Endocrinology has a long and rich history that dates back to ancient times, when different civilizations observed and experimented with the effects of castration, thyroid disorders, and other endocrine phenomena. In this section, we will explore the origins of endocrinology in ancient China, Egypt, Greece, Rome, and Iran and how their discoveries and theories influenced the development of this field. We will also examine the contributions of some of the most prominent endocrinologists and researchers of the ancient world, such as Hippocrates, Galen, and Avicenna.

B. Larijani (✉) · N. Tavasoli
Endocrinology and Metabolism Research Center, Endocrinology and Metabolism Clinical Sciences Institute, Tehran University of Medical Sciences, Tehran, Iran
e-mail: Larijanib@TUMS.ac.ir

H. Gharib et al. (eds.), *Interdisciplinary Advances in Endocrinology*,
https://doi.org/10.1007/978-981-95-2286-6_1

1.1.1 China

Description of endocrine diseases in china dates back to sixteenth century BC, where Chinese physicians used burnt sponges and seaweeds for the treatment of goiter [1]. There are evidence showing that Chinese were aware of existence of sex hormones in urine of pregnant woman and even in 125 BC, they were able to extract these hormones, purify and use them for the treatment of a variety of ailments [2]. Diabetes was known in china and Chang Chung-Ching, referred to as "the Chinese Hippocrates," described polyuria, polydipsia, and loss of weight as symptoms of a specific disease in 200 AD [3].

1.1.2 Egypt

Papyrus scrolls, dating back to more than 4000 years ago, contain detailed information about various aspects of medicine, including surgery, general medicine, and dentistry. One of the most famous papyri is Ebers Papyrus, which contains prescriptions and remedies for various diseases. Some of the endocrine diseases mentioned in these papyri include goiter, diabetes, dwarfism, gigantism, and acromegaly [4]. In this papyrus, goiter is described as swelling of the neck and use of animal thyroid glands, such as those of a fox or a cat, was advised for treatment of this condition [5].

1.1.3 Greece and Rome

The ancient Greeks were the first to coin the term "endocrine," meaning secreting internally, and to propose the concept of hormones as chemical messengers. Even today, modern terms of endocrinology are dominated by the medical language of Corpus Hippocraticum [6].

Ancient Greek and Roman physicians, such as Hippocrates, Galen, and Celsus, wrote extensively about medicine and disease, and their works influenced later generations of medical practitioners.

Hippocrates (460 BC to 370 BC) was one of the first physicians to study the relationship between diet, environment, and health in the time that it was widely believed that disease is a punishment inflicted by "the gods or evil spirits" [7].

He noted that women who were obese and hairy had problems with fertility, which could be related to polycystic ovary syndrome. He also described cases of diabetes, which he called "a melting down of the flesh and limbs into urine." He attributed this disease to excessive consumption of sweet foods and drinks, and recommended a diet of barley, water, and vegetables [8].

Galen was a Greek physician, philosopher, and writer who lived in the second century AD. He is considered to be one of the most influential figures in the history of medicine, especially in the field of endocrinology. He identified seven endocrine glands: the pineal, the pituitary, the thyroid, the thymus, the pancreas, the adrenal, and the gonads. He described their functions and the diseases that resulted from their imbalance. He also performed experiments on animals to demonstrate the effects of nerves on the secretion of hormones. Galen's works on endocrinology were widely accepted and followed by physicians for over a thousand years, until they were challenged by modern discoveries in anatomy and physiology [9].

1.1.4 Iran

Endocrine diseases were known to the ancient Iranians, and during the Sassanid Empire, 4333 diseases were mentioned in the Denkard book, which is a compendium of Zoroastrian beliefs and customs during the time, some of mentioned diseases seem to correspond to Endocrine diseases [10]. These diseases are even mentioned in poetry books, for example, in the Shahnameh (The book of Kings), which is the most important book of epic poetry in Persian literature, a disease called Khajesh is mentioned, which is said to be a swelling of the throat and is consistent with goiter disease. However, the greatest advances in medical science in Iran occurred during the period of Islamic civilization, and among the greatest Iranian physicians of that period, Ibn Sina (Avicenna) and Razi (Rhazes) could be mentioned.

Rhazes

Rhazes (865 AD) was a Persian physician and the first Islamic scholar to document Diabetes as a distinct disease. He had a creative way of diagnosing diabetes; he asked patients to urinate on the sand and diagnosed patients with diabetes if their urine attacks ants. He described complications of diabetes including visual compromise and heart disease. He observed that diabetes was more common among wealthy and sedentary people; therefore, he recommended diet, exercise, moderation in lifestyle, and herbal remedies for treatment of diabetes [11].

Avicenna

Avicenna (980–1037 AD) was a Persian polymath and the most famous and influential physician and philosopher of medieval Islamic world. Avicenna considered principles of all sciences including medicine as a subset of philosophy (Hikmah in Arabic), which could be the reason why physicians at that time were called wise (Hakim in Arabic). As a result, he applied the same philosophical method, based on logical principles, to health and diseases and criticized blind acceptance of traditional ways and was an advocate of observation and experimentation. He believed that although a physician can identify a disease only by recognizing the symptoms, but understanding the cause of a disease can improve diagnosis and treatment [12]. His famous book "The Cannon of Medicine" was the main medical textbook in universities across Europe till seventeenth century [13]. It consists of five books that cover the basic principles of medicine, the properties and effects of drugs, the diagnosis and treatment of diseases, the general pathology and therapeutics, and the preparation and application of compound drugs [14]. He even stated rules and scientific principles for evaluating effectiveness and safety of medications and he can be considered as one of the pioneers of evidence-based medicine and ideological founding father of clinical trials [15]. In the third volume of the canon of medicine, Avicenna examines different organs from top to bottom, and in addition to explaining the function of each organ, he explains the diseases of that organ along with the cause, symptoms, diagnosis, and treatment. He mentions various diseases of endocrine system and suggests treatments, some of which are still useful today [16].

Diabetes mellitus and diabetes insipidus have been mentioned among the differential diagnoses that he proposed for polyuria. Avicenna had provided a detailed description of the symptoms of diabetes mellitus and also recorded the sweet taste of the urine of diabetic patients and diagnosed this disease with the help of these symptoms [17]. Until then, no one had paid attention to the complications of diabetes as much as Avicenna. He identified many complications of this disease, including diabetic gangrene, muscle wasting, and sexual dysfunction. He also discussed the kidney complications of diabetes and considered it to be the result of kidney fatigue caused by renal pores dysfunction [11]. He proposed several treatments for diabetes mellitus, the effectiveness of some of which has been proven even today, and there are even suggestions to add these treatments to the standard treatment of diabetes for better control of the disease [18, 19].

Avicenna had examined numerous other endocrine diseases as well, including obesity and its complications, amenorrhea, infertility, impotence, and orbitopathy related to thyroid disease. He also explained the diseases that could be prevented by exercising in the canon of medicine [20, 21].

1.2 Endocrinology in Modern Times

The modern era of endocrinology began in the nineteenth century. The first period of modern endocrinology was devoted to the description of endocrines. It was during this period that scientists began to describe the chemical messengers that are secreted in the body and cause systemic effects. During this period, many scientists tried to advance the science of endocrinology, and in the following, we will discuss some of the most important scientists and their achievements, which were a turning point in the science of endocrinology [22].

Arnold Berthold: He is known as the first scientist who published an endocrinology experiment. In 1849, he transplanted testes from roosters to capons and observed the morphological and behavioral changes in them, demonstrating that testes produce a substance that could affect other parts of body [23, 24].

Charles Brown-Séquard: He is famous among doctors for discovering spinal cord hemi-section syndrome, but many people are unaware of his contributions to endocrinology. In 1889, he injected himself with the extract obtained from the testicles of animals and reported that after this injection, his physical and mental function was improved. Some people know him as the father of modern endocrinology, and he was among the first to propose the idea of endocrine replacement therapy [25, 26].

George Murray: Inspired by Brown-Séquard, Murray experimented by injecting thyroid extract from a sheep to a woman with severe hypothyroidism in 1891. He reported that this experiment resulted in improvement of symptoms in this patient [27].

Ernest Starling: In 1902, Ernest Starling and William Bayliss discovered secretin and demonstrated its effects on pancreatic secretion. In 1905, Starling coined the term "*Hormone*" [28].

Identification and purification of secretin hormone started a new phase in endocrinology. This period is known as analytical endocrinology. During this period, many hormones were identified, purified, and synthesized. The most influential scientists of this period and their achievements are mentioned below:

Edward Kendall: He was a biochemist who devoted his life to identification of hormones, their structure, and synthesis. He succeeded in isolating thyroxine and cortisone in 1914 and 1936, respectively. In 1948, he and his group succeeded in producing cortisone at a high scale and tested it in clinical trials on patients with rheumatoid arthritis, with dramatic success that revolutionized the treatment of inflammatory diseases [29].

Frederick Banting and Charles Best: In 1921, Banting and Best isolated substances from pancreas extract that was able to prolong the life of diabetic dogs. In 1922, they successfully tried their treatment on a diabetic boy. Fast progression of Insulin project continued and resulted in the availability of insulin in relatively sufficient quantities to treat patients in 1923 and revolutionized diabetes treatment [30].

Edward dosing: He was a biochemist who isolated esrtrone and estriol in 1929 from hundreds of gallons of urine, which he collected from pregnant women [31].

Rosalyn Yalow and Solomon Berson: In 1958, they developed the radioimmunoassay, a technique that allows the measurement of very small amounts of substances in biological fluids, such as hormones, drugs, and antibodies. Their technique helped endocrinology to advance at a fast pace [32].

The third phase of modern endocrinology, synthetic endocrinology, began in the 1970s and continues to the present day, when the use of recombinant DNA technology, gene editing, and stem cell research has opened new possibilities for the manipulation and modulation of the endocrine system. Some of the achievements of this phase are the production of synthetic and biosynthetic hormones, such as human growth hormone, insulin, and erythropoietin; the discovery of new hormones, such as leptin, ghrelin, and adiponectin; the identification of hormone receptors and signaling pathways; and the development of hormone analogs, antagonists, and modulators, such as tamoxifen, flutamide, and somatostatin [33]. In the following, you can see the most influential scientist and discoveries of this period.

Roger Guillemin: He proved that hypothalamus regulates pituitary gland through release of hormones and he was able to discover, isolate, and analyze thyrotropin-releasing hormone (TRH), growth hormone-releasing hormone (GHRH), and somatostatin. His influential discoveries in the neuroendocrine field made him known as one of the founding fathers of this field [34].

Alfred Gilman and Martin Rodbell: In the 1960s, Rodbell discovered that an intermediary molecule functions in cells in order to relay the massage from cell's surface receptor to the amplifier within the cell, and this intermediary molecule is playing an important role in a cell's response to chemical signals. In 1970s, Gilman identified this molecule and named it G protein. Disruption in function of G protein can lead to several diseases such as diabetes. Discovery of this intermediary molecule helped in understanding the pathophysiology of different diseases and finding innovative treatments [35].

Mario Capecchi, Martin Evans, and Oliver Smithies: Their discovery of homologous recombination between DNA sequences known as gene targeting helped in generating any genotype of choice. This technology is now used in many areas of biomedicine [36].

1.3 Future of Endocrinology

The field of endocrinology is constantly evolving with new discoveries and advancements that have profound implications for human health and well-being. Some of the recent breakthroughs in endocrinology include genetic research that reveals the causes and treatments of various endocrine disorders; diabetes management that uses sophisticated technology to monitor and control blood sugar levels; hormonal therapies that offer more natural and individualized options for conditions like PCOS, menopause, and growth hormone deficiencies; and imaging and diagnostic tools that enable earlier and more accurate detection of endocrine abnormalities. These innovations have improved the quality of life and outcomes for millions of people with endocrine problems, and have also opened new avenues for research and practice. The future of endocrinology is bright and promising, as scientists and clinicians continue to explore the complex and fascinating interactions between hormones and the body. We should keep in mind that endocrinology is a dynamic and interdisciplinary field that requires constant learning and adaptation to the changing needs and challenges of the society; the integration of endocrinology with other disciplines, such as neuroscience, immunology, pharmacology, and psychology, helps us to understand the complex interactions between hormones and other biological systems. In the following, we will briefly mention some of the emerging areas in endocrinology that require more focus and research from the experts in this domain as these areas are probably the founders of the future of endocrinology.

Application of digital technologies: The application of machine learning, deep learning, and natural language processing helps us to analyze large and complex data sets, such as electronic health records, imaging, and wearable devices, that can enhance the diagnosis, prognosis, and management of endocrine conditions. Also, innovative models of care can improve the diagnosis, prevention, and treatment of endocrine diseases [37].

Regenerative Medicine: Despite the fact that endocrinologists have been able to treat most of the endocrine diseases and significantly increase the quality of life of patients, there are not many curative treatments in this field and the health of patients depends on the lifelong use of medications. Advances in Regenerative medicine can lead to cure of chronic conditions and negating the lifelong need for treatment [38].

New sources and targets of hormones: The physiological complexity of the human body is so great that there is still a long way to discover its details. New research has been able to find new hormone sources and targets such as the microbiome, the gut, the bone, and the adipose tissue. These new discoveries can help in finding the cause of diseases and new ways of treatment [39].

Personalized and precision medicine: Tailoring of medical interventions to the individual characteristics of each patient, such as genetic, environmental, and lifestyle factors, can influence the response to endocrine therapies, such as hormone replacement, oral contraceptives, and antidiabetic drugs [36]. In achieving this, omics technology, which is a comprehensive analysis of biological molecules, such as genomics, proteomics, metabolomics, and epigenomics, could be very useful by revealing the molecular mechanisms and biomarkers of endocrine diseases [40].

References

1. Niazi AK, Kalra S, Irfan A, Islam A. Thyroidology over the ages. Indian J Endocrinol Metab. 2011;15(Suppl 2):S121–6.
2. Temple R. The autumn mineral: the chinese origins of endocrinology; 1993; 1.
3. Karamanou M, Protogerou A, Tsoucalas G, Androutsos G, Poulakou-Rebelakou E. Milestones in the history of diabetes mellitus: the main contributors. World J Diabetes. 2016;7(1):1–7.
4. Carpenter S, Rigaud M, Barile M, Priest T, Perez L, Ferguson J. An interlinear transliteration and English translation of portions of the Ebers papyrus possibly having to do with diabetes mellitus. Annandale-on-Hudson: Bard College; 1998.
5. Hallmann-Mikołajczak A. Ebers papyrus. The book of medical knowledge of the 16th century B.C. Egyptians. Arch Hist Filoz Med. 2004;67(1):5–14.
6. Poulakou-Rebelakou E, Marketos SG. Endocrine terminology in corpus hippocraticum. Hormones. 2002;1(1):57–8.
7. Hawley JA, Gibala MJ. What's new since Hippocrates? Preventing type 2 diabetes by physical exercise and diet. Diabetologia. 2012;55(3):535–9.
8. Sellers C. 450 health, work, and environment: a Hippocratic turn in medical history. In: Jackson M, editor. The Oxford handbook of the history of medicine. Oxford University Press; 2011.
9. Johnston I. 765 Galen and his system of medicine. In: Keyser PT, Scarborough J, editors. Oxford handbook of science and medicine in the classical world. Oxford University Press; 2018.
10. Gordon BL, Neuburger M. Medicine throughout antiquity: F.A. Davis; 1949.
11. Fleifel M, Fleifel B, El Alam A. Diabetes mellitus across the Arabo-Islamic world: a revolution. Int J Endocrinol. 2023;2023:5541808.
12. Zahabi SA. Avicenna's approach to health: a reciprocal interaction between medicine and Islamic philosophy. J Relig Health. 2019;58(5):1698–712.
13. Moosavi J. The place of avicenna in the history of medicine. Avicenna J Med Biotechnol. 2009;1(1):3–8.
14. Mahdizadeh S, Khaleghi Ghadiri M, Gorji A. Avicenna's canon of medicine: a review of analgesics and anti-inflammatory substances. Avicenna J Phytomed. 2015;5(3):182–202.

15. Shoja MM, Rashidi MR, Tubbs RS, Etemadi J, Abbasnejad F, Agutter PS. Legacy of Avicenna and evidence-based medicine. Int J Cardiol. 2011;150(3):243–6.
16. A Treatise on the Canon of Medicine of Avicenna. Incorporating a translation of the first book; 1984.
17. Nabipour I. Clinical endocrinology in the Islamic civilization in Iran. Int J Endocrinol Metab. 2003;1(1)
18. Boghrati Z, Emami SA, Akaberi M. An evidence-based review of medicinal plants prescribed by Avicenna for management of diabetes. In: Medicinal plants used in traditional persian medicine; 2023. p. 281–7.
19. Sharofova M, Nuraliev Y, Sukhrobov P, Sagdieva S, Dushenkov V. Can Avicenna help manage the diabetes epidemic in Central Asia? 2017.
20. Nabipour I, Burger A, Moharreri M-R, Azizi F. Avicenna, the first to describe thyroid-related orbitopathy. Thyroid. 2009;19(1):7–8.
21. Siahpoosh M, Ebadiani M, Hosseini GS, Isfahani M, Nasrabadi AN, Dadgostar H. Avicenna the first to describe diseases which may be prevented by exercise. Iran J Public Health. 2012;41(11):98.
22. Bahadoran Z, Mirmiran P, Azizi F, Ghasemi A. A brief history of modern endocrinology and definitions of a true hormone. Endocrine Metabolic Immune Disorders-Drug Targets. 2019;19(8):1116–21.
23. Weil ZM, Nelson RJ. Arnold Adolph Berthold. In: Biographical history of behavioral neuroendocrinology. Springer; 2022. p. 1–5.
24. Berthold AA, Quiring D. The transplantation of testes. Bull Hist Med. 1944;16(4):399–401.
25. Rengachary SS, Colen C, Guthikonda M. Charles-Edouard Brown-Séquard: an eccentric genius. Neurosurgery. 2008;62(4):954–64.
26. Brown-Séquard CÉ. On a new therapeutic method consisting in the use of organic liquids extracted from glands and other organs. Br Med J. 1893;1(1693):1212.
27. Murray GR. Note on the treatment of myxoedema by hypodermic injections of an extract of the thyroid gland of a sheep. Br Med J. 1891;2(1606):796.
28. Modlin IM, Kidd M, Farhadi J. Bayliss and Starling and the nascence of endocrinology. Regul Pept. 2000;93(1–3):109–23.
29. Simoni RD, Hill RL, Vaughan M. The isolation of thyroxine and cortisone: the work of Edward C. Kendall. J Biol Chem. 2002;277(21):21–2.
30. Simoni RD, Hill RL, Vaughan M. The discovery of insulin: the work of Frederick banting and Charles best. J Biol Chem. 2002;277(26):e1–2.
31. Simoni RD, Hill RL, Vaughan M. The discovery of estrone, estriol, and estradiol and the biochemical study of reproduction. The work of Edward Adelbert Doisy. J Biol Chem. 2002;277(28):e1–2.
32. Friedman A. Remembrance: the Berson and Yalow Saga. J Clin Endocrinol Metabol. 2002;87(5):1925–8.
33. Kleine B, Rossmanith WG. History of hormones and endocrinology. Hormones and the endocrine system: textbook of endocrinology. Cham: Springer International Publishing; 2016. p. 3–8.
34. Brazeau P, Vale W, Burgus R, Ling N, Butcher M, Rivier J, et al. Hypothalamic polypeptide that inhibits the secretion of immunoreactive pituitary growth hormone. Science. 1973;179(4068):77–9.
35. Gilman AG. G proteins: transducers of receptor-generated signals. Annu Rev Biochem. 1987;56(1):615–49.
36. Capecchi MR. The new mouse genetics: altering the genome by gene targeting. Trends Genet. 1989;5:70–6.
37. Gubbi S, Hamet P, Tremblay J, Koch CA, Hannah-Shmouni F. Artificial intelligence and machine learning in endocrinology and metabolism: the dawn of a new era. Front Endocrinol. 2019;10:185.

38. Zerón HM, Juárez AH, Hernández JV. Stem cells in endocrinology: facts and future. Front Stem Cell Regenerat Med Res. 2018;8:150–67.
39. Neuman H, Debelius JW, Knight R, Koren O. Microbial endocrinology: the interplay between the microbiota and the endocrine system. FEMS Microbiol Rev. 2015;39(4):509–21.
40. Karahalil B. Overview of systems biology and omics technologies. Curr Med Chem. 2016;23(37):4221–30.

Chapter 2
Genetics of Metabolic Diseases

Mahsa M.Amoli, Forough Taheri, Akram Goharifar, Mehri Safari, and Arash Salmaninejad

2.1 Newborn Genetic Screening of Inherited Metabolic Disorders

Newborn screening is a population-wide screening approach used to identify newborns that may have metabolic, endocrine, and other disorders. The purpose is to detect these conditions early on so that prompt treatment can be provided, preventing severe complications and symptoms of the disease. Inclusion of a condition in the screening panel is determined by a set of criteria established by the World Health Organization in 1968, known as the Wilson and Jungner principles. To be included, a condition must have a test available that demonstrates appropriate sensitivity and specificity [5]. Additionally, there must be clear evidence of the benefits that early detection and timely intervention bring. Each criterion must be carefully considered, taking into account its impact on both affected and unaffected individuals. In

M. M.Amoli (✉)
Metabolic Disorders Research Centre, Endocrinology and Metabolism Molecular-Cellular Sciences Institute, Tehran University of Medical Sciences, Tehran, Iran
e-mail: amolimm@tums.ac.ir

F. Taheri
Endocrinology and Metabolism Research Center, Endocrinology and Metabolism Clinical Sciences Institute, Tehran University of Medical Sciences, Tehran, Iran

A. Goharifar
Department of Prosthodontics, School of Dentistry, Islamic Azad University, Isfahan, Iran

M. Safari
Operative Dentistry Specialist, Department of Operative Dentistry, Dental school, Islamic Azad University of Isfahan branch, Isfahan, Iran

A. Salmaninejad
Faculty of Medicine, Department of Medical Genetic, Guilan University of Medical Sciences, Guilan, Iran

H. Gharib et al. (eds.), *Interdisciplinary Advances in Endocrinology*,
https://doi.org/10.1007/978-981-95-2286-6_2

2006, the American College of Medical Genetics put forth a list of 29 core conditions that were endorsed by the Secretary Advisory Committee for Heritable Diseases in Newborns and Children (SACHDNC). These conditions formed the Recommended Uniform Screening Panel (RUSP). The RUSP is regularly updated by the SACHDNC using an evidence-based protocol to propose and approve new conditions. As of now, the RUSP encompasses 35 core conditions and 26 secondary conditions. While newborn screening panels include a variety of disorders, the majority (around 80%) are metabolic disorders [5–7].

Newborn screening programs employ various methods that are designed to directly measure or detect metabolites, assess enzyme activity, or analyze DNA. Typically, these tests are conducted at a centralized laboratory. In addition, screening for certain conditions like critical congenital heart disease and hearing loss requires functional tests that are performed at the birthing facility [8, 9]. The earliest method used for newborn screening can be traced back to the 1960s when screening for phenylketonuria (PKU) began using a bacterial inhibition assay called the Guthrie test. However, technological advancements, particularly in tandem mass spectrometry, have replaced this method and have enabled the expansion of newborn screening programs. Presently, more than 40 metabolic disorders can be screened by using blood samples obtained from a filter paper card, commonly known as a "Guthrie card." This screening method involves measuring a combination of amino acids and acylcarnitines, requiring only 2–4 min of instrument time [10–12].

Earlier studies primarily focused on evaluating the performance of genetic sequencing for inborn errors of metabolism disorders that had already been screened using tandem mass spectrometry [13–15]. However, there has been limited investigation into the clinical impact of genetic sequencing for G6PD deficiency, which is significant in neonates and prevalent in certain regions [16]. These studies provide valuable insights into the performance of genetic screening for commonly occurring metabolic disorders.

Specifically, genetic newborn screening (NBS) exhibited a sensitivity of 100% in detecting G6PD deficiency, surpassing the sensitivity of the fluorometric assay, which was only 96.95%. Notably, the positive predictive value (PPV) of genetic NBS was 47.61%, and it was notably influenced by sex, with a PPV of 99.30% in male patients and 11.36% in female patients. This discrepancy can be attributed to the fact that most female newborns with a heterozygous variant in G6PD exhibit normal G6PD activity due to skewed X-chromosome inactivation [17].

Taken together, these findings suggest that genetic screening has the potential to complement biochemical NBS in terms of detection capability, but it cannot replace it as a universal NBS program, especially for disorders with variable penetrance. Follow-up tests are crucial for the implementation of genetic NBS in clinical practice. Understanding the phase and origin of pathogenic variants is essential for clinical counseling and is valuable for future reproductive planning among family members.

2.2 New Era in Genetic Testing of Metabolic Disorders Using NGS Technology

The identification of nucleotide changes through genomic sequencing serves as the underlying cause of monogenic disorders. This approach holds promise in reducing the false-positive rate of newborn screening (NBS) and expediting case resolution [18]. Furthermore, sequencing-based screening tests have the potential to identify disorders that currently lack an available NBS assay. However, the cost of genomic sequencing has been a subject of criticism [18, 19].

A study conducted in 2020 reported that genomic screening alone could not replace biochemical NBS due to its inadequate sensitivity. However, the potential benefits of incorporating sequencing-based screening as a first-tier test into the existing NBS program remain uncertain [20]. Despite several research groups investigating its utility, these studies had two main limitations. First, genomic screening was always employed as a second-tier test for high-risk infants who initially tested positive in biochemical NBS. The impact of genomic testing as a first-tier screening test for the general population was not determined. Second, these studies suffered from small sample sizes [21]. Given the rarity of monogenic disorders, a sufficiently large sample is necessary, but only a few population-scale studies have been reported. It is important to note that most of these studies utilized whole-exome or genome sequencing, which is not universally applicable in clinical settings due to its high current cost. To strike a balance between cost and the number of genes analyzed, gene panels that target specific genomic regions have emerged as an alternative solution [22]. This approach offers a compromise, allowing for efficient testing of relevant genes. Chen et al. implemented a gene panel as a first-tier screening test, demonstrating a sensitivity of 73.91% and a specificity of 99.98% in screening for amino acid, organic acid, and fatty acid oxidation disorders in a general newborn population. Although the specific disorders screened for may vary across different studies, the performance of the gene panel was comparable to that of whole-exome sequencing, which exhibited an overall sensitivity of 88% and specificity of 98.4% [8, 23].

2.3 Genetic Causes of Diseases of Amino Acid and Peptide Metabolism

Enzyme defects in the pathways involved in the synthesis and breakdown of amino acids are responsible for a group of diseases. These defects result in the accumulation of certain amino acids or their by-products, while causing deficiencies in other amino acids. As a consequence, these accumulated substances enter other metabolic cycles, ultimately leading to the production of various substances like urea and ammonia through decomposition [24]. The excessive build-up of these biological substances adversely affects the growth and development of infants, resulting in varying degrees of mental retardation. Fortunately, many diseases within this group can be identified early through newborn screening, which can help prevent damage to the brain and other vital organs [25, 26]. Amino acids serve as crucial building blocks of proteins, with a total of 20 different types found within protein structures. Additionally, there are other amino acids present in the body that act as metabolic intermediates for other amino acids. Deficiencies in the synthesis and metabolism of these amino acids contribute to the development of certain diseases. Among all amino-acid-related metabolic disorders, phenylketonuria (PKU) holds a prominent position. In 1953, Jervis first identified PKU as the first known disease caused by an enzyme defect [26, 27].

2.4 Metabolism of Side Chain Amino Acids

Within this particular group of diseases, maple syrup urine disease (MSUD) can occur as a result of defects in the metabolism of three essential amino acids: leucine, isoleucine, and valine. MSUD is inherited in an autosomal recessive manner. Autosomal recessive disorders manifest when an individual inherits two nonfunctioning genes for the disease, one from each parent. If an individual inherits one functioning gene and one nonfunctioning gene, they become carriers of the disease but typically do not display symptoms themselves [28, 29].

2.5 Metabolism of Phenylalanine and Tyrosine

Phenylalanine and tyrosine are located in a common biochemical pathway, which can occur as a result of defects in this cycle.

2.5.1 Phenylketonuria (PKU)

Phenylketonuria (PKU), a hereditary metabolic disease, is characterized by an excessive accumulation of a specific amino acid in the bloodstream. The conversion of phenylalanine to tyrosine involves two enzymes: phenylalanine hydroxylase I and II. Enzyme I relies on biopterin, a derivative of folic acid, as a cofactor for hydrogen transfer, while enzyme II requires NADPH [18]. Tetrahydrobiopterin (BH4) plays a crucial role in this metabolic pathway and is oxidized to quinonoid dihydrobiopterin (qBH2) during phenylalanine oxidation and tyrosine formation. Tetrahydrobiopterin is obtained through two routes: biopterin biosynthesis, which involves the enzyme pyruvoyltetrahydropterin synthase converting

7,8-dihydroneopterin triphosphate into biopterin, and biopterin regeneration, which occurs via dihydriopteridine reductase converting quinonoid dihydrobiopterin to tetrahydrobiopterin or dihydrofolate reductase converting dihydrobiopterin to tetrahydrobiopterin. In the normal pathway, phenylalanine is converted to phenylpyruvic acid with the assistance of a transaminase enzyme and alpha-ketoglutaric acid [30, 31]. Excess phenylalanine is then converted to tyrosine, easily eliminated through the kidneys. Phenylpyruvic acid can be transformed into phenylacetic acid through a decarboxylase enzyme or reduced to phenyllactic acid via a dehydrogenase enzyme, and these three acids, known as ketone bodies, are excreted through the kidneys. Classic phenylketonuria arises from a deficiency of phenylalanine hydroxylase I enzyme. Therefore, PKU can be classified into three subgroups: classic phenylketonuria disease caused by the lack of phenylalanine hydroxylase I enzyme, biopterin defect in cofactor biosynthesis (BIOPT-BS) or pyruvoyltetrahydropterin synthase deficiency, which is a very rare disease with a prevalence of 1 in a million, and biopterin defects in cofactor regeneration (BIOPT-REG) or dihydriopteridine reductase deficiency, also a very rare disease with a prevalence of 1 in a million [31–33].

2.5.2 Genetics and Mode of Inheritance of PKU

The assignment of the PAH gene to human chromosome 12 (12q22-12q24.2) was carried out by Lidsky et al. in 1984, and the molecular structure of the gene was finally determined in 1986 [18, 34]. The gene's DNA size is 79.28 kb, and it consists of 13 exons (NG_008690.1, NT_029419.13, NC_018923.2, NC_000012.12). The distribution of exons is uneven, with the second half of the gene having compact exons while the first half has larger introns separating the exons. Transcription occurs on the reverse strand, and only one isoform has been identified. The mature mRNA is 2680 bp in length (NM_000277.1) [35], while the coding sequence (CDS) is 1359 bp [36]. The 5' untranslated region was characterized by Konecki et al. in 1992 [37]. A transcription cap site is located 154 nucleotides upstream of the first ATG codon. The promoter region lacks a proximal TATA box but contains GC boxes, CACCC boxes, CCAAT boxes, activator protein 2 sites, partial glucocorticoid response elements, and partial cyclic AMP response elements consensus sequence. This suggests that the human PAH gene has a TATA-less promoter regulated by multiple transcription factors. The genomic DNA sequence contains three polyadenylation signals [AATAAA] in exon 13. The PAH gene has the ID 5053 [37]. This disease is inherited as an autosomal recessive trait. That is, for the baby to have this disease, he must have received a defective gene from each of his parents (in other words, the parents of this baby each have a copy of the defective gene, but because they also have a copy of the healthy gene, therefore they do not show symptoms) [18, 38, 39].

2.5.3 *Prevalence of Phenylketonuria*

The prevalence of PKU disease in the United States is approximately one out of every 10,000 to 15,000 babies born. However, due to universal screening for PKU in newborns since the 1960s, the number of cases with symptoms has decreased. Among specific countries, the highest reported prevalence of PKU is in Turkey, with a rate of 1 in 2600. Ireland follows with a prevalence of 1 in 4500, and Scotland with a prevalence of 1 in 5300. In Iran, the prevalence of PKU is 1 in 5000, resulting in an annual occurrence of approximately 300 to 400 babies born with PKU in the country [39, 40].

2.5.4 *Alkaptonuria*

Alkaptonuria is a hereditary metabolic disease resulting from a deficiency of the enzyme homogentisic acid oxidase in the phenylalanine-tyrosine metabolic pathway. This disorder follows an autosomal recessive pattern of inheritance. The absence of homogentisic acid oxidase disrupts the metabolism of phenylalanine and tyrosine during the homogentisic acid stage, leading to the accumulation of homogentisic acid in the body [4, 41, 42].

2.6 Types Metabolism of Sulfur-Containing Amino Acids

Homocystinuria is a disorder belonging to this group of diseases. It is inherited in an autosomal recessive manner and is characterized by various symptoms and complications. Individuals with homocystinuria may experience learning disabilities, sudden neurological attacks, increased blood clotting tendency (thrombophilia), osteoporosis, scoliosis, and elongated fingers and toes (arachnodactyly). These clinical features are commonly associated with this condition [43, 44].

2.7 Carbohydrate Metabolism Disorders

Congenital disorders of carbohydrate metabolism encompass various subgroups. These subgroups include intolerance diseases such as lactose intolerance and rarer disaccharide intolerance diseases, as well as the large group of glycogen storage diseases. Intolerance diseases involve deficiencies in enzymes responsible for digesting specific sugars like lactose or disaccharides. Glycogen storage diseases, on the other hand, are characterized by defects in enzymes or transport proteins related to glycogen metabolism. Galactosemia is another subgroup where individuals cannot metabolize galactose properly. Disorders of fructose metabolism involve difficulties in processing fructose, leading to severe symptoms upon consumption. Pentose phosphate pathway disorders encompass abnormalities in the metabolism of pentose phosphate pathway intermediates. Each subgroup represents a distinct set of congenital abnormalities with unique biochemical, genetic, and clinical characteristics [45–47].

2.7.1 Classical Galactosomia

Galactosomia is an autosomal recessive disease caused by a defect in the enzyme galactose 1-phosphate uridyltransferase. This enzyme is needed by the body for the metabolism and digestion of oral galactose sugar. People who have a defect in the gene responsible for making this enzyme have increased amounts of galactose in their blood and body fluids. Affected infants show symptoms such as vomiting, lethargy, growth failure, and jaundice during the second week after birth. Without treatment, eventually the disease will lead to mental retardation, cataracts and liver cirrhosis. To treat these babies, it is necessary to use lactose-free milk. Lactose breaks down in the body into glucose and galactose. The presence of galactosemia can be detected in newborn screening [48, 49].

2.7.2 Hereditary Fructose Intolerance

Hereditary fructose intolerance is an autosomal recessive disease caused by a defect in the fructose 1-phosphate aldolase enzyme. Fructose sugar is found in abundance in honey, fruits, and vegetables. Affected people are identified at different ages and depending on when this sugar is introduced into their diet. The symptoms are usually mild, but they can be more severe in some cases and include vomiting, jaundice, and convulsions. By controlling the amount of fructose in the patient's food, the disease can be managed well [50].

2.7.3 Glycogen Storage Disorders

Glycogen is a storage form of glucose in muscles and liver, which is formed as a polymer (chain) of glucose molecules. This substance is broken down when needed by the body and turns into glucose and is used by muscles and other tissues. Several different enzymes are involved in the production and breakdown of glycogen, and the disruption of any of them can lead to one of the types of glycogen storage diseases (GSD). In total, about 30 types of glycogen storage disease are known, the most important of which are Von Gierke's disease, Pompe disease, Cori disease, McArdle disease, and hepatic phosphorylase deficiency [46, 51, 52].

2.8 Steroid Metabolism Disorders

Steroid metabolism disorders include a number of autosomal recessive congenital disorders related to cortisol biosynthesis pathways. These disorders can cause masculinization (virilization) along with the loss of solutes in both male and female patients due to aldosterone hormone deficiency. Also, in this group, androgen receptor defects lead to the absence of male reproductive organs in embryos with 46, XY karyotype, and their appearance will be female [53].

2.8.1 Congenital Adrenal Hyperplasia (CAH)

Congenital adrenal hyperplasia (CAH) is a group of hereditary disorders that occurs due to a defect in one of the enzymes that produce sex hormones and is the most common cause of genital ambiguity. More than 90% of the cases of this disease occur due to the lack of 21-hydroxylase enzyme, which leads to a decrease in cortisol production with or without a decrease in aldosterone and ultimately an increase in male sex hormones from the adrenal cortex [54].

2.8.2 Types of 21-Hydroxylase Enzyme Defects

Depending on the severity of 21-hydroxylase enzyme deficiency, there is a wide range of clinical symptoms, ranging from classic or severe types to non-classic or mild types. The CYP21 gene, located on the short arm of chromosome 6, encodes the enzyme 21 hydroxylase, and so far, more than 60 different types of disease-causing mutations have been identified on it [55].

2.8.3 Molecular Diagnosis of CAH Disease

The primary objective of molecular analysis for congenital adrenal hyperplasia (CAH) is to enable prenatal diagnosis and prevent complications associated with the disease, such as genital ambiguity and potentially fatal adrenal hematoma. To achieve this, families with a first-born child are initially screened for the disease-causing mutation in family members. Once a subsequent pregnancy is confirmed, treatment with dexamethasone is initiated in the mother starting from the 5th to 6th week of pregnancy. Additionally, chorionic villus sampling (CVS) is performed between the 10th and 12th week of pregnancy. If the fetus is determined to be female, treatment continues until the end of the pregnancy. Another target group for molecular diagnosis includes patients with nonclassic forms of CAH. Unfortunately, due to the disorder's high prevalence, delayed manifestations, and symptom similarity with other causes of hyperandrogenism, it often does not receive adequate attention. By considering the specific disease and identifying the responsible mutations, prenatal diagnosis for the children of these patients can also be facilitated [55–57].

2.8.4 *Androgen Insensitivity (Feminization of the Testicles)*

Androgen insensitivity syndrome (AIS) is a condition in which an individual, who is genetically male, with one X chromosome and one Y chromosome, is resistant to male hormones known as androgens. Consequently, the person possesses some physical characteristics of a woman despite having the genetic makeup of a man [58]. AIS is caused by a genetic defect on the X chromosome, impairing the body's ability to respond to androgen hormones responsible for male development. The syndrome is categorized into two main types: complete AIS and partial AIS. In complete AIS, the individual does not develop a penis or other male reproductive organs. At birth, they typically appear as female [59]. The incidence of complete AIS is approximately 1 in 20,000 live births. On the other hand, individuals with partial AIS exhibit varying degrees of male traits. Partial AIS can also present with additional abnormalities, such as undescended testicles (cryptorchidism), hypospadias (abnormally placed urethral opening), and other associated features. Individuals with partial AIS may display a combination of masculine and feminine physical characteristics, including a partially closed external vagina, an enlarged clitoris, and a shortened vagina. Some may have a vagina but lack a cervix or uterus, while others may exhibit testicles in the abdomen or uncommon locations. Inguinal hernia, where the testicles can be felt during physical examination and normal development of female breasts may also be observed [60, 61]. Diagnostic tests for AIS include blood tests to assess testosterone, luteinizing hormone (LH), and follicle-stimulating hormone (FSH) levels. Genetic testing, such as karyotyping, is performed to determine the individual's specific genetic makeup. Pelvic ultrasound may be conducted, and additional blood tests might be employed to differentiate between AIS and androgen deficiency. It is important to note that the features and manifestations of AIS can vary among individuals, and a multidisciplinary approach involving medical professionals from various specialties is often necessary for diagnosis and management [58, 60, 62].

2.9 Disorders of Lipoprotein and Lipid (Fat) Metabolism

The group of disorders involving the metabolism of lipids (fats) and lipoproteins encompasses a diverse array of diseases in which the processing of cholesterol, triglycerides, and lipoproteins is disrupted. These conditions are significant, because their impact is closely associated with the development of cardiovascular diseases [63, 64].

2.9.1 Familial Hypercholesterolemia

Familial hypercholesterolemia is the most common disorder associated with lipid metabolism, characterized by significantly elevated levels of LDL (bad cholesterol). Since this condition is inherited, it manifests from birth and can increase the risk of heart attacks even at a young age, particularly for individuals who inherit the defective gene from both parents [65]. Prompt treatment of familial hypercholesterolemia is crucial as untreated cases may result in premature death by the age of 20. The primary approaches for managing this condition involve drug therapy and lifestyle modifications under the supervision of a cardiologist. Genetic testing can aid in diagnosing familial hypercholesterolemia, although it may not always be necessary and is usually recommended for at-risk family members. In cases where one parent has familial hypercholesterolemia, there is a 50% chance of their child inheriting the defective gene, while inheriting the altered gene from both parents increases the likelihood of a more severe form of the disease [66, 67]. It is advisable for individuals diagnosed with familial hypercholesterolemia to have their first-degree relatives, such as siblings, parents, and children, assessed for the condition to initiate appropriate treatment. The LDLR, APOB, and PCSK9 genes are commonly associated with familial hypercholesterolemia, although researchers have identified over 2000 gene mutations responsible for causing this condition [67].

2.10 Disorders of Fatty Acid Metabolism and Ketobodies and Lipids

This category of diseases primarily encompasses a range of disorders related to the transfer and metabolism of carnitine, a molecule essential for the transportation of long-chain fatty acids into or out of mitochondria. Numerous significant diseases fall within this group, each characterized by specific defects in carnitine-related processes [68, 69].

2.10.1 *Deficiency of Carnitine Palmitoyl Transferase ll (CPTll)*

Carnitine palmitoyl transferase (CPT) deficiency is a disorder that hinders the body's ability to utilize specific fats for energy, particularly during fasting periods [70, 71]. There are three types of CPT II defects: fatal neonatal type, severe hepatocardiomuscular neonatal type, and myopathic type. The fatal neonatal form of the disease typically emerges shortly after birth, with affected infants experiencing respiratory failure, seizures, liver failure, cardiomyopathy (weakened heart muscle), arrhythmia (irregular heartbeat), hypoglycemia (low blood sugar), and reduced ketone production. These symptoms collectively referred to as hypoctotic hypoglycemia. Structural abnormalities may also affect the brain and kidneys, and babies with the fatal neonatal type typically have a lifespan of a few days to a few months. The severe hepatocardiomuscular neonatal type primarily affects the liver, heart, and muscles, and symptoms typically manifest in the first year of life [72, 73]. This type involves recurring episodes of hypoglycemia, hypoctotic, seizures, hepatomegaly (enlarged liver), cardiomyopathy, and arrhythmia. Fasting periods or viral infections can trigger problems related to this type, and individuals with this form of the disease are at risk of liver failure, nervous system damage, coma, and sudden death. The myopathic type is the most severe form of CPT deficiency and is characterized by frequent episodes of muscle pain (myalgia) and weakness. It is associated with the breakdown of muscle tissue (rhabdomyolysis) [74–76]. The destruction of muscle tissue leads to the release of myoglobin, a protein processed by the kidneys and excreted in the urine (myoglobinuria). This causes the urine to turn red or brown. Myoglobin can also harm the kidneys and potentially result in life-threatening kidney failure. Episodes of myalgia and rhabdomyolysis can be triggered by factors such as exercise, stress, extreme temperatures, infections, or fasting. The first episode typically occurs during childhood or adolescence, and individuals with the myopathic type may be asymptomatic between episodes [76]. CPT deficiency is a rare disease, with the fatal neonatal variant reported in at least 18 families, the severe hepatocardiomuscular neonatal variant identified in at least 30 families, and the myopathic type reported in over 300 cases. CPT2 gene mutations are responsible for CPT II defects. The CPT2 gene provides instructions for producing an enzyme called carnitine palmitoyl transferase 2, which is crucial for the oxidation of fatty acids—a multi-step process involved in breaking down fatty acids and converting them into energy. This disease follows an autosomal recessive inheritance pattern, meaning that both copies of the gene in each cell have mutations. Parents of individuals with this autosomal recessive disease each carry one copy of the mutated gene, but they typically do not exhibit symptoms of the disease [71, 77].

2.11 Diseases of Energy Metabolism

Two crucial reactions in the body that play a significant role in energy production primarily take place within the mitochondria, which are cellular organelles. These reactions involve the pyruvate dehydrogenase complex and the mitochondrial respiratory chain. Disorders affecting these processes can lead to various conditions, including certain forms of blindness, deafness, paralysis, epilepsy, and convulsions [78, 79].

2.11.1 Carnitine-Acylcarnitine Translocase Deficiency

Carnitine-acylcarnitine translocase (CACT) deficiency is a disorder that impairs the body's ability to utilize specific fats for energy production, particularly during periods of fasting or inadequate nutrition. The symptoms of this disease typically manifest shortly after birth and may include respiratory difficulties, seizures, and irregular heart rhythm (arrhythmia) [80]. Affected individuals often experience low blood sugar (hypoglycemia) and reduced production of ketones, which are byproducts of fat breakdown used for energy. These symptoms combined are referred to as hypoctotic hypoglycemia [81, 82]. CACT deficiency is also associated with elevated levels of ammonia in the blood (hyperammonemia), an enlarged liver (hepatomegaly), and weakened heart muscle (cardiomyopathy). Mutations in the SLC25A20 gene are responsible for causing CACT defects [82, 83].

2.11.2 Hartnup Disease

Hartnup disease results from the body's inability to effectively absorb certain amino acids from the diet, which are essential building blocks for producing various substances like vitamins and proteins. Consequently, individuals with Hartnup disease are unable to utilize these amino acids properly. Most people with Hartnup disease can obtain the necessary vitamins and nutrients through a well-balanced diet. However, they exhibit increased levels of various amino acids in their urine, a condition known as aminoaciduria [84, 85]. Periodically, individuals with Hartnup disease may experience additional symptoms, including skin rashes, coordination difficulties (cerebellar ataxia), and psychological manifestations such as depression or psychosis. It is estimated that Hartnup disease affects approximately 1 in 30,000 individuals. Hartnup disease is caused by mutations in the SLC6A19 gene [84]. This gene provides instructions for producing a protein called BAT1, which is embedded in the membranes of intestinal and kidney cells. The primary role of this protein is to facilitate the transport of specific amino acids into the cells. The disease follows an autosomal recessive inheritance pattern, meaning that both copies of the gene in each cell must have mutations for the disease to manifest. The parents of an individual with an autosomal recessive disease each carry one copy of the mutated gene, but typically do not exhibit any symptoms of the disease [84].

2.12 Diseases of Purine, Pyrimidine, and Nucleotide Metabolism

Nucleotides are the building blocks of DNA and RNA molecules that are responsible for maintaining genetic information in the human body. This group includes diseases such as gout (primary and secondary) and Lesch-Nyhan syndrome and a number of other nucleotide defects [86, 87].

2.12.1 Lesch-Nyhan Syndrome

Lesch-Nyhan syndrome occurs mostly in men and is a rare inherited disorder caused by hypoxanthine guanine phosphoribosyl enzyme deficiency and is considered a behavioral and neurological abnormality in which the production of uric acid increases greatly. Uric acid is a product of normal chemical processes and is found in blood and urine. The frequency of this syndrome is about 1 in 380,000 people. It is seen in almost all populations with the same frequency [88, 89].

2.12.2 Cause of Lesch-Nyhan Disease

Lesch-Nyhan syndrome is attributed to a mutation in the HGPRT gene located on the X chromosome. This gene mutation typically arises in the mother and is passed down to her sons. Symptoms of the disease typically manifest within the first year of life. The excessive accumulation of uric acid is a characteristic feature of Lesch-Nyhan syndrome [89, 90]. Uric acid can be cleared from the bloodstream but instead accumulates beneath the skin, leading to the development of gouty arthritis. Moreover, the buildup of uric acid can result in the formation of bladder and kidney stones. Nervous system and behavioral abnormalities are prevalent in individuals with Lesch-Nyhan syndrome. These include sudden involuntary and abnormal muscle movements, movement disorders affecting the eyes, and rhythmic limb twitching. Mobility is severely compromised, often necessitating wheelchair assistance [91, 92]. One distinctive behavioral issue among Lesch-Nyhan syndrome individuals is self-injury, commonly involving biting and head banging. This self-destructive behavior is a prominent manifestation of the syndrome. Lesch-Nyhan syndrome follows an X-linked recessive inheritance pattern, wherein the mutated gene is situated on the X chromosome. Males are typically more severely affected as they possess a single X chromosome. Females can carry the gene mutation without exhibiting significant symptoms due to the presence of a normal copy of the gene on their other X chromosome [92].

2.12.3 Porphyrin and Metabolism Diseases

The heme molecule is a critical component of hemoglobin found in red blood cells, facilitating the proper transport of oxygen and carbon dioxide within and outside the body. Disorders related to porphyrins, as well as defects in enzymes involved in their production, can lead to various congenital porphyria diseases [93, 94]. Two common types of porphyria include:

Acute porphyria: This form primarily affects the nervous system. Symptoms are typically intermittent and may reoccur over time. Seizures can cause nerve damage and long-lasting muscle weakness. This condition arises from a deficiency in the enzyme porphobilinogen deaminase, resulting in the accumulation of toxic porphyrins in the body [94].

Cutaneous porphyria: This type of porphyria manifests as skin symptoms upon exposure to sunlight. The areas typically affected include the face, back of the hands, ears, neck, and forearms [94].

Most porphyria types are genetic disorders, meaning they are inherited when an abnormal gene is passed down from parents to their offspring. In some cases, a single defective gene from one parent can result in the condition (autosomal dominant pattern), while in others, both parents contribute defective genes (autosomal recessive pattern) [94, 95].

2.12.4 Lysosomal Diseases

Lysosomes are organelles located inside cells that have important functions in storing and distributing essential nutrients required for cell function. They also participate in the digestion of food particles. Within this group of diseases, a malfunction or deficiency in one of the enzymes present within lysosomes results in the accumulation of substances within these organelles [96]. This accumulation leads to the development of a diverse array of conditions known as lysosomal storage diseases. Examples of these diseases include Hunter syndrome, Hurler syndrome, and various types of mucopolysaccharidoses [96, 97]. The specific lysosomal storage disease that occurs depends on the particular enzyme deficiency involved. These diseases can cause a range of symptoms and complications, affecting multiple organ systems. Treatment approaches for lysosomal storage diseases may involve enzyme replacement therapy, supportive care, and other targeted interventions [97, 98].

2.12.5 Mucopolysaccharidosis Type I or Horler Syndrome

The disease under discussion affects multiple aspects of the human body and presents in two forms, severe and mild, among patients. Newborns with the condition often do not display any immediate signs, although some may present with umbilical or inguinal hernias. The severe form of the disease typically manifests symptoms by the age of one, while the mild form may exhibit milder symptoms that appear later in childhood. Individuals with this condition, known as Horler syndrome, may experience various physical manifestations. These include macrocephaly (an enlarged head), hydrocephaly (accumulation of fluid in the brain), heart valve abnormalities, coarse facial features, hepatosplenomegaly (enlarged liver and spleen), macroglossia (enlarged tongue), and elongated vocal cords resulting in hoarseness of voice [99, 100]. Additionally, the clear outer layer of the eye (cornea) becomes cloudy in affected individuals, leading to significant vision impairment. Hearing loss and recurrent ear infections are also common. The severe form of the disease occurs in approximately 1 in every 100,000 births, while the mild form is less common, affecting about 1 in every 500,000 births [99, 101]. MPS1 disease is caused by a mutation in the IDUA gene, which provides instructions for producing an enzyme responsible for breaking down large sugar molecules called glycosaminoglycans. The disease follows an autosomal recessive inheritance pattern, meaning that both copies of the gene must be mutated for a person to be affected. Therefore, the parents of an affected individual are carriers of the mutated gene [101, 102]. Another variant of this disease is Hurler-Scheie syndrome, which falls between the severe Hurler syndrome and the milder Scheie syndrome. It is a rare lysosomal storage disease characterized by skeletal deformities and motor development delay [102].

2.12.6 Hunter Syndrome (MPS II)

Hunter syndrome, also known as mucopolysaccharidosis type II (MPS II), is a rare genetic disorder characterized by the accumulation of large sugar molecules called glycosaminoglycans or mucopolysaccharides in the body's tissues. This condition belongs to a group of disorders known as lysosomal storage disorders. The symptoms of Hunter syndrome can vary in severity, ranging from severe to milder forms, and are similar to those seen in MPS I (Hurler syndrome). At birth, individuals with MPS II typically do not display any immediate signs of the disease [103]. However, Hunter syndrome can cause abnormalities in various organs, including the skeletal system, heart, and respiratory system. Affected individuals may experience hearing problems during childhood, skin changes, frequent ear, nose, and throat infections, breathing difficulties, enlarged liver and spleen, and, in advanced cases, growth delay [103, 104]. The underlying cause of Hunter syndrome is a deficiency in the enzyme lysosomal iduronate 2 sulfatase (IDS). The lack of this enzyme leads to the accumulation of heparan sulfate and dermatan sulfate in tissues throughout the body

[105]. The gene associated with Hunter syndrome is located on the X chromosome, which is one of the two sex chromosomes. As a result, Hunter syndrome follows an X-linked recessive inheritance pattern. In males (who have only one X chromosome), a single altered copy of the gene in each cell is sufficient to cause the disease. In females (who have two X chromosomes), both copies of the gene must be mutated to develop the disorder [106].

Other Mucopolysaccharidosis are [107]:

- MPS III A, B, C, and D (Sanfillipo syndrome)
- MPS I S (Scheie syndrome)
- MPS IV A and B (Morquio syndrome)
- MPS IX (hyaluronidase deficiency)
- MPS VII (Sly syndrome)
- MPS VI (Maroteaux-Lamy syndrome)

2.13 Peroxisomal Diseases

Peroxisomes are organelles found in all cells that possess a lipid membrane composed of fat. They are particularly important in liver cells and kidney parenchyma, where they play a vital role in fatty acid oxidation reactions and cholesterol metabolism. Peroxisome disorders can be classified into two categories: disorders affecting peroxisome biogenesis, such as Zellweger syndrome, which is characterized by a significant reduction in the number of peroxisomes, and disorders resulting from enzyme deficiencies within peroxisomes, such as adrenoleukodystrophy [108, 109].

2.13.1 Zellweger Syndrome

Zellweger syndrome belongs to a group of disorders known as Zellweger spectrum, with Zellweger syndrome being the most severe form. It is characterized by the onset of signs and symptoms during infancy. Common features include muscle weakness (hypotonia), feeding difficulties, seizures, impaired vision, distinct facial characteristics, and skeletal abnormalities. The facial features often include a flat face, prominent forehead, and large fontanelles. Additionally, affected children may experience life-threatening complications involving the liver, heart, and kidneys. Unfortunately, most children with Zellweger syndrome do not survive beyond their first year of life. The occurrence of Zellweger syndrome is associated with mutations in at least 12 different genes [110]. The most common cause is a mutation in the PEX1 gene, and the inheritance pattern is autosomal recessive. Currently, there is no cure for Zellweger syndrome, and treatment primarily focuses on providing supportive and symptomatic care to manage the various aspects of the disease [111].

2.13.2 Adrenoleukodystrophy

Adrenoleukodystrophy (ALD) is a type of adrenocortical dystrophy, which is a group of neurological disorders. ALD is characterized by abnormalities in the myelin, the protective substance that surrounds nerve fibers in the brain and spinal cord. It is also known as X-linked adrenoleukodystrophy (X-ALD) because it is caused by a defective gene located on the X chromosome [112, 113]. Individuals with ALD experience an accumulation of very-long-chain saturated fatty acids (VLCFAs) in their nervous system and the adrenal cortex, which is the largest part of the adrenal gland. The adrenal glands are located above each kidney. The disease is characterized by the loss of myelin and progressive dysfunction of the adrenal glands, which are early features of ALD [113].

2.14 Metabolic Diseases of Elements and Metals

Certain elements, including iron, copper, manganese, molybdenum, and other types of metals and rare elements, are essential for various biological processes. However, defects in the metabolism of these elements can lead to a wide range of different diseases. One of the most common disorders related to element metabolism is Wilson's disease, which is characterized by the abnormal accumulation of copper in the body [114].

2.14.1 Wilson's Disease

Wilson's disease is a rare genetic disorder characterized by copper poisoning in the body. It is caused by a disruption in the ATP7B gene, which is responsible for copper transport within the body [115, 116]. This disorder was first identified by Dr. Wilson in 1912 and is known as the underlying cause of the disease. In a healthy individual, excess copper is normally eliminated through the liver, filtered, and excreted in urine. However, in patients with Wilson's disease, the liver does not function properly, resulting in the retention of copper in organs such as the brain, liver, and eyes [117]. Copper is obtained through daily dietary intake, with certain foods like oysters, liver, mushrooms, chocolate, and nuts being rich sources of copper. Approximately half of the copper ingested is absorbed through the stomach and intestines, entering the bloodstream and eventually reaching the liver cells via the hepatic vein [118]. Once inside liver cells, the copper is converted into different forms. Some is utilized for enzyme production, while another portion binds to a protein called ceruloplasmin. The remainder is excreted into the bile and eliminated through feces. In Wilson's disease, problems arise with the last two forms of copper metabolism, leading to the accumulation of copper within the liver cells [119]. As the disease progresses, copper can also accumulate in other organs such as the kidneys, brain, and cornea of the eye. Additionally, there can be instances where copper is abruptly released from the liver, causing severe damage to the liver, kidneys, and red blood cells [117–119].

2.14.2 *Menkes Disease*

Menkes disease, also known as kinky hair disease, is an inherited genetic disorder that affects the transfer and absorption of copper in the body. A low level of copper in the brain leads to dysfunction of the nervous system and impacts the structure of bones, hair, and skin [120, 121]. It is a rare condition, with an incidence rate of approximately 1 case in 35,000 live births in Melbourne, Australia, and 1 case in every 250,000 live births in Europe. The underlying cause of Menkes disease is a mutation in the ATP7A gene. This mutation results in defects in the production of the adenosine triphosphatase enzyme, which is responsible for transporting copper throughout the body [121]. Menkes disease follows an X-linked recessive inheritance pattern, meaning it is passed from one generation to the next through the X chromosome. If a mother carries the defective gene, each of her sons has a 50% chance of being affected, while her daughters also have a 50% chance of being carriers of the gene. As a result, the disease is more commonly observed in males [122].

References

1. Hoffmann GF, Nyhan WL, Zschocke J, Mayatepek E, Kahler SG, Hoffmann N, et al. Inherited metabolic diseases. Springer; 2002.
2. Matalon KM. Introduction to genetics and genetics of inherited metabolic disorders. In: Nutrition management of patients with inherited metabolic disorders; 2009. p. 1.
3. Prasad C, Galbraith P. Sir Archibald Garrod and Alkaptonuria–'story of metabolic genetics'. Clin Genet. 2005;68(3):199–203.
4. Mistry JB, Bukhari M, Taylor AM. Alkaptonuria. Rare Diseases. 2013;1(1):e27475.
5. Patel K, Master SR. Newborn screening and inborn errors of metabolism. In: Contemporary practice in clinical chemistry. Elsevier; 2020. p. 865–83.
6. Pasquali M, Longo N, editors. Newborn screening and inborn errors of metabolism. American journal of medical genetics Part C, Seminars in medical genetics; 2011.
7. Trotter TL, Fleischman AR, Howell RR, Lloyd-Puryear M. Secretary's advisory committee on heritable disorders in newborns and children response to the president's council on bioethics report: the changing moral focus of newborn screening. Genet Med. 2011;13(4):301–4.
8. Adhikari AN, Gallagher RC, Wang Y, Currier RJ, Amatuni G, Bassaganyas L, et al. The role of exome sequencing in newborn screening for inborn errors of metabolism. Nat Med. 2020;26(9):1392–7.
9. Dunne E, O'Reilly D, Murphy CA, Howard C, Kelleher G, Suttie T, et al. Biochemical testing for inborn errors of metabolism: experience from a large tertiary neonatal Centre. Eur J Pediatr. 2022;181(10):3725–32.

10. Ma S, Guo Q, Zhang Z, He Z, Yue A, Song Z, et al. Expanded newborn screening for inborn errors of metabolism by tandem mass spectrometry in newborns from Xinxiang city in China. J Clin Lab Anal. 2020;34(5):e23159.
11. Mukherjee S, Ray SK. Inborn errors of metabolism screening in neonates: current perspective with diagnosis and therapy. Curr Pediatr Rev. 2022;18(4):274–85.
12. Mordaunt D, Cox D, Fuller M. Metabolomics to improve the diagnostic efficiency of inborn errors of metabolism. Int J Mol Sci. 2020;21(4):1195.
13. Frazier D, Millington D, McCandless S, Koeberl D, Weavil S, Chaing S, et al. The tandem mass spectrometry newborn screening experience in North Carolina: 1997–2005. J Inherit Metab Dis. 2006;29(1):76–85.
14. Kasper DC, Ratschmann R, Metz TF, Mechtler TP, Möslinger D, Konstantopoulou V, et al. The national Austrian newborn screening program-eight years experience with mass spectrometry. Past, present, and future goals. Wien Klin Wochenschr. 2010;122:122.
15. Lindner M, Gramer G, Haege G, Fang-Hoffmann J, Schwab KO, Tacke U, et al. Efficacy and outcome of expanded newborn screening for metabolic diseases-report of 10 years from south-West Germany. Orphanet J Rare Dis. 2011;6(1):1–10.
16. Chace DH, Kalas TA, Naylor EW. Use of tandem mass spectrometry for multianalyte screening of dried blood specimens from newborns. Clin Chem. 2003;49(11):1797–817.
17. Lindner M, Hoffmann GF, Matern D. Newborn screening for disorders of fatty-acid oxidation: experience and recommendations from an expert meeting. J Inherit Metab Dis. 2010;33(5):521–6.
18. van Spronsen FJ, Blau N, Harding C, Burlina A, Longo N, Bosch AM. Phenylketonuria. Nat Rev Dis Prim. 2021;7(1):36.
19. Woerner AC, Gallagher RC, Vockley J, Adhikari AN. The use of whole genome and exome sequencing for newborn screening: challenges and opportunities for population health. Front Pediatr. 2021;9:652.
20. Chace DH, Kalas TA, Naylor EW. The application of tandem mass spectrometry to neonatal screening for inherited disorders of intermediary metabolism. Annu Rev Genomics Hum Genet. 2002;3:17–45.
21. Kwon C, Farrell PM. The magnitude and challenge of false-positive newborn screening test results. Arch Pediatr Adolesc Med. 2000;154(7):714–8.
22. Biesecker LG, Green RC. Diagnostic clinical genome and exome sequencing. N Engl J Med. 2014;370(25):2418–25.
23. Schwarze K, Buchanan J, Taylor JC, Wordsworth S. Are whole-exome and whole-genome sequencing approaches cost-effective? A systematic review of the literature. Genet Med. 2018;20(10):1122–30.
24. Bröer S, Palacin M. The role of amino acid transporters in inherited and acquired diseases. Biochem J. 2011;436(2):193–211.
25. Wu G. Amino acids: metabolism, functions, and nutrition. Amino Acids. 2009;37:1–17.
26. Bender DA. Amino acid metabolism. Wiley; 2012.
27. Palacín M, Nunes V, Font-Llitjós M, Jiménez-Vidal M, Fort J, Gasol E, et al. The genetics of heteromeric amino acid transporters. Physiology. 2005;20(2):112–24.
28. Puckett R, Lorey F, Rinaldo P, Lipson M, Matern D, Sowa M, et al. Maple syrup urine disease: further evidence that newborn screening may fail to identify variant forms. Mol Genet Metab. 2010;100(2):136–42.
29. Chen T, Lu D, Xu F, Ji W, Zhan X, Gao X, et al. Newborn screening of maple syrup urine disease and the effect of early diagnosis. Clin Chim Acta. 2023;548:117483.
30. Kim HK, Han J. Tetrahydrobiopterin in energy metabolism and metabolic diseases. Pharmacol Res. 2020;157:104827.
31. Vasquez-Vivar J, Shi Z, Tan S. Tetrahydrobiopterin in cell function and death mechanisms. Antioxid Redox Signal. 2022;37(1–3):171–83.
32. Himmelreich N, Blau N, Thöny B. Molecular and metabolic bases of tetrahydrobiopterin (BH4) deficiencies. Mol Genet Metab. 2021;133(2):123–36.

33. Chatre L, Ducat A, Spradley FT, Palei AC, Chéreau C, Couderc B, et al. Increased NOS coupling by the metabolite tetrahydrobiopterin (BH4) reduces preeclampsia/IUGR consequences. Redox Biol. 2022;55:102406.
34. Carducci C, Amayreh W, Ababneh H, Mahasneh A, Al Rababah B, Al Qaqa K, et al. Molecular genetics of phenylketonuria and tetrahydrobiopterin deficiency in Jordan. JIMD reports. 2020;55(1):59–67.
35. Paul DB, Brosco JP. The PKU paradox: a short history of a genetic disease. JHU Press; 2013.
36. Pujar S, O'Leary NA, Farrell CM, Loveland JE, Mudge JM, Wallin C, et al. Consensus coding sequence (CCDS) database: a standardized set of human and mouse protein-coding regions supported by expert curation. Nucleic Acids Res. 2018;46(D1):D221–D8.
37. Konecki DS, Wang Y, Trefz FK, Lichter-Konecki U, Woo SL. Structural characterization of the 5'regions of the human phenylalanine hydroxylase gene. Biochemistry. 1992;31(35):8363–8.
38. Nyhan WL. Inborn errors of amino acid metabolism phenylketonuria and disorders of biopterin metabolism. In: Rosenberg's molecular and genetic basis of neurological and psychiatric disease. Elsevier; 2020. p. 817–26.
39. Hillert A, Anikster Y, Belanger-Quintana A, Burlina A, Burton BK, Carducci C, et al. The genetic landscape and epidemiology of phenylketonuria. Am J Hum Genet. 2020;107(2):234–50.
40. Shoraka HR, Haghdoost AA, Baneshi MR, Bagherinezhad Z, Zolala F. Global prevalence of classic phenylketonuria based on neonatal screening program data: systematic review and meta-analysis. Clin Exp Pediatrics. 2020;63(2):34.
41. Introne WJ, Perry M, Chen M. Alkaptonuria; 2021.
42. Zatkova A, Ranganath L, Kadasi L. Alkaptonuria: current perspectives. Appl Clin Genet. 2020;Volume 13:37–47.
43. Brosnan JT, Brosnan ME. The sulfur-containing amino acids: an overview. J Nutr. 2006;136(6):1636S–40S.
44. Oda H. Functions of sulfur-containing amino acids in lipid metabolism. J Nutr. 2006;136(6):1666S–9S.
45. Herman MA, Birnbaum MJ. Molecular aspects of fructose metabolism and metabolic disease. Cell Metab. 2021;33(12):2329–54.
46. Molares-Vila A, Corbalán-Rivas A, Carnero-Gregorio M, González-Cespón JL, Rodríguez-Cerdeira C. Biomarkers in glycogen storage diseases: an update. Int J Mol Sci. 2021;22(9):4381.
47. Gümüş E, Özen H. Glycogen storage diseases: an update. World J Gastroenterol. 2023;29(25):3932.
48. Delnoy B, Coelho AI, Rubio-Gozalbo ME. Current and future treatments for classic galactosemia. J Pers Med. 2021;11(2):75.
49. Welsink-Karssies MM, Ferdinandusse S, Geurtsen GJ, Hollak CE, Huidekoper HH, Janssen MC, et al. Deep phenotyping classical galactosemia: clinical outcomes and biochemical markers. Brain Commun. 2020;2(1):fcaa006.
50. Singh SK, Sarma MS. Hereditary fructose intolerance: a comprehensive review. World J Clin Pediatr. 2022;11(4):321.
51. Marion RW, Paljevic E. The glycogen storage disorders. Pediatr Rev. 2020;41(1):41–4.
52. Hannah WB, Derks TG, Drumm ML, Grünert SC, Kishnani PS, Vissing J. Glycogen storage diseases. Nat Rev Dis Primers. 2023;9(1):46.
53. Miller WL. Disorders in the initial steps of steroid hormone synthesis. J Steroid Biochem Mol Biol. 2017;165:18–37.
54. Merke DP, Bornstein SR. Congenital adrenal hyperplasia. Lancet. 2005;365(9477):2125–36.
55. Arriba M, Ezquieta B. Molecular diagnosis of steroid 21-hydroxylase deficiency: a practical approach. Front Endocrinol. 2022;13:834549.
56. Wang W, Han R, Yang Z, Zheng S, Li H, Wan Z, et al. Targeted gene panel sequencing for molecular diagnosis of congenital adrenal hyperplasia. J Steroid Biochem Mol Biol. 2021;211:105899.

57. Espinosa Reyes TM, Collazo Mesa T, Lantigua Cruz PA, Agramonte Machado A, Domínguez Alonso E, Falhammar H. Molecular diagnosis of patients with congenital adrenal hyperplasia due to 21-hydroxylase deficiency. BMC Endocr Disord. 2020;20(1):1–8.
58. Hornig NC, Holterhus P-M. Molecular basis of androgen insensitivity syndromes. Mol Cell Endocrinol. 2021;523:111146.
59. Tyutyusheva N, Mancini I, Baroncelli GI, D'Elios S, Peroni D, Meriggiola MC, et al. Complete androgen insensitivity syndrome: from bench to bed. Int J Mol Sci. 2021;22(3):1264.
60. Liu Q, Yin X, Li P. Clinical, hormonal and genetic characteristics of androgen insensitivity syndrome in 39 Chinese patients. Reprod Biol Endocrinol. 2020;18:1–9.
61. Sultan C, Gaspari L, Kalfa N, Paris F. Androgen insensitivity syndrome. In: Genetic steroid disorders; 2023. p. 327–41.
62. Delli Paoli E, Di Chiano S, Paoli D, Lenzi A, Lombardo F, Pallotti F. Androgen insensitivity syndrome: a review. J Endocrinol Investig. 2023;1-9:2237.
63. Di Donato S, Taroni F. Disorders of lipid metabolism. In: Rosenberg's molecular and genetic basis of neurological and psychiatric disease. Elsevier; 2015. p. 559–76.
64. Morigny P, Boucher J, Arner P, Langin D. Lipid and glucose metabolism in white adipocytes: pathways, dysfunction and therapeutics. Nat Rev Endocrinol. 2021;17(5):276–95.
65. Khera AV, Hegele RA. What is familial hypercholesterolemia, and why does it matter? Am Heart Assoc. 2020;141:1760–3.
66. Harada-Shiba M, Ohtake A, Sugiyama D, Tada H, Dobashi K, Matsuki K, et al. Guidelines for the diagnosis and treatment of pediatric familial hypercholesterolemia 2022. J Atheroscler Thromb. 2023;30(5):531–57.
67. Lui DT, Lee AC, Tan KC. Management of familial hypercholesterolemia: current status and future perspectives. J Endocr Soc. 2021;5(1):bvaa122.
68. Cantrell CB, Mohiuddin SS. Biochemistry, ketone metabolism; 2020.
69. Chandel NS. Lipid metabolism. Cold Spring Harb Perspect Biol. 2021;13(9):a040576.
70. Duran M. Disorders of mitochondrial fatty acid oxidation and ketone body handling. In: Physician's guide to the laboratory diagnosis of metabolic diseases. Springer; 2003. p. 309–34.
71. Joshi PR, Zierz S. Muscle carnitine palmitoyltransferase II (CPT II) deficiency: a conceptual approach. Molecules. 2020;25(8):1784.
72. Mccormick BJ, Chirila RM. Carnitine palmitoyltransferase-II deficiency: case presentation and review of the literature. Rom J Intern Med. 2021;59(4):420–4.
73. Parimbelli M, Pezzotti E, Negro M, Calanni L, Allemano S, Bernardi M, et al. Nutrition and exercise in a case of carnitine palmitoyl-transferase II deficiency. Front Physiol. 2021;12:238.
74. Bonnefont J-P, Djouadi F, Prip-Buus C, Gobin S, Munnich A, Bastin J. Carnitine palmitoyltransferases 1 and 2: biochemical, molecular and medical aspects. Mol Asp Med. 2004;25(5–6):495–520.
75. Joshi PR, Deschauer M, Zierz S. Carnitine palmitoyltransferase II (CPT II) deficiency: genotype–phenotype analysis of 50 patients. J Neurol Sci. 2014;338(1–2):107–11.
76. Corti S, Bordoni A, Ronchi D, Musumeci O, Aguennouz M, Toscano A, et al. Clinical features and new molecular findings in carnitine palmitoyltransferase II (CPT II) deficiency. J Neurol Sci. 2008;266(1–2):97–103.
77. IJlst L, Mandel H, Oostheim W, Ruiter J, Gutman A, Wanders R. Molecular basis of hepatic carnitine palmitoyltransferase I deficiency. J Clin Invest. 1998;102(3):527–31.
78. Wallace DC. Mitochondrial DNA mutations in diseases of energy metabolism. J Bioenerg Biomembr. 1994;26:241–50.
79. Yang S, Lian G. ROS and diseases: role in metabolism and energy supply. Mol Cell Biochem. 2020;467:1–12.
80. Corado JAM, Lee CU, Enns GM. Carnitine-Acylcarnitine Translocase Deficiency. GeneReviews®[Internet]; 2022.

81. Ryder B, Inbar-Feigenberg M, Glamuzina E, Halligan R, Vara R, Elliot A, et al. New insights into carnitine-acylcarnitine translocase deficiency from 23 cases: management challenges and potential therapeutic approaches. J Inherit Metab Dis. 2021;44(4):903–15.
82. Ja MC, Lee C, Enns G. Carnitine-acylcarnitine translocase deficiency; 2022.
83. Zhang L, Hu Y, Xie M, Zhang Y, Cen K, Chen L, et al. Carnitine-acylcarnitine translocase deficiency caused by SLC25A20 gene heterozygous variants in twins: a case report. J Int Med Res. 2023;51(4):03000605231163811.
84. Hashmi MS, Gupta V. Hartnup disease; 2020.
85. Wang X, Li XY, Piao Y, Yuan G, Lin Y, Chen H, et al. Hartnup disease presenting as hereditary spastic paraplegia and severe peripheral neuropathy. Am J Med Genet A. 2022;188(1):237–42.
86. Kamatani N, Jinnah H, Hennekam RC, van Kuilenburg AB. Purine and pyrimidine metabolism. In: Emery and Rimoin's principles and practice of medical genetics and genomics. Elsevier; 2021. p. 183–234.
87. Chandel NS. Nucleotide metabolism. Cold Spring Harb Perspect Biol. 2021;13(7):a040592.
88. Micheli V, Jacomelli G, Santucci A, Bernardini G. Animal and cell models for Lesch-Nyhan syndrome. Drug Discov Today Dis Model. 2020;31:45–57.
89. Bell S, Kolobova I, Crapper L, Ernst C. Lesch-Nyhan syndrome: models, theories, and therapies. Mol Syndromol. 2016;7(6):302–11.
90. Harris JC. Lesch–Nyhan syndrome and its variants: examining the behavioral and neurocognitive phenotype. Curr Opin Psychiatry. 2018;31(2):96–102.
91. Torres RJ, Puig JG. Hypoxanthine-guanine phosophoribosyltransferase (HPRT) deficiency: Lesch-Nyhan syndrome. Orphanet J Rare Dis. 2007;2:1–10.
92. Rami E, Bhatt N, Wadhwani N, Sharma A. Metabolic disorders: lesch-nyhan syndrome. J Adv Sci Res. 2020;11(Suppl 04):31–7.
93. Tortorelli S, White AL, Raymond K. Disorders of porphyrin metabolism. In: Biochemical and molecular basis of pediatric disease. Elsevier; 2021. p. 503–28.
94. Goldberg A, McColl KE, Moore M, Rimington C. Disorders of porphyrin metabolism. Springer Science & Business Media; 2013.
95. Wang X, Cai Y, Li W, Jia Y, Fu J, Ni Y, et al. Research Progress on serum porphyrin and chronic liver disease. J Clin Nurs Res. 2022;6(3):221–8.
96. Breiden B, Sandhoff K. Mechanism of secondary ganglioside and lipid accumulation in lysosomal disease. Int J Mol Sci. 2020;21(7):2566.
97. Leal AF, Espejo-Mojica AJ, et al. Lysosomal storage diseases: current therapies and future alternatives. J Mol Med. 2020;98(7):931–46.
98. Mehta AB, Winchester B. Lysosomal storage disorders: a practical guide. Wiley; 2022.
99. Hampe CS, Wesley J, Lund TC, Orchard PJ, Polgreen LE, Eisengart JB, et al. Mucopolysaccharidosis type I: current treatments, limitations, and prospects for improvement. Biomolecules. 2021;11(2):189.
100. Clarke LA. Mucopolysaccharidosis type I; 2021.
101. Khalid N, Abdullah M, et al. Hurler Syndrome (Mucopolysaccharidosis Type); 2023.
102. Hampe CS, Eisengart JB, Lund TC, Orchard PJ, Swietlicka M, Wesley J, et al. Mucopolysaccharidosis type I: a review of the natural history and molecular pathology. Cells. 2020;9(8):1838.
103. Mohamed S, He QQ, Singh AA, Ferro V. Mucopolysaccharidosis type II (hunter syndrome): clinical and biochemical aspects of the disease and approaches to its diagnosis and treatment. Adv Carbohydr Chem Biochem. 2020;77:71–117.
104. D'Avanzo F, Rigon L, Zanetti A, Tomanin R. Mucopolysaccharidosis type II: one hundred years of research, diagnosis, and treatment. Int J Mol Sci. 2020;21(4):1258.
105. Wraith JE, Scarpa M, Beck M, Bodamer OA, De Meirleir L, Guffon N, et al. Mucopolysaccharidosis type II (hunter syndrome): a clinical review and recommendations for treatment in the era of enzyme replacement therapy. Eur J Pediatr. 2008;167:267–77.
106. Sestito S, Falvo F, Scozzafava C, Apa R, Pensabene L, Bonapace G, et al. Genetics and gene therapy in hunter disease. Curr Gene Ther. 2018;18(2):90–5.

107. Kobayashi H. Recent trends in mucopolysaccharidosis research. J Hum Genet. 2019;64(2):127–37.
108. Aubourg P, Wanders R. Peroxisomal disorders. Handb Clin Neurol. 2013;113:1593–609.
109. Shimozawa N. Molecular and clinical aspects of peroxisomal diseases. J Inherit Metab Dis. 2007;30(2):193–7.
110. Lee PR, Raymond GV. Child neurology: Zellweger syndrome. Neurology. 2013;80(20):e207–e10.
111. Steinberg SJ, Raymond GV, Braverman NE, Moser AB. Zellweger spectrum disorder; 2020.
112. Zhu J, Eichler F, Biffi A, Duncan CN, Williams DA, Majzoub JA. The changing face of adrenoleukodystrophy. Endocr Rev. 2020;41(4):577–93.
113. Switzky HN, Van Haneghan JP, Baxter A. Adrenoleukodystrophy; 2023.
114. Ferreira CR, Gahl WA. Disorders of metal metabolism. Transl Sci Rare Dis. 2017;2(3–4):101–39.
115. Ala A, Walker AP, Ashkan K, Dooley JS, Schilsky ML. Wilson's disease. Lancet. 2007;369(9559):397–408.
116. Chang IJ, Hahn SH. The genetics of Wilson disease. Handb Clin Neurol. 2017;142:19–34.
117. Pfeiffer RF. Wilson's disease. In: Seminars in neurology, vol. 27. Thieme Medical Publishers, Inc; 2007.
118. Shribman S, Poujois A, Bandmann O, Czlonkowska A, Warner TT. Wilson's disease: update on pathogenesis, biomarkers and treatments. J Neurol Neurosurg Psychiatry. 2021;92:1053.
119. Mulligan C, Bronstein JM. Wilson disease: an overview and approach to management. Neurol Clin. 2020;38(2):417–32.
120. Fujisawa C, Kodama H, Sato Y, Mimaki M, Yagi M, Awano H, et al. Early clinical signs and treatment of Menkes disease. Mol Genetics Metab Rep. 2022;31:100849.
121. Tümer Z, Møller LB. Menkes disease. Eur J Hum Genet. 2010;18(5):511–8.
122. Parad RB, Kaler SG, Mauceli E, Sokolsky T, Yi L, Bhattacharjee A. Targeted next generation sequencing for newborn screening of Menkes disease. Mol Genetics Metab Rep. 2020;24:100625.

Chapter 3
Artificial Intelligence (AI) in Medicine and Endocrinology

Sassan Sharghi and Bagher Larijani

3.1 Introduction

Artificial intelligence (AI) refers to the use of computers and related technologies to simulate intelligent behavior and critical thinking similar to that of humans. The application of AI in medicine dates back to the 1970s, although early models faced numerous challenges and limitations that hindered widespread adoption for many years.

The emergence of deep learning in the early 2000s marked a turning point, allowing many of these obstacles to be overcome. Over the past two decades, AI has undergone significant development and continues to evolve. Modern AI systems are now capable of analyzing complex algorithms and learning autonomously, ushering in a new era in which AI is increasingly applied in clinical practice. These applications include risk assessment models, improved diagnostic accuracy, and enhanced workflow efficiency.

This new era is characterized by promising results in the diagnosis, prediction, and management of various diseases. AI supports personalized treatment planning, accelerates drug discovery, enables predictive analytics, and enhances the reach and effectiveness of telemedicine.

In the field of endocrinology, AI technologies are also showing great promise. They assist in diagnosing endocrine disorders such as diabetes mellitus, thyroid cancer, and osteoporosis. Looking ahead, AI is expected to bring substantial improvements in the treatment of endocrine and metabolic diseases, offer new insights in research, support continuous patient monitoring, and enable

S. Sharghi (✉) · B. Larijani
Endocrinology and Metabolism Research Center, Endocrinology and Metabolism Clinical Sciences Institute, Tehran University of Medical Sciences, Tehran, Iran
e-mail: ssharghi@tums.ac.ir

H. Gharib et al. (eds.), *Interdisciplinary Advances in Endocrinology*,
https://doi.org/10.1007/978-981-95-2286-6_3

personalized medical recommendations. These advancements could reduce healthcare costs and improve operational efficiency.

However, challenges remain. Regulatory approval of newly developed AI-powered medical devices is essential to ensure that the benefits of AI are safe, equitable, and accessible to all. Continued research is necessary to optimize AI's effectiveness in healthcare settings.

It is important to emphasize that, despite its advances, AI cannot replace the clinical judgment and expertise of healthcare professionals. Beyond technical capability, AI lacks the empathy, compassion, and human connection that are fundamental to patient care.

Although a universally accepted definition remains elusive, artificial intelligence (AI) is generally understood as the development of complex systems—both hardware and software—designed to replicate algorithmic human thinking and problem-solving processes, particularly those grounded in logical principles. One of the earliest and most cited definitions was provided by John McCarthy, a Stanford professor widely regarded as the father of AI, who described it as the "science and engineering of making intelligent machines" in his proposal for the seminal Dartmouth Conference in the summer of 1956 [1].

Since that time, a broad array of tools and systems have been developed to support data integration and analysis, with the aim of assisting human decision-making across diverse domains of life. These systems are built to mirror general principles of reasoning and judgment, drawing on human expertise to address emerging problems and identify optimal solutions. As such, they are expected to be intelligent, adaptive, and purpose-driven.

A notable feature of these systems is their capacity for continuous evolution and refinement in decision-making processes. In other words, they are dynamic tools capable of self-training based on cumulative experience, thereby improving over time [2]. By identifying patterns within data, computers can reorganize information into structured, applicable schemes that can be used to address current and future scenarios. This ongoing refinement process enables AI to function as a constantly evolving, highly adaptable algorithm [3].

This self-improvement capability—often referred to as machine learning—enables AI systems to enhance their performance by utilizing models and networks. Machine learning may occur through several approaches: (i) unsupervised learning, which involves spontaneous pattern detection; (ii) supervised learning, in which algorithms are trained using prelabeled data; and (iii) reinforcement learning, which relies on reward and punishment strategies to achieve desired outcomes. A hybrid model combining supervised and unsupervised learning most closely resembles traditional human reasoning, incorporating both empirical data and a trial-and-error approach [4].

Some scholars have introduced a fourth category: semisupervised learning. This model represents a pragmatic combination of supervised and unsupervised learning and is particularly valuable for datasets that include both labeled and unlabeled data [5–8].

Machine learning is typically implemented through two principal architectures: artificial neural networks (ANNs) and deep learning. ANNs attempt to replicate the signal processing pathways of the human brain [4]. In contrast, deep learning processes data through multiple layered structures, with each layer utilizing the output of the previous one to refine and generate increasingly accurate representations [9].

Far from being a futuristic ideal, AI has become an integral part of modern life. It is already being applied in diverse sectors such as finance, national security, criminal justice, transportation, healthcare, and the development of smart cities [10].

Among the drivers of AI's rapid advancement is its significant economic potential. Evidence suggests that AI could substantially boost global GDP, prompting many nations to make strategic investments in this field. Notably, AI systems themselves can offer analyses, generate investment strategies, and construct portfolios with an efficiency and speed that rival or even surpass traditional financial advisors [11–13].

Despite its many advantages, AI also raises critical challenges related to policy, ethics, and regulation. Issues such as data accessibility, prevention of misleading data integration, transparency of data sources, and accountability for erroneous or harmful outputs require careful oversight by experts, policymakers, and regulatory bodies [14].

Given that AI is expected to process data in real time for problem-solving, one of the most urgent concerns is the creation of standardized and shareable data platforms. However, issues related to data ownership may restrict access and hinder both economic and academic innovation. Addressing this will require clear national—and possibly international—strategies [15, 16].

Ethical considerations focus largely on the transparency of embedded value judgments and the criteria for data inclusion in algorithm development. Understanding the functional pathways of these systems is also critical. Neglecting these aspects, or incorporating biased or unfair criteria, could result in harmful outcomes, such as discrimination or ethical violations [17]. As a response, various regulatory frameworks, guidelines, and oversight mechanisms are being established to mitigate these risks [18]. Moreover, there is a growing consensus that accountability mechanisms must be in place to sanction those responsible for algorithmic harms [19, 20].

In conclusion, we are witnessing a technological revolution wherein intelligent systems—employing both physical and virtual components—can emulate human reasoning to solve complex problems with remarkable speed and adaptability. While the advantages of such advancements are profound, they are accompanied by significant ethical, legal, and societal challenges. It is therefore imperative that we prepare for the responsible integration of AI into all aspects of life, maximizing its benefits while safeguarding against its potential risks [21, 22].

3.2 AI in Medicine

Initially conceived as a simple series of "if-then" rules, artificial intelligence (AI) has now evolved into systems that emulate key aspects of human brain function. Through the integration of advanced methodologies such as machine learning (ML),[1] deep learning (DL),[2] and computer vision (CV),[3] AI systems now possess the ability to recognize complex patterns, analyze diverse situations, learn from data, and apply learned models to future, similar cases [3].

Leveraging ML and DL techniques, AI in medicine (AIM) has, over the past five decades, become a highly accurate and efficient tool in the realm of personalized medicine. Predictive models generated through these methods now support diagnostic, prognostic, and potentially preventive clinical applications [23].

The evolution of AIM can be broadly categorized into three phases. The initial phase was marked by the development of systems capable of reasoning and decision-making in ways closely aligned with human cognitive processes. An illustrative milestone from this era is the creation of PubMed by the US National Library of Medicine in the 1960s, which served as an early demonstration of information retrieval and AI-supported inference in healthcare [24–27].

This was followed by a prolonged period—often referred to as the "AI winter"—characterized by a decline in both interest and investment. Technical limitations and economic constraints led to slowed development during this era. Nevertheless, foundational progress continued in the form of collaborations and early medical AI events, such as the advent of time-shared computing systems. The first workshop on AI in medicine was held in 1975, and domain-specific models like CASNET for glaucoma were introduced during this time, setting important precedents for disease-focused AI systems [28, 29].

A notable advancement of the 1970s was MYCIN, a rule-based system employing "backward chaining" logic. Built on approximately 600 rules, MYCIN supported clinicians in the diagnosis and treatment of bacterial infections by recommending antibiotic regimens based on patient data [30]. MYCIN later led to the development of derivative systems such as EMYCIN and INTERNIST-1 [27].

In 1986, the University of Massachusetts introduced DXplain, a decision support system that generated differential diagnoses and functioned as an electronic medical knowledge base [31]. More recently, the development of IBM's Watson marked a significant milestone. Created in 2007, Watson gained public recognition when it won the television quiz show Jeopardy! in 2011 against human competitors [32, 33]. Watson subsequently laid the groundwork for AI-driven, evidence-based medical

[1] Machine learning (ML): Pattern identification and analysis; machines improve through experience using provided datasets

[2] Deep learning (DL): Composed of multilayer neural networks, enabling systems to independently learn and make decisions

[3] Computer vision (CV): Enables systems to extract and interpret information from visual inputs such as images or videos

decision-making. In 2017, Bakkar et al. effectively used Watson to identify novel RNA-binding proteins implicated in amyotrophic lateral sclerosis, highlighting the potential of AI in advancing biomedical research [34].

Progress in AI-based clinical applications continued with the development of tools such as Pharmabot (2015), a medication education chatbot for pediatric patients and their caregivers, modeled after earlier virtual assistants like Siri (2011) and Alexa (2014). In 2017, Mandy was introduced as an automated patient intake system for primary care settings [35, 36]. These innovations represent notable developments in the application of deep learning within AIM [33].

The exponential growth of AIM has been further fueled by advances in computational hardware and software, as well as the emergence of foundational theories such as Bayesian inference, artificial neural networks, and hybrid intelligence. These factors have facilitated the widespread adoption and integration of AI technologies across diverse areas of medicine [37].

From genomic mapping to chatbot-based communication, robotic and remote surgeries, risk assessment applications, online appointment scheduling, digital check-ins, electronic health record systems, follow-up and immunization reminders, to dosage optimization and drug interaction alerts—AI has permeated virtually every corner of medical practice. Ongoing research continues to explore and validate these applications, underscoring the need for medical professionals to adopt and adapt to this rapidly advancing paradigm [3, 37, 38].

3.3 AI in Endocrine Diseases

The application of artificial intelligence (AI) in endocrinology holds significant promise due to the inherent complexity of the endocrine system. Comprising a network of glands dispersed throughout the body and interacting with numerous hormones, receptors, signaling pathways, and feedback loops, the endocrine system also intertwines closely with the nervous system to regulate physiological balance. This complexity, including distant hormone action and multilayered metabolic regulation, often exceeds the cognitive capacity of human reasoning [39, 40].

Further complicating this already intricate system are elements such as autocrine and paracrine signaling, circadian and seasonal hormonal variations, autonomous hormonal activity, and the involvement of clock genes and other regulatory pathways—some of which remain only partially understood. These factors collectively position endocrinology as a prime candidate for AI-driven analysis and decision-making [41, 42].

Given this, the use of AI and machine learning (ML) is steadily increasing in the field of endocrine disorders. The integration of these technologies offers transformative potential for improving diagnostic precision, enhancing predictive capabilities, and facilitating personalized therapeutic strategies [43].

The global surge in endocrine disorders—particularly diabetes—necessitates tools for prediction, early detection, and ongoing monitoring. AI is already contributing to this domain with technologies such as biosensors, continuous glucose monitoring (CGM) systems, and automated insulin delivery platforms, all of which support proactive and data-driven diabetes management [44].

Over recent years, AI has gained traction in endocrinology due to its capacity to improve patient care and revolutionize clinical workflows. Studies demonstrate its utility in nearly all aspects of endocrine practice—from screening and diagnosis to risk assessment, treatment optimization, and translational research. Publications in this field have grown rapidly, with approximately 2000 studies published by the end of the previous decade [45].

An analysis of 66 articles from the past 5 years showed that among 2115 total words in the titles, "diabetes" or "diabetic" appeared most frequently (52%), followed by terms like "retinopathy" (14%), "thyroid" (14%), "carcinoma" (8%), and "osteoporosis" (7%). Regarding AI-related tasks, predictive modeling accounted for 31%, while terms like "detection," "classification," "identification," and "diagnosis" comprised 40% of mentions, with additional references to "segmentation" (5%) and "bioinformatics" (7%) [46, 47].

AI has significantly improved screening strategies in endocrinology by enabling more accurate, rapid, and data-rich assessments of medical records, images, and laboratory findings. Its pattern recognition capabilities allow for the identification of disease clusters and relationships that were previously undetectable through conventional methods. AI can unearth novel interactions within biological systems and between individuals and their environments—offering insights into disease mechanisms that shape clinical presentation and progression.

AI algorithms can process large, heterogeneous datasets—including patient demographics, laboratory tests, imaging results, and genomic data—to construct precise models that forecast disease risk, progression, and therapeutic outcomes. This supports more tailored clinical decisions, from adjusting medication dosages to selecting optimal therapeutic approaches.

In addition, the advent of multiomics has further empowered machine learning in translational research. By analyzing genomic, proteomic, and other biological data, AI offers the potential to predict disease onset and evolution, advancing the goal of preemptive and personalized medicine. In the near future, AI may allow clinicians to anticipate individual disease trajectories and implement timely interventions to prevent disease progression [47].

3.4 AI in Diabetes Mellitus

Numerous studies have affirmed the effectiveness of ML and DL approaches in diabetes screening, a disease projected by the International Diabetes Federation (IDF) to affect 700 million people globally by 2045 [48].

Giorgini et al. demonstrated the potential of AI in the early detection of diabetes and in devising therapeutic strategies to delay or prevent complications [49]. Trained neural networks, by analyzing a range of patient-specific parameters, can predict diabetes onset and assess individual risk levels. These models offer a powerful tool for personalized medical decision-making [50].

Other investigations have applied deep neural networks—specifically, semisupervised, multitask long short-term memory (LSTM) architectures—to analyze electronic health records and accurately predict diabetes development [51]. On the genetic front, AI has been used to examine single-nucleotide polymorphisms (SNPs), which number in the millions per individual. These models can identify high-risk variants associated with diabetes susceptibility [52–60].

Artzi et al. employed machine learning to develop gestational diabetes screening tools using large electronic health record (EHR) datasets. Their model, based on only nine self-reported variables and a gradient boosting algorithm, achieved fair predictive accuracy even without prior lab results [61].

AI models are also proving beneficial in forecasting diabetes-related complications. For instance, Nicolucci et al. focused on six major complications—ocular, cardiovascular, cerebrovascular, peripheral vascular, renal, and neuropathic—and demonstrated high accuracy in predicting early versus late onset of these conditions using ML techniques [62]. Similar efforts using large diabetes datasets have aimed at developing AI applications for individualized treatment planning and complication prevention [63].

Diabetic retinopathy (DR), the most prevalent microvascular diabetes complication, is a target for routine AI-enabled screening. Recommended by the American Diabetes Association (ADA), early detection is crucial to prevent vision loss [64]. AI-based tools—including deep learning (DL) and artificial neural networks (ANN)—have shown high sensitivity and specificity in grading the severity of DR [65–67]. These models can accurately detect various DR stages and predict progression using retinal image datasets [68, 69].

Notably, IDx-DR, developed by IDx Technologies, became the first AI system approved by the FDA in 2018 for autonomous DR diagnosis, with a reported 87% sensitivity and 97% specificity [70].

An unsupervised clustering approach using clinical data and coronary computed tomography angiography (CCTA) has been used to differentiate subgroups of type 2 diabetes patients based on coronary atherosclerosis risk—revealing heterogeneity in plaque formation and stenosis patterns [71]. Whole-genome sequencing, analyzed through AI/ML platforms, further aids in identifying individuals predisposed to subclinical atherosclerosis [72].

In terms of treatment response, ML models have been used to classify patients with painful diabetic peripheral neuropathy (pDPN). Teh et al. developed a 3D convolutional neural network (3D-CNN) model using resting-state fMRI data to distinguish responders from nonresponders to lidocaine therapy [73].

AI has also been applied to insulin dose optimization. A reinforcement learning algorithm was designed to recommend personalized long-acting insulin doses for type 1 diabetes patients based on clinical input, with promising results that still require validation in broader trials [74].

DreaMed Diabetes, an AI-driven remote diabetes management tool with FDA approval, supports personalized insulin therapy by analyzing data from insulin pumps, glucometers, and lifestyle inputs [75].

In the ACCORD trial, machine learning methods helped identify factors contributing to all-cause mortality in type 2 diabetes [76]. Based on this trial, the WATCH-DM score was developed, incorporating variables like weight, age, blood pressure, renal and lipid profiles, and cardiovascular history to estimate heart failure risk [77].

Chao et al. employed risk-factor-based clustering using demographic and clinical variables to identify six distinct population clusters with significantly varying diabetes prevalence and metabolic characteristics [78].

Several dosing algorithms for automated insulin delivery systems have been developed and evaluated in clinical trials. The Cambridge algorithm has consistently demonstrated improved glycemic control, while algorithms from the University of Virginia and Medtronic also showed efficacy in randomized trials [79–81]. Medtronic's second-generation algorithm, assessed in a four-week trial, yielded improved glucose outcomes [82].

The iPancreas system—featuring closed-loop insulin delivery using sensor-augmented pump therapy in outpatient settings—demonstrated increased time-in-range glucose levels and reduced hypoglycemia in a randomized trial, highlighting the potential of unsupervised AI platforms in real-world scenarios [83].

3.5 AI in Adrenal Disorders

Artificial intelligence is playing a transformative role in the diagnosis and management of adrenal diseases. One of the notable advancements is the use of supervised machine learning in conjunction with comprehensive urine multisteroid profiling via mass spectrometry, known as urine steroid metabolomics (USM). This combination has proven effective in distinguishing malignant from benign adrenal tumors. When integrated with imaging parameters, diagnostic accuracy improves further. Additionally, USM has shown potential for early detection of adrenocortical carcinoma (ACC) recurrence post-surgery [84, 85].

AI applications also extend to the interpretation of imaging data. Machine learning techniques—particularly logistic regression (LR), support vector machines (SVM), and random forests (RF)—have been successfully used to differentiate between subclinical pheochromocytoma and lipid-poor adrenal adenomas based on CT imaging, with enhanced precision compared to traditional methods [86].

The diagnosis of Cushing's syndrome, which is often clinically complex, has been streamlined using random forest algorithms, which can differentiate between its various subtypes. Studies have also shown that steroidomic profiles can help characterize autonomous cortisol secretion and identify patients at elevated cardiometabolic risk, even among those with seemingly benign adrenal tumors [84, 85, 87–89].

Yang et al. utilized machine learning to analyze gene expression data for differentiating multiple adrenal and neuroendocrine tumors, including pheochromocytomas, paragangliomas, adrenal adenomas, hyperplasias, and carcinomas, demonstrating AI's capability in molecular tumor classification [90].

In the context of primary aldosteronism (PA), a predictive model developed by Shi et al. uses ten clinical parameters to subclassify PA without the need for CT imaging or adrenal vein sampling (AVS), thereby simplifying the identification of aldosterone-producing adenomas suitable for surgical treatment [91]. Moreover, integrating plasma steroid profiling with machine learning can help identify unilateral adenomas harboring somatic KCNJ5 mutations, further guiding surgical decision-making [92].

AI has also been used to replicate expert clinical judgment in analyzing steroid profiles for diagnosing forms of congenital adrenal hyperplasia (CAH) [93]. Baranowski et al. extended this concept to identify inborn errors of steroidogenesis using steroid metabolomics, validated with genetic data [94]. Machine learning may even assist in tailoring glucocorticoid therapy in CAH patients by predicting individual treatment responses based on unique steroid fingerprints [95].

In another significant development, RNA sequencing data from The Cancer Genome Atlas (TCGA) were used by Aruardt et al. to cluster adrenocortical tumors via unsupervised machine learning. This analysis revealed two distinct subgroups with differing survival outcomes and identified new biomarker genes linked to each cluster [96].

Collaborative efforts among clinicians, statisticians, and data scientists are expected to further advance AI applications in adrenal disease, especially in the integration of multisteroid profiling and mechanistic stratification.

3.6 AI in Thyroid Disorders

AI has emerged as a valuable tool in managing thyroid diseases, particularly in evaluating thyroid nodules. Several studies have validated the ability of machine learning models to assist clinicians in determining the need for invasive biopsies based on ultrasound findings, performing on par with experienced radiologists [97, 98].

Despite the presence of standardized classification systems like TIRADS for sonography and the Bethesda system for cytology, interpretation can still be subjective and inconsistent. AI-based models, such as the "ThyNet" system developed by Peng et al., have been designed to improve diagnostic accuracy by analyzing ultrasound images and supporting decision-making on whether to proceed with fine-needle aspiration [99].

AI models have also demonstrated superiority over clinicians in integrating sonographic, cytologic, and molecular data to estimate malignancy risk more precisely [100–102]. Furthermore, automated analysis of thyroid fine-needle aspiration

(FNA) cytology slides has produced results comparable to those of expert pathologists, offering a promising tool for preliminary diagnosis [103].

In thyroid function testing, AI can optimize both test utilization and result interpretation. This can address the widespread issue of thyroid function test overuse in clinical practice [104, 105]. Deep learning algorithms have also been employed to recommend appropriate lab tests and avoid unnecessary testing [106]. With access to electronic health records, AI tools can help establish personalized reference ranges and interpret thyroid hormone variability with greater precision [107–109].

Deep neural networks have proven effective in early identification of conditions like Graves' disease and Graves' orbitopathy by synthesizing imaging, laboratory, and clinical data [110–112]. A novel ML-based model introduced by Zaborek et al. has improved levothyroxine dose predictions following thyroidectomy, outperforming conventional weight-based dosing strategies [113]. Similarly, HU et al. utilized protein-protein interaction networks to analyze differential gene expression in anaplastic thyroid carcinoma [114].

In papillary thyroid carcinoma (PTC), individualized treatment planning has been supported through AI-based analysis of the BRAFV600E mutation, the most frequently detected genetic alteration in PTC [115, 116]. AI techniques have also enabled preoperative identification of this mutation in FNA cytology samples, enhancing diagnostic precision [117].

3.7 AI in Osteoporosis and Calcium Metabolism Disorders

The diagnostic potential of AI in osteoporosis and calcium metabolism disorders is increasingly recognized. Radiomics—converting medical images into high-dimensional data for advanced analysis—enables extraction of detailed bone features from traditional DXA scans, potentially revealing structural heterogeneity not apparent to the human eye [118].

Rastegar et al. have been working on ML models that integrate radiomic features and DXA data to distinguish between normal bone density and various stages of bone loss [119]. Similarly, AI-based radiomic models utilizing lumbar spine CT images have been used to identify vertebral fragility and fracture risk independently of bone mineral density [120].

Somnay et al. developed a supervised ML model to differentiate primary hyperparathyroidism from osteoporosis and other calcium-related disorders in diagnostically challenging cases [121]. An unsupervised hierarchical clustering approach applied by Kruse et al. to a large Danish dataset uncovered high-risk fracture clusters that responded differently to treatment, despite having similar BMD values. This revealed new insights into medication responses and screening strategies [122].

A simplified model created by Su et al. using only age and BMD via classification and regression trees showed performance similar to the widely used FRAX tool for predicting hip fracture risk in elderly men [123]. In another development, a supervised ML algorithm trained on CT scans was able to identify vertebral fractures by incorporating density and texture features, outperforming models that relied solely on volumetric bone mineral density [124].

3.8 AI in Pituitary Disorders

Artificial intelligence (AI) and machine learning (ML) have shown great promise in the early identification of pituitary disorders such as acromegaly and Cushing's disease. These technologies are particularly adept at detecting subtle facial changes that often go unnoticed in the early stages of these conditions, thus facilitating timely diagnosis and reducing the risk of disease progression and complications. The use of 3D facial imaging in combination with ML techniques has yielded diagnostic performance comparable to that of experienced clinicians and has proven useful for patient follow-up as well [125, 126].

Kong et al. developed a similar ML model designed to recognize facial features of acromegaly from photographs, which also demonstrated potential in aiding early diagnosis of the condition [127].

Predicting the aggressiveness of pituitary adenomas—based on parameters such as rapid growth, local invasion, and elevated Ki-67 proliferation index—has traditionally been difficult through clinical and radiological assessments alone. However, AI is beginning to offer viable solutions in this domain. For instance, ML-based histogram analysis has been utilized to predict tumor consistency, which is critical for determining the most appropriate surgical approach. An artificial neural network (ANN) classifier outperformed traditional methods in this application [128].

Fan et al. introduced a radiomics model that aids neurosurgeons in assessing tumor consistency in acromegalic patients preoperatively. This model was user-friendly and demonstrated strong predictive accuracy in a multicenter prospective validation study [129]. Similarly, a linear support vector machine (SVM) has been successfully applied to preoperatively predict cavernous sinus invasion in pituitary adenomas [130].

ML algorithms have also been employed to differentiate nonfunctioning pituitary adenomas—particularly those that may benefit from neoadjuvant radiotherapy—from other tumor subtypes, aiding presurgical planning [131].

In another study, Kocak et al. demonstrated that high-dimensional quantitative texture analysis (qTA) using ML could be useful in predicting the therapeutic response to somatostatin analogs in patients with GH-secreting adenomas [132]. Moreover, diffusion tensor imaging (DTI), when integrated with predictive models, offers valuable information about potential tumor regrowth and visual pathway damage, thereby informing treatment decisions [132].

Similar ML-based strategies have been proposed for predicting the likelihood of achieving gross total resection during transsphenoidal surgery [133]. In the context of acromegaly, combining anthropometric, biochemical, and imaging data into an ML framework has led to superior treatment response prediction compared to traditional tools [134, 135].

Shomoish et al. demonstrated the feasibility of predicting adult height in children under 6 years using ML. Their model not only exhibited improved accuracy but also offered insights into key predictive variables and areas for refinement [136].

3.9 Ethical and Practical Considerations

Despite the growing potential of AI, there remains a lack of level 1 evidence to support its widespread adoption as a clinical decision-making tool [137]. In addition, AI-driven healthcare presents several challenges. Concerns around data privacy are significant, particularly as AI systems collect and analyze detailed patient data, including facial and genetic information. This can lead to data availability issues, especially if patients are reluctant to share sensitive information, potentially introducing bias into datasets [138, 139].

Moreover, the unstructured and heterogeneous nature of many medical datasets limits the direct applicability of ML methods. Access to large volumes of data alone does not guarantee meaningful AI outcomes without adequate data quality and standardization [140].

Ethical limitations also persist. AI systems, by their nature, lack the capacity for empathy and moral judgment—qualities that are fundamental in patient care. Without human oversight, the use of AI in sensitive clinical contexts could give rise to legal and ethical dilemmas [141].

A compassionate and ethically sound AI-supported healthcare system should include six key components: recognizing suffering, understanding its context, connecting with patients, assessing the need for action, responding empathetically, and evaluating the effectiveness of interventions. These principles must operate at both the individual and systemic levels to ensure that AI enhances, rather than diminishes, the quality of care [142].

AI systems, no matter how advanced, cannot replace the moral discernment and emotional intelligence intrinsic to human clinicians. While AI can be programmed to simulate human behavior, it remains a tool devoid of consciousness and true empathy. As such, AI must be guided and monitored by healthcare professionals to prevent misuse and ensure that decisions remain ethically grounded [143–145].

3.10 Outlook and Future Directions

Despite these challenges, the future of AI in endocrinology is highly promising. AI technologies are being developed for tasks such as transcribing clinical notes, organizing patient data, supporting diagnoses, offering second opinions, facilitating follow-up care, and even aiding in drug development. These advancements may help extend healthcare access to underserved regions and assist in diagnosing and managing neglected diseases [146].

AI is already being applied across various endocrine subspecialties, where it has improved clinical outcomes, optimized operations, and reduced healthcare costs.

Personalized care strategies are becoming increasingly feasible through AI-supported analysis [45].

To fully realize the benefits of AI in endocrinology, several key steps are necessary:

- Conduct timely, expert-driven clinical studies.
- Prioritize standardized methods for data quality control.
- Foster strong collaboration between clinicians and ML developers.
- Design interpretable, transparent ML models.
- Create supportive ecosystems with contributions from governments, private and nonprofit sectors, and patient communities.

These steps are critical to integrating human expertise with artificial intelligence in a way that enhances care while maintaining ethical and clinical integrity [30].

Ultimately, endocrinologists will continue to play a pivotal role as domain experts—validating the clinical utility of AI solutions, upholding scientific rigor, and ensuring that technological innovations translate into tangible benefits for patients with endocrine disorders [147].

References

1. McCarthy J, Minsky ML, Rochester N, Shannon CE. A proposal for the Dartmouth summer research project on artificial intelligence, august 31, 1955. AI Mag. 2006;27(4):12.
2. Shukla Shubhendu S, Vijay J. Applicability of artificial intelligence in different fields of life. Int J Sci Eng Res. 2013;1(1):28–35.
3. Kaul V, Enslin S, Gross SA. History of artificial intelligence in medicine. Gastrointest Endosc. 2020;92(4):807–12.
4. Choi RY, Coyner AS, Kalpathy-Cramer J, Chiang MF, Campbell JP. Introduction to machine learning, neural networks, and deep learning. Transl Vis Sci Technol. 2020;9(2):14.
5. Hamet P, Tremblay J. Artificial intelligence in medicine. Metab Clin Exp. 2017;69:S36–40.
6. Bishop CM, Nasrabadi NM. Pattern recognition and machine learning. Springer; 2006.
7. Krittanawong C, Zhang H, Wang Z, Aydar M, Kitai T. Artificial intelligence in precision cardiovascular medicine. J Am Coll Cardiol. 2017;69(21):2657–64.
8. Salian I. NVIDIA Blog: Supervised Vs. Unsupervised Learning. The Official NVIDIA Blog; 2018.
9. Esteva A, Robicquet A, Ramsundar B, Kuleshov V, DePristo M, Chou K, et al. A guide to deep learning in healthcare. Nat Med. 2019;25(1):24–9.
10. West DM. The future of work: robots, AI, and automation. Brookings Institution Press; 2018.
11. Rao AS, Verweij G. Sizing the prize: What's the real value of AI for your business and how can you capitalise? 2017.
12. Lewis M. Flash boys: a wall street revolt. WW Norton & Company; 2014.
13. Metz C. In quantum computing race, Yale professors Battle tech giants. New York Times. 2017;B3
14. Osoba OAWW. The risks of artificial intelligence to security and the future of work. Santa Monica: RAND; 2017.
15. Barton D WJ, Seong J, Tian Q. Artificial intelligence: implications for China. 2017.
16. West DM, Allen JR. How artificial intelligence is transforming the world. Report April. 2018;24:2018.
17. Accenture P. Why Artificial Intelligence is the Future of Growth; 2016.
18. Kuang C. Can AI be taught to explain itself. The New York Times. 2017;21.

19. Governing Machine Learning. Exploring the IntersectionBetween Machine Learning L, and Regulation. Yale Law School Information Society Project. 2017.
20. Benner K. Airbnb vows to fight racism, but its users can't sue to prompt fairness. New York Times. 2016;19.
21. Poole DI, Goebel RG, Mackworth AK. Computational intelligence. New York: Oxford University Press; 1998.
22. Cleophas TJ, Zwinderman AH, Cleophas-Allers HI. Machine learning in medicine. Springer; 2013.
23. Ruffle JK, Farmer AD, Aziz Q. Artificial intelligence-assisted gastroenterology- promises and pitfalls. Am J Gastroenterol. 2019;114(3):422–8.
24. Moran ME. Evolution of robotic arms. J Robot Surg. 2007;1(2):103–11.
25. Weizenbaum J. ELIZA – a computer program for the study of natural language communication between man and machine. Commun ACM. 1966;9(1):36–45.
26. Kuipers B, Feigenbaum EA, Hart PE, Nilsson NJ. Shakey: from conception to history. AI Mag. 2017;38(1):88–103.
27. Kulikowski CA. Beginnings of artificial intelligence in medicine (AIM): computational artifice assisting scientific inquiry and clinical art–with reflections on present AIM challenges. Yearb Med Inform. 2019;28(01):249–56.
28. Kulikowski CA. An opening chapter of the first generation of artificial intelligence in medicine: the first Rutgers AIM workshop, June 1975. Yearb Med Inform. 2015;10(1):227–33.
29. Weiss S, Kulikowski CA, Safir A. Glaucoma consultation by computer. Comput Biol Med. 1978;8(1):25–40.
30. Shortliffe EH, Davis R, Axline SG, Buchanan BG, Green CC, Cohen SN. Computer-based consultations in clinical therapeutics: explanation and rule acquisition capabilities of the MYCIN system. Comput Biomed Res Int J. 1975;8(4):303–20.
31. Using decision support to help explain clinical manifestations of disease can be mentioned as the landmarks of that freezing period. The Massachusetts General Hospital Laboratory of Computer Science; 2020.
32. Ferrucci D, Levas A, Bagchi S, Gondek D, Mueller ET. Watson: beyond jeopardy! Artif Intell. 2013;199:93–105.
33. Mintz Y, Brodie R. Introduction to artificial intelligence in medicine. Minim Invasive Ther Allied Technol. 2019;28(2):73–81.
34. Bakkar N, Kovalik T, Lorenzini I, Spangler S, Lacoste A, Sponaugle K, et al. Artificial intelligence in neurodegenerative disease research: use of IBM Watson to identify additional RNA-binding proteins altered in amyotrophic lateral sclerosis. Acta Neuropathol. 2018;135(2):227–47.
35. Comendador BEV, Francisco BMB, Medenilla JS, Mae S. Pharmabot: a pediatric generic medicine consultant chatbot. J Automation Control Eng. 2015;3(2):137.
36. Ni L, Lu C, Liu N, Liu J. Mandy: towards a smart primary care chatbot application. In: International symposium on knowledge and systems sciences. Springer; 2017.
37. Amisha MP, Pathania M, Rathaur VK. Overview of artificial intelligence in medicine. J Family Med Prim Care. 2019;8(7):2328–31.
38. Bianconi G, Mehra R, Yeung S, Salipur F, Jopling J, Downing L, et al. Vision-based prediction of ICU mobility care activities using recurrent neural networks. NIPS workshop on Machine Learning for Health; 2017.
39. Ashwell E. The endocrine system and associated disorders. Br J Nurs. 2022;31(6):316–20.
40. Oikonomakos IT, Steenblock C, Bornstein SR. Artificial intelligence in diabetes mellitus and endocrine diseases – what can we expect? Nat Rev Endocrinol. 2023;19(7):375–6.
41. Oikonomakos IT, Steenblock C, Bornstein SR. Artificial intelligence in diabetes mellitus and endocrine diseases – what can we expect? Nat Rev Endocrinol. 2023;19:1–2.
42. Gardiner LJ, Rusholme-Pilcher R, Colmer J, Rees H, Crescente JM, Carrieri AP, et al. Interpreting machine learning models to investigate circadian regulation and facilitate exploration of clock function. Proc Natl Acad Sci USA. 2021;118(32)

43. Gubbi S, Hamet P, Tremblay J, Koch CA, Hannah-Shmouni F. Artificial intelligence and machine learning in endocrinology and metabolism: the Dawn of a new era. Front Endocrinol. 2019;10:185.
44. Rigla M, García-Sáez G, Pons B, Hernando ME. Artificial intelligence methodologies and their application to diabetes. J Diabetes Sci Technol. 2018;12(2):303–10.
45. Aziz S. The use of artificial intelligence in endocrinology. A review article. J Rehman Med Instit. 2023;9(2):26–9.
46. Hong N, Park H, Rhee Y. Machine learning applications in endocrinology and metabolism research: an overview. Endocrinol Metab. 2020;35(1):71–84.
47. Giorgini F, Di Dalmazi G, Diciotti S. Artificial intelligence in endocrinology: a comprehensive review. J Endocrinol Investig. 2023;47:1067.
48. Federation ID. The IDF Diabetes Atlas, 10th edn; 2021.
49. Giorgini F, Di Dalmazi G, Diciotti S. Artificial intelligence in endocrinology: a comprehensive review. J Endocrinol Investig. 2023;47:1–16.
50. Agliata A, Giordano D, Bardozzo F, Bottiglieri S, Facchiano A, Tagliaferri R. Machine learning as a support for the diagnosis of type 2 diabetes. Int J Mol Sci. 2023;24(7)
51. Ballinger B, Hsieh J, Singh A, Sohoni N, Wang J, Tison G, et al. DeepHeart: semi-supervised sequence learning for cardiovascular risk prediction. In: Proceedings of the AAAI conference on artificial intelligence, vol. 32; 2018.
52. Erfani T, Sarhangi N, Afshari M, Abbasi D, Meybodi HRA, Hasanzad M. KCNQ1 common genetic variant and type 2 diabetes mellitus risk. J Diabetes Metab Disord. 2020;19(1):47–51.
53. Azizi SM, Sarhangi N, Afshari M, Abbasi D, Aghaei Meybodi HR, Hasanzad M. Association analysis of the HNF4A common genetic variants with type 2 diabetes mellitus risk. Int J Mol Cell Med. 2019;8(Suppl1):56–62.
54. Saki N, Sarhangi N, Afshari M, Bandarian F, Meybodi HRA, Hasanzad M. MTNR1B common genetic variant is associated with type 2 diabetes mellitus risk. Gene Reports. 2020;20:100695.
55. Scott LJ, Mohlke KL, Bonnycastle LL, Willer CJ, Li Y, Duren WL, et al. A genome-wide association study of type 2 diabetes in Finns detects multiple susceptibility variants. Science (New York, NY). 2007;316(5829):1341–5.
56. Saxena R, Voight BF, Lyssenko V, Burtt NP, de Bakker PI, Chen H, et al. Genome-wide association analysis identifies loci for type 2 diabetes and triglyceride levels. Science (New York, NY). 2007;316(5829):1331–6.
57. Cirelli T, Nepomuceno R, Goveia JM, Orrico SRP, Cirelli JA, Theodoro LH, et al. Association of type 2 diabetes mellitus and periodontal disease susceptibility with genome-wide association-identified risk variants in a southeastern Brazilian population. Clin Oral Investig. 2021;25(6):3873–92.
58. Dietrich K, Birkmeier S, Schleinitz D, Breitfeld J, Enigk B, Müller I, et al. Association and evolutionary studies of the melatonin receptor 1B gene (MTNR1B) in the self-contained population of sorbs from Germany. Diabet Med. 2011;28(11):1373–80.
59. Rapakoulia T, Theofilatos K, Kleftogiannis D, Likothanasis S, Tsakalidis A, Mavroudi S. EnsembleGASVR: a novel ensemble method for classifying missense single nucleotide polymorphisms. Bioinf (Oxf). 2014;30(16):2324–33.
60. Hasanzad M, Aghaei Meybodi HR, Sarhangi N, Larijani B. Artificial intelligence perspective in the future of endocrine diseases. J Diabetes Metab Disord. 2022;21(1):971–8.
61. Artzi NS, Shilo S, Hadar E, Rossman H, Barbash-Hazan S, Ben-Haroush A, et al. Prediction of gestational diabetes based on nationwide electronic health records. Nat Med. 2020;26(1):71–6.
62. Nicolucci A, Romeo L, Bernardini M, Vespasiani M, Rossi MC, Petrelli M, et al. Prediction of complications of type 2 diabetes: a machine learning approach. Diabetes Res Clin Pract. 2022;190:110013.

63. Musacchio N, Giancaterini A, Guaita G, Ozzello A, Pellegrini MA, Ponzani P, et al. Artificial intelligence and big data in diabetes care: a position statement of the Italian Association of Medical Diabetologists. J Med Internet Res. 2020;22(6):e16922.
64. American Diabetes Association (ADA). Available from: https://www.Diabetiesorg/ (2020).
65. Gulshan V, Peng L, Coram M, Stumpe MC, Wu D, Narayanaswamy A, et al. Development and validation of a deep learning algorithm for detection of diabetic retinopathy in retinal fundus photographs. JAMA. 2016;316(22):2402–10.
66. Ting DSW, Cheung CY, Lim G, Tan GSW, Quang ND, Gan A, et al. Development and validation of a deep learning system for diabetic retinopathy and related eye diseases using retinal images from multiethnic populations with diabetes. JAMA. 2017;318(22):2211–23.
67. Sahlsten J, Jaskari J, Kivinen J, Turunen L, Jaanio E, Hietala K, et al. Deep learning fundus image analysis for diabetic retinopathy and macular edema grading. Sci Rep. 2019;9(1):10750.
68. Van Der Heijden AA, Abramoff MD, Verbraak F, van Hecke MV, Liem A, Nijpels G. Validation of automated screening for referable diabetic retinopathy with the IDx-DR device in the Hoorn diabetes care system. Acta Ophthalmol. 2018;96(1):63–8.
69. Raju M, Pagidimarri V, Barreto R, Kadam A, Kasivajjala V, Aswath A. Development of a deep learning algorithm for automatic diagnosis of diabetic retinopathy. Stud Health Technol Inform. 2017;245:559–63.
70. Abràmoff MD, Lavin PT, Birch M, Shah N, Folk JC. Pivotal trial of an autonomous AI-based diagnostic system for detection of diabetic retinopathy in primary care offices. NPJ Digital Med. 2018;1:39.
71. Jiang Y, Yang ZG, Wang J, Shi R, Han PL, Qian WL, et al. Unsupervised machine learning based on clinical factors for the detection of coronary artery atherosclerosis in type 2 diabetes mellitus. Cardiovasc Diabetol. 2022;21(1):259.
72. Zekavat SM, Ruotsalainen S, Handsaker RE, Alver M, Bloom J, Poterba T, et al. Deep coverage whole genome sequences and plasma lipoprotein(a) in individuals of European and African ancestries. Nat Commun. 2018;9(1):2606.
73. Teh K, Armitage P, Tesfaye S, Selvarajah D. Deep learning classification of treatment response in diabetic painful neuropathy: a combined machine learning and magnetic resonance neuroimaging methodological study. Neuroinformatics. 2023;21(1):35–43.
74. Oroojeni Mohammad Javad M, Agboola SO, Jethwani K, Zeid A, Kamarthi S. A reinforcement learning-based method for Management of Type 1 diabetes: exploratory study. JMIR Diabetes. 2019;4(3):e12905.
75. Benjamens S, Dhunnoo P, Meskó B. The state of artificial intelligence-based FDA-approved medical devices and algorithms: an online database. NPJ Digital Med. 2020;3:118.
76. Basu S, Raghavan S, Wexler DJ, Berkowitz SA. Characteristics associated with decreased or increased mortality risk from glycemic therapy among patients with type 2 diabetes and high cardiovascular risk: machine learning analysis of the ACCORD trial. Diabetes Care. 2018;41(3):604–12.
77. Segar MW, Vaduganathan M, Patel KV, McGuire DK, Butler J, Fonarow GC, et al. Machine learning to predict the risk of incident heart failure hospitalization among patients with diabetes: the WATCH-DM risk score. Diabetes Care. 2019;42(12):2298–306.
78. Cho SB, Kim SC, Chung MG. Identification of novel population clusters with different susceptibilities to type 2 diabetes and their impact on the prediction of diabetes. Sci Rep. 2019;9(1):3329.
79. Tauschmann M, Hovorka R. Technology in the management of type 1 diabetes mellitus – current status and future prospects. Nat Rev Endocrinol. 2018;14(8):464–75.
80. Kovatchev BP, Raghinaru D, Lum JW, Kudva YC, Laffel LM, Levy CJ, et al. Six-month randomized, multicenter trial of closed-loop control in type 1 diabetes; 2019.
81. Kovatchev B, Anderson SM, Raghinaru D, Kudva YC, Laffel LM, Levy C, et al. Randomized controlled trial of mobile closed-loop control. Diabetes Care. 2020;43(3):607–15.
82. Collyns O, Meier R, Betts Z, Chan D, Frampton C, Frewen CM, et al. 199-OR: improved glycemic outcomes with Medtronic MiniMed advanced hybrid closed-loop delivery: results from a randomized crossover trial comparing automated insulin delivery with predictive low glucose suspend in people with type 1 diabetes. Diabetes. 2020;69:69(Supplement_1).

83. Haidar A, Legault L, Raffray M, Gouchie-Provencher N, Jacobs PG, El-Fathi A, et al. Comparison between closed-loop insulin delivery system (the artificial pancreas) and sensor-augmented pump therapy: a randomized-controlled crossover trial. Diabetes Technol Ther. 2021;23(3):168–74.
84. Bancos I, Taylor AE, Chortis V, Sitch AJ, Jenkinson C, Davidge-Pitts CJ, et al. Urine steroid metabolomics for the differential diagnosis of adrenal incidentalomas in the EURINE-ACT study: a prospective test validation study. Lancet Diabetes Endocrinol. 2020;8(9):773–81.
85. Chortis V, Bancos I, Nijman T, Gilligan LC, Taylor AE, Ronchi CL, et al. Urine steroid metabolomics as a novel tool for detection of recurrent adrenocortical carcinoma. J Clin Endocrinol Metabol. 2020;105(3):e307–e18.
86. Liu H, Guan X, Xu B, Zeng F, Chen C, Yin HL, et al. Computed tomography-based machine learning differentiates adrenal Pheochromocytoma from lipid-poor adenoma. Front Endocrinol. 2022;13:833413.
87. Prete A, Abdi L, Canducci M, van den Brandhof E, Zhang Y, Tino P, et al., editors. Combining steroid and global metabolome profiling by mass spectrometry with machine learning to investigate metabolic risk in benign adrenal tumours with mild autonomous cortisol secretion. Endocrine Abstracts; 2022: Bioscientifica.
88. Arlt W, Biehl M, Taylor AE, Hahner S, Libe R, Hughes BA, et al. Urine steroid metabolomics as a biomarker tool for detecting malignancy in adrenal tumors. J Clin Endocrinol Metabol. 2011;96(12):3775–84.
89. Louie P, Wilkes R. Representations of race and skin tone in medical textbook imagery. Soc Sci Med. 2018;202:38–42.
90. Yang JY, Yang MQ, Luo Z, Ma Y, Li J, Deng Y, et al. A hybrid machine learning-based method for classifying the Cushing's syndrome with comorbid adrenocortical lesions. BMC Genomics. 2008;9(Suppl 1):S23.
91. Shi S, Tian Y, Ren Y, Li Q, Li L, Yu M, et al. A new machine learning-based prediction model for subtype diagnosis in primary aldosteronism. Front Endocrinol. 2022;13:1005934.
92. Eisenhofer G, Durán C, Cannistraci CV, Peitzsch M, Williams TA, Riester A, et al. Use of steroid profiling combined with machine learning for identification and subtype classification in primary Aldosteronism. JAMA Netw Open. 2020;3(9):e2016209.
93. Wilkes EH, Rumsby G, Woodward GM. Using machine learning to aid the interpretation of urine steroid profiles. Clin Chem. 2018;64(11):1586–95.
94. Baranowski ES, Ghosh S, Shackleton CH, Taylor AE, Hughes BA, Gilligan LC, et al., editors. Steroid metabolomics: a rapid computational approach for accurate differentiation of inborn disorders of steroidogenesis. Endocrine Abstracts; 2019: Bioscientifica.
95. Kamrath C, Hartmann MF, Pons-Kühnemann J, Wudy SA. Urinary GC–MS steroid metabotyping in treated children with congenital adrenal hyperplasia. Metab Clin Exp. 2020;112:154354.
96. Marquardt A, Landwehr LS, Ronchi CL, di Dalmazi G, Riester A, Kollmannsberger P, et al. Identifying new potential biomarkers in adrenocortical tumors based on mRNA expression data using machine learning. Cancer 2021;13(18)
97. Buda M, Wildman-Tobriner B, Hoang JK, Thayer D, Tessler FN, Middleton WD, et al. Management of Thyroid Nodules Seen on US images: deep learning may match performance of radiologists. Radiology. 2019;292(3):695–701.
98. Akkus Z, Cai J, Boonrod A, Zeinoddini A, Weston AD, Philbrick KA, et al. A survey of deep-learning applications in ultrasound: artificial intelligence-powered ultrasound for improving clinical workflow. J Am Coll Radiol. 2019;16(9 Pt B):1318–28.
99. Peng S, Liu Y, Lv W, Liu L, Zhou Q, Yang H, et al. Deep learning-based artificial intelligence model to assist thyroid nodule diagnosis and management: a multicentre diagnostic study. Lancet Digital Health. 2021;3(4):e250–e9.
100. Cordes M, Götz TI, Lang EW, Coerper S, Kuwert T, Schmidkonz C. Advanced thyroid carcinomas: neural network analysis of ultrasonographic characteristics. Thyroid Res. 2021;14(1):16.

101. Thomas J, Ledger GA, Mamillapalli CK. Use of artificial intelligence and machine learning for estimating malignancy risk of thyroid nodules. Curr Opin Endocrinol Diabetes Obes. 2020;27(5):345–50.
102. Wang Y, Yue W, Li X, Liu S, Guo L, Xu H, et al. Comparison study of radiomics and deep learning-based methods for thyroid nodules classification using ultrasound images. IEEE Access. 2020;8:52010–7.
103. Girolami I, Marletta S, Pantanowitz L, Torresani E, Ghimenton C, Barbareschi M, et al. Impact of image analysis and artificial intelligence in thyroid pathology, with particular reference to cytological aspects. Cytopathology. 2020;31(5):432–44.
104. Crampton N, Kalia S, Del Giudice ME, Wintemute K, Sullivan F, Aliarzadeh B, et al. Over-use of thyroid testing in Canadian and UK primary care in frequent attenders: a cross-sectional study. Int J Clin Pract. 2021;75(6):e14144.
105. Islam MM, Poly TN, Yang HC, Li YC. Deep into laboratory: an artificial intelligence approach to recommend laboratory tests. Diagnostics. 2021;11(6):990.
106. Harmon E, Blackwell JN, Pan JA, Miller M, Laja O, Brock L, et al. Implementation of a novel order set to improve baseline pulmonary, hepatic, and thyroid function testing at time of inpatient amiodarone initiation. Am J Cardiol. 2020;136:173–5.
107. Ma C, Cheng X, Xue F, Li X, Yin Y, Wu J, et al. Validation of an approach using only patient big data from clinical laboratories to establish reference intervals for thyroid hormones based on data mining. Clin Biochem. 2020;80:25–30.
108. Wang D, Cheng X, Yu S, Qiu L, Lian X, Guo X, et al. Data mining: seasonal and temperature fluctuations in thyroid-stimulating hormone. Clin Biochem. 2018;60:59–63.
109. Mairesse A, Wauthier L, Courcelles L, Luyten U, Burlacu MC, Maisin D, et al. Biological variation and analytical goals of four thyroid function biomarkers in healthy European volunteers. Clin Endocrinol. 2021;94(5):845–50.
110. Choi B, Jang JH, Son M, Lee MS, Jo YY, Jeon JY, et al. Electrocardiographic biomarker based on machine learning for detecting overt hyperthyroidism. Eur Heart J Digital Health. 2022;3(2):255–64.
111. Hanai K, Tabuchi H, Nagasato D, Tanabe M, Masumoto H, Miya S, et al. Automated detection of enlarged extraocular muscle in graves' ophthalmopathy with computed tomography and deep neural network. Sci Rep. 2022;12(1):16036.
112. Moon JH, Shin K, Lee GM, Park J, Lee MJ, Choung H, et al. Machine learning-assisted system using digital facial images to predict the clinical activity score in thyroid-associated orbitopathy. Sci Rep. 2022;12(1):22085.
113. Zaborek NA, Cheng A, Imbus JR, Long KL, Pitt SC, Sippel RS, et al. The optimal dosing scheme for levothyroxine after thyroidectomy: a comprehensive comparison and evaluation. Surgery. 2019;165(1):92–8.
114. Hu S, Liao Y, Chen L. Identification of key pathways and genes in anaplastic thyroid carcinoma via integrated bioinformatics analysis. Med Sci Monitor. 2018;24:6438–48.
115. Zhao CK, Zheng JY, Sun LP, Xu RY, Wei Q, Xu HX. BRAFV600E mutation analysis in fine-needle aspiration cytology specimens for diagnosis of thyroid nodules: the influence of false-positive and false-negative results. Cancer Med. 2019;8(12):5577–89.
116. Haugen BR, Alexander EK, Bible KC, Doherty GM, Mandel SJ, Nikiforov YE, et al. 2015 American Thyroid Association management guidelines for adult patients with thyroid nodules and differentiated thyroid cancer: the American Thyroid Association guidelines task force on thyroid nodules and differentiated thyroid cancer. Thyroid. 2016;26(1):1–133.
117. Diggans J, Kim SY, Hu Z, Pankratz D, Wong M, Reynolds J, et al. Machine learning from concept to clinic: reliable detection of BRAF V600E DNA mutations in thyroid nodules using high-dimensional RNA expression data. Pacific symposium on biocomputing. Pac Symp Biocomput. 2015:371–82.
118. Gillies RJ, Kinahan PE, Hricak H. Radiomics: images are more than pictures, they are data. Radiology. 2016;278(2):563–77.

119. Rastegar S, Vaziri M, Qasempour Y, Akhash MR, Abdalvand N, Shiri I, et al. Radiomics for classification of bone mineral loss: a machine learning study. Diagn Interv Imaging. 2020;101(9):599–610.
120. Krenz H, Sansone A, Fujarski M, Krallmann C, Zitzmann M, Dugas M, et al. Machine learning based prediction models in male reproductive health: development of a proof-of-concept model for Klinefelter syndrome in azoospermic patients. Andrology. 2022;10(3):534–44.
121. Somnay YR, Craven M, McCoy KL, Carty SE, Wang TS, Greenberg CC, et al. Improving diagnostic recognition of primary hyperparathyroidism with machine learning. Surgery. 2017;161(4):1113–21.
122. Kruse C, Eiken P, Vestergaard P. Clinical fracture risk evaluated by hierarchical agglomerative clustering. Osteoporos Int. 2017;28(3):819–32.
123. Su Y, Kwok TC, Cummings SR, Yip BH, Cawthon PM. Can classification and regression tree analysis help identify clinically meaningful risk groups for hip fracture prediction in older American men (the MrOS cohort study)? JBMR Plus. 2019;3(10):e10207.
124. Valentinitsch A, Trebeschi S, Kaesmacher J, Lorenz C, Löffler M, Zimmer C, et al. Opportunistic osteoporosis screening in multi-detector CT images via local classification of textures. Osteoporos Int. 2019;30:1275–85.
125. Meng T, Guo X, Lian W, Deng K, Gao L, Wang Z, et al. Identifying facial features and predicting patients of acromegaly using three-dimensional imaging techniques and machine learning. Front Endocrinol. 2020;11:492.
126. Wei R, Jiang C, Gao J, Xu P, Zhang D, Sun Z, et al. Deep-learning approach to automatic identification of facial anomalies in endocrine disorders. Neuroendocrinology. 2020;110(5):328–37.
127. Kong X, Gong S, Su L, Howard N, Kong Y. Automatic detection of acromegaly from facial photographs using machine learning methods. EBioMedicine. 2018;27:94–102.
128. Zeynalova A, Kocak B, Durmaz ES, Comunoglu N, Ozcan K, Ozcan G, et al. Preoperative evaluation of tumour consistency in pituitary macroadenomas: a machine learning-based histogram analysis on conventional T2-weighted MRI. Neuroradiology. 2019;61:767–74.
129. Fan Y, Hua M, Mou A, Wu M, Liu X, Bao X, et al. Preoperative noninvasive radiomics approach predicts tumor consistency in patients with acromegaly: development and multicenter prospective validation. Front Endocrinol. 2019;10:403.
130. Niu J, Zhang S, Ma S, Diao J, Zhou W, Tian J, et al. Preoperative prediction of cavernous sinus invasion by pituitary adenomas using a radiomics method based on magnetic resonance images. Eur Radiol. 2019;29:1625–34.
131. Zhang S, Song G, Zang Y, Jia J, Wang C, Li C, et al. Non-invasive radiomics approach potentially predicts non-functioning pituitary adenomas subtypes before surgery. Eur Radiol. 2018;28:3692–701.
132. Kocak B, Durmaz ES, Kadioglu P, Polat Korkmaz O, Comunoglu N, Tanriover N, et al. Predicting response to somatostatin analogues in acromegaly: machine learning-based high-dimensional quantitative texture analysis on T2-weighted MRI. Eur Radiol. 2019;29:2731–9.
133. Staartjes VE, Serra C, Muscas G, Maldaner N, Akeret K, van Niftrik CH, et al. Utility of deep neural networks in predicting gross-total resection after transsphenoidal surgery for pituitary adenoma: a pilot study. Neurosurg Focus. 2018;45(5):E12.
134. Zhang H, Kahlert U, Shi W. Application of machine learning in the diagnosis and treatment of endocrine disorders. Front Endocrinol. 14:1305897.
135. Fan Y, Li Y, Li Y, Feng S, Bao X, Feng M, et al. Development and assessment of machine learning algorithms for predicting remission after transsphenoidal surgery among patients with acromegaly. Endocrine. 2020;67(2):412–22.
136. Shmoish M, German A, Devir N, Hecht A, Butler G, Niklasson A, et al. Prediction of adult height by machine learning technique. J Clin Endocrinol Metab. 2021;106(7):e2700–e10.
137. Yin J, Ngiam KY, Teo HH. Role of artificial intelligence applications in real-life clinical practice: systematic review. J Med Internet Res. 2021;23(4):e25759.
138. Grus J. Data science from scratch: first principles with python: O'Reilly Media; 2019.

139. Lucas GM, Gratch J, King A, Morency L-P. It's only a computer: virtual humans increase willingness to disclose. Comput Hum Behav. 2014;37:94–100.
140. Kim HS, Kim DJ, Yoon KH. Medical big data is not yet available: why we need realism rather than exaggeration. Endocrinol Metab. 2019;34(4):349–54.
141. Montemayor C, Halpern J, Fairweather A. In principle obstacles for empathic AI: why we can't replace human empathy in healthcare. AI & Soc. 2022;37(4):1353–9.
142. Morrow E, Zidaru T, Ross F, Mason C, Patel KD, Ream M, et al. Artificial intelligence technologies and compassion in healthcare: a systematic scoping review. Front Psychol. 2022;13:971044.
143. Leyen VD. The President of European Commission unveiled EU's plans to regulate AI; 2020.
144. Joseph W. Computer power and human reason. New York: Freeman; 1976.
145. Tai MC. The impact of artificial intelligence on human society and bioethics. Tzu Chi Med J. 2020;32(4):339–43.
146. Basu K, Sinha R, Ong A, Basu T. Artificial intelligence: how is it changing medical sciences and its future? Indian J Dermatol. 2020;65(5):365–70.
147. Topol EJ. High-performance medicine: the convergence of human and artificial intelligence. Nat Med. 2019;25(1):44–56.

Chapter 4
Regenerative Medicine and Endocrinology: Advanced Cell Therapies for Diabetes

Zahra Ghezelayagh, Yaser Tahamtani, Mahsa Valizadeh, and Hamid Reza Aghayan

4.1 Introduction

Diabetes mellitus (DM) is a complex and multifactorial metabolic disease characterized by hyperglycemia and disrupted glucose homeostasis. The inability to produce insulin causes type 1 diabetes (T1D), while type 2 diabetes (T2D) is due to insulin- resistance. The destruction of endogenous insulin-producing cells results in T1D, and T2D develops when organs such as muscle, liver, and adipose tissue become insulin resistant. Consequently, all T1D and long-standing T2D patients require exogenous insulin administration. Despite advancements in the formulation and manufacturing of numerous insulin analogs, and the introduction of ultra-rapid-acting and ultra-long-acting insulins, there are still significant challenges to achieving persistent normoglycemia with exogenous insulin injection [1–3]. Long-term hyperglycemia increases the risk of diabetes complications such as ischemic heart disease, stroke, neuropathy, ulcers, retinopathy, renal failure, and liver disease. Recently, regenerative medicine (RM) has opened new horizons for the treatment of

Z. Ghezelayagh · Y. Tahamtani
Department of Basic and Population-Based Studies in NCD, Reproductive Epidemiology Research Center, Rayan Institute, ACECR, Tehran, Iran

Department of Stem Cells and Developmental Biology, Cell Science Research Center, Royan Institute for Stem Cell Biology and Technology, ACECR, Tehran, Iran

M. Valizadeh
Department of Basic and Population-Based Studies in NCD, Reproductive Epidemiology Research Center, Rayan Institute, ACECR, Tehran, Iran

Department of Developmental Biology, Faculty of Basic Sciences and Advanced Technologies in Biology, University of Science and Culture, ACECR, Tehran, Iran

H. R. Aghayan (✉)
Cell Therapy and Regenerative Medicine Research Center, Endocrinology and Metabolism Molecular-Cellular Sciences Institute, Tehran University of Medical Sciences, Tehran, Iran

H. Gharib et al. (eds.), *Interdisciplinary Advances in Endocrinology*, https://doi.org/10.1007/978-981-95-2286-6_4

chronic and incurable diseases, including DM and its complications. RM is a promising branch of biomedical sciences that offers new therapeutic opportunities based on cell therapy, gene therapy, and tissue engineering. In recent decades, various cell types have been proposed as potential sources of transplantable insulin-producing cells (IPCs) [1, 2]. Stem cells can be sourced from adult tissues, fetal tissues, and embryos with varying potencies (from unipotent to totipotent) [4, 5]. To increase the accessibility of cell-based therapies, a readily available supply of IPCs or pancreatic islets must be developed. Furthermore, transplantation methods and graft rejection prevention strategies should be improved. Recent advancements in the differentiation and clinical applications of human pluripotent stem cells (hPSCs) suggest that this field can be a transformative treatment for incurable diseases like diabetes [6–8]. This chapter summarizes various cell-based approaches for β-cell replacement in diabetes and discusses the potential of organoid technology in diabetes treatment.

4.2 Human Islet Transplantation

Whole pancreas transplantation has been performed since 1966 in T1D patients, routinely after or simultaneously with a kidney transplant. This model of pancreas transplantation effectively manages blood glucose and achieves insulin-independence in 76% of transplanted patients 5 years after transplantation. However, the mortality rate after 5 years exceeds 10%. As the endocrine tissue represents only 2% of the whole pancreas, and the whole-pancreas transplantation procedure is frequently associated with surgical complications such as graft thrombosis and pancreatitis, pancreatic islet transplantation has been developed to provide a less invasive procedure, rescue metabolic homeostasis, and avoid these life-threatening complications [9–11]. In 1894, Williams et al. transplanted fragmented sheep pancreatic tissue subcutaneously in a T1D patient [12]. The first allotransplantation of sliced human pancreatic tissue was conducted on two patients in 1924 [13]. A shift from pancreatic tissue transplantation to the transplantation of purified islets was achieved in the 1960s after improvements in methods of islet isolation such as enzymatic digestion, density gradient separation, and tissue dissociation [14]. In 1973, a study in a rat model suggested that the liver could be the most appropriate place for engraftment of the transplanted islets [15]. The first human islet transplantation was reported in 1977 by Najarian et, al [16]. In 1980, it was reported that ten patients underwent islet auto-transplantation, with some patients successfully avoiding pancreatogenic diabetes after surgery [17, 18]. The first successful results of intrahepatic allogeneic islet transplantation in T1D patients were reported in 1990 [19, 20]. Up to the year 2000, several islet transplantations were done worldwide, but the results showed that only about 11% of patients achieved insulin independence beyond 1-year post-transplant [14]. Shapiro et al. (2000) was the first group to show insulin independence in all patients during the first year after allogeneic islet transplantation [21]. This milestone, known as the Edmonton Protocol, was conducted in seven patients with T1D who received a complementary glucocorticoid-free immunosuppressive regime. Afterward, several centers around the world tried to reproduce the Edmonton Protocol, which led to a significant increase in the number of islet-processing facilities. However, substantial variability in success rates between centers was reported. Long-term follow-up of seven patients enrolled in the multicenter international Edmonton Protocol islet transplantation program revealed continued islet function for over a decade in all subjects. One patient remained insulin-free for 12 years post-islet transplantation. Another subject who had been insulin-independent for over 8 years experienced graft failure about 11 years after islet transplantation [22, 23]. In the next decade, several modifications of the original Edmonton protocol have improved the rates of insulin independence [24, 25]. The TRIMECO trial was the first multicentral randomized clinical trial comparing islet transplant to a reference treatment of optimal insulin therapy, which was conducted in 2016 [26]. Recent data on islet transplantation in T1D patients show that insulin independence is gained in approximately 54% of the patients after the first-year follow-up, while at the end of the second year, 20% of the patients remain insulin-free, and eventually, they return to using some form of exogenous insulin within a few years after the transplantation [27]. These studies have provided proof of concept that human pancreatic islets can restore β-cell function and achieve insulin independence immediately after transplantation. A global survey on islet transplantation revealed that between 2000 and 2020, a total of 4365 allogenic islet transplantations were conducted. 2608 were in Europe, 1475 in North America, 135 in Asia, 119 in Oceania, and 28 in South America. These procedures were performed on a total of 2170 patients [28]. Clinical islet transplantation has become one of the safest and least invasive transplant procedures, restoring hypoglycemia awareness and protecting against severe hypoglycemic events. However, major challenges include lifelong immunosuppression, the decline of insulin independence over time, and the limited pool of pancreas donors [27, 29, 30]. The limited availability of allogenic islets of Langerhans necessitates the development of new and large-scale sources of insulin-producing cells such as xenogeneic islets or stem-cell-derived β-cells [31]. Promising results from hPSCs-derived progenitors in various clinical and preclinical studies have encouraged scientists to optimize protocols for generating IPCs or islet organoids from hPSCs in vitro [5, 8, 32].

4.3 Xenogeneic Islet Transplantation

In the past two decades, four clinical trials have been conducted using different sources of porcine islets. These sources include fetal porcine islet cell clusters, neonatal porcine pancreatic cell clusters, and adult porcine islets. In 2005, Valdes-Gonzalez et al. from Mexico reported the 4-year follow-up of 12 patients who received cotransplantation of neonatal porcine pancreatic cell clusters and neonatal porcine Sertoli cells in a collagen-covered device subcutaneously in a pre-vascularized site with no immunosuppressive regimen. During the follow-up period, no serious adverse events occurred. Two patients became insulin-independent for several months, half of the patients showed a significant reduction in daily insulin dosage, and porcine insulin was detected in three patients. The second report noted the presence of porcine C-peptide in all urine samples under basal conditions with an increase post-stimulation with L-arginine [33–37]. Intraperitoneal transplantation of alginate-encapsulated fetal porcine islets in a T1D patient was reported in New Zealand in 2007. A one-year follow-up demonstrated a mild decrease in HbA1c and evidence of porcine C-peptide in the urine [38]. Two other clinical trials (NCT00940173, NCT01739829) were performed in Argentina where alginate-encapsulated neonatal porcine pancreatic cell clusters were transplanted in the peritoneal cavity of T1D patients. A two-year follow-up showed a lasting impact on HbA1c [39, 40]. It should be noted that all of these trials were conducted with encapsulated devices and without immunosuppressive drugs. However, none of the patients achieved insulin independence [31].

4.4 Mesenchymal Stem Cells (MSCs)

MSCs possess characteristics such as immunomodulatory and regenerative capacity, potential for differentiation into insulin-producing cells, display of an immunosuppressive effect on stimulated lymphocytes, and low immunogenicity under certain biological conditions. These cells can be derived from various tissues such as bone marrow, fat, placenta, umbilical cord, amnion, and endometrial tissue [41, 42]. Many clinical studies have explored the efficacy of MSC transplantation in diabetic patients and suggested different mechanisms of action, including protection of existing β-cells, immunomodulatory effects, and differentiation/trans-differentiation into β-cells. It has been demonstrated that MSCs can ameliorate or reverse the manifestation of diabetes in animal models. The majority of clinical trials have utilized various sources of adult MSCs to understand the protective mechanisms provided by MSCs and evaluate their efficacy in modulating the immune response. From preclinical and clinical research data, it appears that MSC transplantation may represent a safe and effective treatment for T1D patients. However, a clear interpretation of early MSC-based clinical trials for T1D has been challenged by the small sample size and short follow-up period that do not allow for proper statistical analysis [5, 32]. Due to the various properties of MSCs, they have also been used for T2D treatment. Clinical trial data of MSC transplantation in T2D patients have shown a significant increase in stimulated C-peptide and fasting C-peptide levels, improvement in HbA1c values, and reductions in the required insulin dosage [5]. Studies have focused on transplanting MSC-derived IPCs to overcome the underlying T-cell-mediated autoimmune dysfunction, restore immune homeostasis, preserve residual β-cells, and replace damaged β-cells. However, clear evidence supporting this hypothesis is currently lacking [41, 42]. Two clinical trials have reported positive outcomes of in vitro-generated MSC-derived pancreatic progenitor transplantation in T1D. However, these studies lack clear evidence for the presence of mature functioning MSC-derived β-cells. The ability of MSCs to differentiate into functional β-cells is poor, and in vivo, trans-differentiation does not seem to occur. In conclusion, it can be assumed that the use of MSCs can be supportive for islet cell survival in T2D patients. However, the therapeutic efficacy of MSCs in T1D remains controversial [5].

4.5 hPSCs-Derived Pancreatic Progenitors or β-Like Cells

The advantages of unlimited self-renewability, accessibility, and the extensive potential to generate an alternative source of insulin-secreting cells in vitro make hPSCs an important source to overcome major challenges of clinical islet transplantation [43, 44]. Several studies have demonstrated the potential of hESCs and human induced pluripotent stem cells (h-iPSCs) to form mature, functional insulin-producing β-cells [5]. However, only a few clinical trials have used differentiated hESCs for β-cell replacement therapy to evaluate their safety and efficacy in T1D [32, 45]. The first-in-human clinical trial (NCT02239354) was initiated by the company ViaCyte in 2014. In the first cohort, 19 T1D patients received hESC-derived pancreatic progenitor cells (PEC-01) encapsulated into an immunoprotective device (PEC-Encap). The study demonstrated the potential for prolonged cell survival during a 24-month follow-up period. Furthermore, the product was safe and well tolerated without any signs of immunogenicity or off-target growth of donor cells. Despite the detection of positive pancreatic islet cell markers NKX6-1, insulin, and glucagon in the transplanted cells, the trial was discontinued due to a foreign body reaction and fibrosis of the implanted device [46]. After optimizing the device material and construction, ViaCyte initiated two further clinical trials (NCT03162926 and NCT03163511) implanting the new device named VC-02 containing the same type of cells (PEC-01). The outcomes showed that PEC-01 cells were able to survive, mature, and produce measurable C-peptide levels. Additionally, patients developed meal-response C-peptide production 26 weeks post implantation. They suggested that hPSCs may offer a scalable, renewable alternative to pancreatic islet transplants [8, 47]. Vertex Pharmaceuticals and Sigilon Therapeutics implemented a different approach in terms of cell type and immune protection in phase 1/2 clinical trials. They used hESC-derived, fully differentiated β-cells (SC-β-cells), while PEC-01 consists of a mixture of hESC-derived pancreatic progenitors and immature hormone-producing cells. Vertex transplanted the VX-880 cells intraportally with an immunosuppressive regimen (NCT04786262). SC-β-cells transplanted into patients with hypoglycemia unawareness syndrome were able to achieve glucose-responsive insulin secretion, reduce exogenous insulin requirements, improve glycemic control, and improve HbA1c in two diabetic patients without any serious adverse events [5, 31, 43]. The company Kadimastem has recently announced the effectiveness of their microencapsulated hESC-derived islet-like clusters (IsletRx) in immunocompetent diabetic mice [45]. Patient-specific iPSCs potentially offer a promising source for developing autologous IPCs. A clinical trial conducted in Japan showed the safety and feasibility of autologous iPSCs-derived pancreatic endoderm transplantation in a T1DM patient [44].

4.6 Islet Organoids

Recent advances in three-dimensional (3D) culture methods have led to the development of organoids, which are 3D cellular structures created through the self-organization of tissue-specific cells. Organoids can mimic the structure and function of the original organ [48]. Due to the better simulation of the natural pancreatic islet structure, islet organoids provide more favorable conditions than conventionally differentiated IPCs. Islet organoids can be created from pancreatic tissue or the in vitro differentiation of PSCs [49, 50]. The use of disease-specific pancreatic organoids facilitates an understanding of the molecular mechanisms of diseases (disease modeling), the identification of potential biomarkers, drug screening, new drug development, toxicology studies, and personalized medicine [51].

4.6.1 Adult Pancreatic-Tissue-Derived Organoids

Adult tissues have more sources of stem cells than was originally predicted. The success in tissue culture of adult cells was due to the discovery of Lgr5-positive adult stem cells in mouse intestinal crypts, which led to the in vitro production of intestinal organoids [52]. Since then, organoid culture methods have been developed for organs such as the stomach, liver, pancreas, brain, and lungs [53]. These achievements have led to the hypothesis that deriving organoids from adult pancreas stem cells could be suitable for pancreatic regeneration studies and β-cell replacement therapy. Human pancreatic ductal cells can proliferate and expand in vitro, forming hollow 3D structures when cultured in collagen or Matrigel, making them a promising source for regenerative therapies [54]. Initially, the proliferation and short-term differentiation of mouse and human adult pancreas cells in suspension culture showed that each cell of the pancreatic ducts or islets formed spheres expressing both neural and progenitor markers, capable of differentiation into neurons and β-like cells. This suggests the existence of a proliferative clonogenic progenitor source in the adult pancreas of mice and humans [55, 56]. Several groups have successfully generated pancreatic organoids from the adult human pancreas. These organoids include hollow spheres, which, unlike organoids derived from embryonic tissue, cannot form complex apical-truncal structures or spontaneously differentiate towards endocrine cells [57, 58]. By overexpressing the main transcription factors that regulate the formation of β-cells, organoids derived from adult human tissue can be induced to differentiate into a pseudo-β-cell phenotype. Researchers are working on producing complex organoids from the residues of human pancreas islet isolation procedures. These organoids showed increased aldehyde dehydrogenase (ALDH) expression in their budding structures without any genetic modification. Additionally, insulin-expressing cells were observed in these organoids after transplantation into immunodeficient mice [59]. The first reported attempt to develop GMP-compliant large-scale human adult pancreatic organoids for clinical application came from Dossena et al. The islet-depleted pancreatic tissue derived from a single cadaver donor was expanded up to 250 × 10^6 pancreatic organoids, reaching a total number of approximately 250 × 10^9 cells [60]. However, more research is necessary to develop a truly efficient and safe approach. Currently, pancreatic organoids are far from being applied as a source of cell-based therapy for diabetes. Drawbacks of organoid formation from the adult pancreas include complicated access to this potential source, the doubtful existence of adult pancreatic bipotential progenitors, the inaccessibility of the proper pancreatic niche, the inherent variability among different donors, safety concerns, and the technical difficulties associated with up-scaling organoid culture [45].

4.6.2 *PSC-Derived Pancreatic Organoids*

In 2015, hESC-derived PDX1- and NKX6.1-positive pancreatic progenitor cells were successfully cultivated in a 3D format using Matrigel. The culture medium was supplemented with B27, ascorbic acid, insulin, hydrocortisone, FGF2, retinoic acid, and a Rock inhibitor. The resulting spheroids could be passaged and maintained for 12 days in culture, continuing to express progenitor cell markers such as SOX9, PDX1, and NKX6.1 [61]. Another study showed that inhibiting the TGFβ and Notch pathways, and removing EGF and FGF7 from the culture composition resulted in the differentiation of 10–15% of cells into ductal cells and more than 1% of cells into acinar cells [62]. The production of islet organoids through targeted differentiation of pluripotent cells in 3D culture conditions has seen many successes. However, the use of suspension and air-interfaced culture systems led to the creation of immature β-cells unable to secrete insulin [63, 64]. Conversely, 3D islet-like organoids generated from human embryonic stem cells or through spontaneous accumulation of endocrine cells were able to secrete insulin in response to glucose both in vitro and in vivo [65, 66].

4.6.3 *Strategies for the Development of Pancreatic Organoids*

4.6.3.1 Coculture Systems

Simulating the cell interactions of the development process in vitro provides a suitable model for organoid formation. Analyses of signaling pathways have shown the important role of tissue-specific stromal cells. Therefore, by applying these cells, the niche of pancreatic development is better mimicked [67–69]. The cocultivation of ESC-derived pancreatic progenitors with pancreatic-derived endothelial or mesenchymal cells increases the possibility of their proliferation and self-renewal, which can be differentiated into insulin-secreting cells after transplantation. Cocultivation of endothelial cells with hESC-derived pancreatic progenitor cells accompanied by the removal of chemical inducers and through signaling pathways is effective in the maturation and differentiation of pancreatic progenitor cells into insulin-secreting cells [70]. The cocultivation of PSC-derived pancreatic endoderm cells with pancreatic islets or islet cells conditioned medium led to an increase in β-cell markers. Transplantation of the cells obtained from this co-cultivation into nude diabetic mice induced euglycemia, C-peptide, and insulin secretion. These results show that mature islet cells are effective in increasing the differentiation efficiency of pancreatic endoderm into insulin-secreting cells through the secretion of stimulating factors [71, 72]. Through the cocultivation of umbilical cord endothelial cells with human adipose-tissue-derived stem cells (ADSCs) and differentiated pancreatic progenitor cells on a Gellan gum substrate, 3D spheroids of pancreatic pseudo-islets were generated after a few days, showing an increase in the secretion of human C-peptide after being transplanted into diabetic mice [73]. Using a polydimethylsiloxane (PDMS) microwell, researchers were able to create a 3D coculture system of rat pancreatic islets and hepatocytes to produce functional spheroids of the same size and shape. They used different cell ratios of these two cell types to determine the effect of each cell on the other. This construct was more viable and stable after 7 days of cultivation compared to the structures obtained from the culture of each cell type individually [74]. In 2015, Takebe and his colleagues produced various types of organoids, including the pancreas. In their first attempt, mouse insulinoma (MIN6) cells were cocultured with bone-marrow-derived mesenchymal stem cells (BM-MSCs) and umbilical cord endothelial cells on Matrigel to form pancreatic buds. As a result, the cells spontaneously aggregated and created a 3D structure that could be manipulated. In this structure, after transplantation, revascularization occurred rapidly, and the newly formed blood vessels were linked with the recipient's vascular system, which is crucial for rapid oxygen supply to cells prone to insulin production [75]. Subsequent studies have also emphasized the importance of mimicking pancreas development and recapitulating pancreatic cell-cell interactions to generate more mature pancreatic organoids through pancreatic non-epithelial cell coculture [76, 77]. Therefore, 3D coculture of the pancreas is a suitable method for studies in various fields such as tissue development, disease modeling, drug testing, small- molecule screening, and β-cell regeneration. They also provide evidence for mimicking in vivo developmental processes to differentiate ESC-derived β-like cells. However, there are still gaps in understanding the actual effects of pancreatic epithelial and non-epithelial cells in human pancreas development, particularly regarding their contributions to producing pancreatic organoids that faithfully mimic the structure of the islets of Langerhans.

4.6.3.2 Tissue Engineering-Based Approaches

Despite the progress made in the production of pancreatic organoids, this knowledge is still subject to improvement, and the application of new technologies can lead to advancements in this field. During organ development, cells can be influenced by various environmental factors, including soluble factors (such as small molecules, cytokines, and growth factors), the extracellular matrix, intercellular interactions, and mechanical forces. This highlights the necessity of using 3D coculture systems for the formation of multicellular structures. Various bioengineering approaches, such as extracellular matrix design, engineered vascularization, genetic manipulation of signaling molecules at the cell level, bioprinting, and microfluidic methods, can engineer cellular interactions to generate pancreatic organoids or produce mature and functional pseudo-β-cells [78]. 3D multicellular structures are designed for the coculture or encapsulation of epithelial or nonepithelial cells on polymer substrates or biological materials such as polyethylene glycol (PEG), amikagel, gelatin, fibrin, laminin, and Matrigel. Encapsulation in a hydrogel with specific proportions of different cells can facilitate and control the signals created by each cell in the coculture system. Studies have shown that when epithelial and mesenchymal cells are placed in the vicinity of each other in the collagen gel, the extracellular matrix provides an environment for cell interactions [79]. In a study in 2018, a new hydrogel substrate called amikagel was used to spontaneously produce homogeneous aggregates of pancreatic progenitor cells derived from human pluripotent stem cells. These structures were differentiated into mature β-like cells with high expression of the INS1 gene and the C-peptide protein [80]. Bioprinting is a computerized printing system that creates or assembles different cell-based constructs in a 3D format. The resulting bio-engineered 3D structures can be applied in regenerative medicine, pharmacokinetics assays, and cell-based studies. In 2020, Hakobyan et al. used this method to produce pancreatic exocrine cancer spheroids with high precision and the ability to control the number of organoids. Methacrylated gelatin was used as a cell substrate, and the desired 3D pattern was formed by laser bioprinting. The authors suggest that the spheres obtained from this method, which consisted of ductal and acinar cells, can be a suitable model for the reconstruction of the initial stages of pancreatic ductal adenocarcinoma (PDAC) tumor formation and provide new hope in the study and treatment of this aggressive cancer [81]. Microfluidic methods use small channels to deliver precise volumes of liquids that allow controlled physical and chemical analyses. This technology has been applied to PDAC organoid formation. In a study using a microchannel sheet, organoids derived from PDAC cells were cocultured with pluripotent stem cells. This sheet contained three chambers, one for organoids and two for pluripotent stem cells, surrounded by four channels. This system helps to study the activation and maturation of these organoids by pluripotent stem cells. It also analyzes the number of migrating cells and the expression of epithelial-mesenchymal transition markers [82]. A microfluidic system provides an osmotic flow at a lower speed than the interstitial flow in a living organism. Therefore, the islets can be cultured in concave microwells for a month with a low-speed flow without the negative effect of shear force. Additionally, it provides oxygen and nutrients to the islets. This model helps study the function of islets after isolation and can be used for antidiabetic drug screening. Physical protection of islets from the flow inside the chip by enclosing them in a micromesh sheet has also been reported as a strategy to prevent islet damage by shear force while allowing oxygen and nutrients to reach the islets within the chip [83]. Pancreas-on-a-chip technology is rapidly advancing as a platform for modeling islet physiology and studying the endocrine part of the pancreas in vitro. In

2020, Lun Lai et al. created a 3D PDAC tissue on a chip to investigate the interaction between pancreatic ductal adenocarcinoma tumors and surrounding stromal cells. They produced pancreatic ductal adenocarcinoma tissue on a 3D permeable structure in a triple culture system consisting of patient-derived pancreatic organoids, human fibroblasts, and endothelial cells. The demonstration of pancreatic tumor organoid expansion by monitoring changes in tissue metabolic activity validated this system. Examining the tumor environment highlighted the role of fibroblasts in relation to patient-derived organoids, showing that collagen deposition increased up to six times. This system facilitates the examination of the interaction between cancer cells and stromal cells and the introduction of drugs through a vessel-like structure in the center of the chip [84].

4.7 Gene Therapy as a New Approach

Gene therapy provides therapeutic benefits by modifying genes through the replacement, disruption, or correction of the host genes. This is a new therapeutic strategy that involves transferring DNA to a patient's cells to correct defective genes or introduce a new gene to treat incurable diseases [85, 86]. Gene delivery can be achieved through the administration of viral vectors, non-viral vectors, or the transplantation of in vitro gene-manipulated stem cells. Gene therapy has made significant progress in modern medicine and has entered clinical trials and the market. The first gene therapy product approved by the United States Food and Drug Administration (US-FDA) entered the US market as a drug for inherited retinal dystrophy. Many genetic disorders and life-threatening diseases are currently being evaluated for gene and cell-based gene therapy [87]. Gene therapy for diabetes management has shown preliminary evidence of safety and efficacy. Researchers have utilized viral and non-viral techniques in recent decades for insulin gene delivery to various tissues such as the pancreas, liver, adipocytes, and muscle [88, 89]. The CRISPR/Cas9 system is a valuable therapeutic strategy for gene therapy. CRISPR Therapeutics and ViaCyte have recently launched the first-in-human clinical trial (NCT05565248) based on gene-edited immune-evasive hPSCs-derived pancreatic progenitors (VCTX211) in T1D. This trial allows for the allotransplantation of pancreatic progenitors without the administration of immunosuppressive drugs [5]. The combination of gene editing with pancreatic islets or hESC-derived IPCs could be a new therapeutic approach for diabetes. However, this technology is still in its early stages of development for diabetes, and further studies are needed to confirm its clinical safety and efficacy.

4.8 Summary

Several ongoing clinical studies have focused on stem-cell-derived β or progenitor cells for treating diabetes. Alongside significant advancements in islet transplantation, new regenerative approaches such as PSC-derived islet progenitors or β-like cell transplantation, gene manipulation, immunotherapy, immunoisolation, and organoid formation have also opened new avenues for treating diabetes. With improvements in pancreatic islet cell engraftment and progenitor cell differentiation protocols, the number of IPCs required for transplantation can be reduced. PSC-derived islets offer a potentially limitless resource for islet transplantation, making this therapy more accessible for patients. Progress in the generation of immune-evading PSC-derived IPCs may enhance the safety and efficacy of their application and reduce the need for immunosuppressive drugs. It should be considered that there is no single solution for diabetes treatment and that a combination of therapeutic approaches may be necessary for achieving optimal outcomes. Nevertheless, the rapid progress in regenerative medicine makes it a promising area of research for finding a cure for diabetes.

References

1. Ashe S, Hebrok M. Role of cell-based therapies in T2D. In: Seminars in nephrology. Elsevier; 2023. p. 43.
2. Singh A, Afshan N, Singh A, Singh SK, Yadav S, Kumar M, et al. Recent trends and advances in type 1 diabetes therapeutics: a comprehensive review. Eur J Cell Biol. 2023;151329:151329.
3. Wilson LM, Castle JR. Recent advances in insulin therapy. Diabetes Technol Ther. 2020;22(12):929–36.
4. Jarrige M, Frank E, Herardot E, Martineau S, Darle A, Benabides M, et al. The future of regenerative medicine: cell therapy using pluripotent stem cells and acellular therapies based on extracellular vesicles. Cells. 2021;10(2):240.
5. De Klerk E, Hebrok M. Stem cell-based clinical trials for diabetes mellitus. Front Endocrinol. 2021;12:631463.
6. Cochrane VA, Hebrok M. Stem cell-derived islet therapy: is this the end of the beginning? Nat Rev Endocrinol. 2023;19(12):681–2.
7. Hogrebe NJ, Ishahak M, Millman JR. Developments in stem cell-derived islet replacement therapy for treating type 1 diabetes. Cell Stem Cell. 2023;30(5):530–48.
8. Shapiro AMJ, Thompson D, Donner TW, Bellin MD, Hsueh W, Pettus J, et al. Insulin expression and C-peptide in type 1 diabetes subjects implanted with stem cell-derived pancreatic endoderm cells in an encapsulation device. Cell Rep Med. 2021;2(12):100466.
9. Perez-Basterrechea M, Esteban MM, Vega JA, Obaya AJ. Tissue-engineering approaches in pancreatic islet transplantation. Biotechnol Bioeng. 2018;115(12):3009–29.
10. Sharples E, Mittal S, Friend P. Challenges in pancreas transplantation. Acta Diabetol. 2016;53:871–8.
11. Takaki T, Shimoda M. Pancreatic islet transplantation: toward definitive treatment for diabetes mellitus. Global Health Med. 2020;2(4):200–11.
12. PW W. Notes on diabetes treated with grafts of sheeps' pancreas. Br Med J. 1894;19:1303–4.
13. Shapiro AJ. A historical perspective on experimental and clinical islet transplantation. In: Islet transplantation and beta cell replacement therapy. CRC Press; 2007. p. 15–42.
14. Marfil-Garza BA, Shapiro AMJ, Kin T. Clinical islet transplantation: current progress and new frontiers. J Hepatobiliary Pancreat Sci. 2021;28(3):243–54.
15. Kemp CB, Knight MJ, Scharp DW, Lacy PE, Ballinger WF. Transplantation of isolated pancreatic islets into the portal vein of diabetic rats. Nat Rev Endocrinol. 1973;244(5416):447.
16. Najarian J. Human islets transplantation. A preliminary report. Transplant Proc. 1977;9:233–6.
17. Ricordi C, Lacy PE, Finke EH, Olack BJ, Scharp DWJD. Automated method for isolation of human pancreatic islets. Diabetes. 1988;37(4):413–20.

18. Najarian JS, Sutherland D, Baumgartner D, Burke B, Rynasiewicz JJ, Matas AJ, et al. Total or near total pancreatectomy and islet autotransplantation for treatment of chronic pancreatitis. Ann Surg. 1980;192(4):526.
19. Scharp DW, Lacy PE, Santiago JV, McCullough CS, Weide LG, Falqui L, et al. Insulin independence after islet transplantation into type I diabetic patient. Diabetes. 1990;39(4):515–8.
20. Tzakis AG, Zeng Y, Fung J, Todo S, Demetris A, Starzl T, et al. Pancreatic islet transplantation after upper abdominal exeriteration and liver replacement. Lancet. 1990;336(8712):402–5.
21. Shapiro AJ, Lakey JR, Ryan EA, Korbutt GS, Toth E, Warnock GL, et al. Islet transplantation in seven patients with type 1 diabetes mellitus using a glucocorticoid-free immunosuppressive regimen. N Engl J Med. 2000;343(4):230–8.
22. Matsumoto S, Shimoda MJ. Current situation of clinical islet transplantation from allogeneic toward xenogeneic. J Diabetes. 2020;12(10):733–41.
23. Brennan DC, Kopetskie HA, Sayre PH, Alejandro R, Cagliero E, Shapiro AM, et al. Long-term follow-up of the Edmonton protocol of islet transplantation in the United States. Am J Transplant. 2016;16(2):509–17.
24. Bellin MD, Kandaswamy R, Parkey J, Zhang HJ, Liu B, Ihm S-H, et al. Recent advancements in the differentiation and clinical applications of human pluripotent stem cells (hPSCs) suggests that this field can be a transformative treatment for incurable disease like diabetes (6, 7). This book chapter summarizes different cell-based approaches for beta cell replacement and pancreatic organoid technologies. Am J Transplant. 2008;8(11):2463–70.
25. Vantyghem M-C, Kerr-Conte J, Arnalsteen L, Sergent G, Defrance F, Gmyr V, et al. Primary graft function, metabolic control, and graft survival after islet transplantation. Diabetes Care. 2009;32(8):1473–8.
26. Lablanche S, Vantyghem M-C, Kessler L, Wojtusciszyn A, Borot S, Thivolet C, et al. Islet transplantation versus insulin therapy in patients with type 1 diabetes with severe hypoglycaemia or poorly controlled glycaemia after kidney transplantation (TRIMECO): a multicentre, randomised controlled trial. Lancet Diabetes Endocrinol. 2018;6(7):527–37.
27. Kabakchieva P, Assyov Y, Gerasoudis S, Vasilev G, Peshevska-Sekulovska M, Sekulovski M, et al. Islet transplantation-immunological challenges and current perspectives. World J Transplant. 2023;13(4):107–21.
28. Berney T, Andres A, Bellin MD, de Koning EJP, Johnson PRV, Kay TWH, et al. A worldwide survey of activities and practices in clinical islet of Langerhans transplantation. Transpl Int. 2022;35:10507.
29. Khan K, Desai CS. Islet transplantation in children. Curr Gastroenterol Rep. 2019;21:1–7.
30. Cayabyab F, Nih LR, Yoshihara E. Advances in pancreatic islet transplantation sites for the treatment of diabetes. Front Endocrinol. 2021;12:732431.
31. Berney T, Wassmer CH, Lebreton F, Bellofatto K, Fonseca LM, Bignard J, et al. From islet of Langerhans transplantation to the bioartificial pancreas. Presse Med. 2022;51(4):104139.
32. Chen S, Du K, Zou CJSCR. Current progress in stem cell therapy for type 1 diabetes mellitus. Stem Cell Res Ther. 2020;11(1):1–13.
33. Vizzardelli C, Molano RD, Pileggi A, Berney T, et al. Neonatal porcine pancreatic cell clusters as a potential source for transplantation in humans: characterization of proliferation, apoptosis, xenoantigen expression and gene delivery with recombinant AAV. Xenotransplantation. 2002;9(1):14–24.
34. Valdés-González RA, Dorantes LM, Garibay GN, Bracho-Blanchet E, Mendez AJ, Dávila-Pérez R, et al. Xenotransplantation of porcine neonatal islets of Langerhans and Sertoli cells: a 4-year study. Eur J Endocrinol. 2005;153(3):419–27.
35. Kemter E, Wolf E. Recent progress in porcine islet isolation, culture and engraftment strategies for xenotransplantation. Curr Opin Organ Transplant. 2018;23(6):633–41.
36. Valdés-González R, Silva-Torres L, Ramírez-González B, Ormsby CE, Terán-Ortiz L, Ayala-Sumuano JT. Method for evaluating quality of cultured neonatal pig Sertoli cells. Xenotransplantation. 2005;12(4):316–23.
37. Valdes-Gonzalez R, Rodriguez-Ventura A, White D, Bracho-Blanchet E, Castillo A, Ramírez-González B, et al. Long-term follow-up of patients with type 1 diabetes transplanted with neonatal pig islets. Clin Exp Immunol. 2010;162(3):537–42.

38. Elliott RB, Escobar L, Tan PL, Muzina M, Zwain S, Buchanan C. Live encapsulated porcine islets from a type 1 diabetic patient 9.5 yr after xenotransplantation. Xenotransplantation. 2007;14(2):157–61.
39. Matsumoto S, Abalovich A, Wechsler C, Wynyard S, Elliott RB. Clinical benefit of islet xenotransplantation for the treatment of type 1 diabetes. EBioMedicine. 2016;12:255–62.
40. Matsumoto S, Tan P, Baker J, Durbin K, Tomiya M, Azuma K, et al. Clinical porcine islet xenotransplantation under comprehensive regulation. In: Transplantation proceedings, vol. 46. Elsevier; 2014.
41. Stiner R, Alexander M, Liu G, Liao W, Liu Y, Yu J, et al. Transplantation of stem cells from umbilical cord blood as therapy for type I diabetes. Cell Tissue Res. 2019;378:155–62.
42. Pavathuparambil Abdul Manaph N, Sivanathan KN, Nitschke J, Zhou X-F, Coates PT, Drogemuller CJ. An overview on small molecule-induced differentiation of mesenchymal stem cells into beta cells for diabetic therapy. Stem Cell Res Ther. 2019;10(1):1–18.
43. Jiang H, Jiang F-X. Human pluripotent stem cell-derived β cells: truly immature islet β cells for type 1 diabetes therapy? World J Stem Cells. 2023;15(4):182.
44. Dadheech N, James Shapiro AM. Human induced pluripotent stem cells in the curative treatment of diabetes and potential impediments ahead. In: Cell biology and translational medicine, volume 5: stem cells: translational science to therapy; 2018. p. 25–35.
45. Bittenglova K, Habart D, Saudek F, Koblas T. The potential of pancreatic organoids for diabetes research and therapy. Islets. 2021;13(5–6):85–105.
46. Henry RR, Pettus J, Wilensky JON, et al. Initial clinical evaluation of VC-01TM combination product – a stem cell–derived islet replacement for type 1 diabetes (T1D). Diabetes. 2018;67(Supplement_1)
47. Ramzy A, Thompson DM, Ward-Hartstonge KA, Ivison S, Cook L, Garcia RV, et al. Implanted pluripotent stem-cell-derived pancreatic endoderm cells secrete glucose-responsive C-peptide in patients with type 1 diabetes. Cell Stem Cell. 2021;28(12):2047–61.e5.
48. Balak JRA, Juksar J, Carlotti F, Lo Nigro A, de Koning EJP. Organoids from the human fetal and adult pancreas. Curr Diab Rep. 2019;19(12):160.
49. Chen H, Zhuo Q, Ye Z, Xu X, Ji S. Organoid model: a new hope for pancreatic cancer treatment? Biochim Biophys Acta Rev Cancer. 2021;1875(1):188466.
50. Tsakmaki A, Fonseca Pedro P, Bewick GA. Diabetes through a 3D lens: organoid models. Diabetologia. 2020;63(6):1093–102.
51. Funata M, Nio Y, Erion DM, Thompson WL, Takebe T. The promise of human organoids in the digestive system. Cell Death Differ. 2021;28(1):84–94.
52. Sato T, Vries RG, Snippert HJ, van de Wetering M, Barker N, Stange DE, et al. Single Lgr5 stem cells build crypt-villus structures in vitro without a mesenchymal niche. Nature. 2009;459(7244):262–5.
53. Fatehullah A, Tan SH, Barker N. Organoids as an in vitro model of human development and disease. Nat Cell Biol. 2016;18(3):246–54.
54. Kerr-Conte J, Pattou F, Lecomte-Houcke M, Xia Y, Boilly B, Proye C, et al. Ductal cyst formation in collagen-embedded adult human islet preparations. A means to the reproduction of nesidioblastosis in vitro. Diabetes. 1996;45(8):1108–14.
55. Smukler SR, Arntfield ME, Razavi R, Bikopoulos G, Karpowicz P, Seaberg R, et al. The adult mouse and human pancreas contain rare multipotent stem cells that express insulin. Cell Stem Cell. 2011;8(3):281–93.
56. Seaberg RM, Smukler SR, Kieffer TJ, Enikolopov G, Asghar Z, Wheeler MB, et al. Clonal identification of multipotent precursors from adult mouse pancreas that generate neural and pancreatic lineages. Nat Biotechnol. 2004;22(9):1115–24.
57. Lee J, Sugiyama T, Liu Y, Wang J, Gu X, Lei J, et al. Expansion and conversion of human pancreatic ductal cells into insulin-secreting endocrine cells. elife. 2013;2:e00940.
58. Boj SF, Hwang CI, Baker LA, Chio II, Engle DD, Corbo V, et al. Organoid models of human and mouse ductal pancreatic cancer. Cell. 2015;160(1–2):324–38.
59. Loomans CJM, Williams Giuliani N, Balak J, Ringnalda F, van Gurp L, Huch M, et al. Expansion of adult human pancreatic tissue yields organoids harboring progenitor cells with endocrine differentiation potential. Stem Cell Rep. 2018;10(3):712–24.

60. Dossena M, Piras R, Cherubini A, Barilani M, Dugnani E, Salanitro F, et al. Standardized GMP-compliant scalable production of human pancreas organoids. Stem Cell Res Ther. 2020;11(1):1–12.
61. Huang L, Holtzinger A, Jagan I, BeGora M, Lohse I, Ngai N, et al. Ductal pancreatic cancer modeling and drug screening using human pluripotent stem cell- and patient-derived tumor organoids. Nat Med. 2015;21(11):1364–71.
62. Zhou Q, Law AC, Rajagopal J, Anderson WJ, Gray PA, Melton DA. A multipotent progenitor domain guides pancreatic organogenesis. Dev Cell. 2007;13(1):103–14.
63. Pagliuca FW, Millman JR, Gürtler M, Segel M, Van Dervort A, Ryu JH, et al. Generation of functional human pancreatic β cells in vitro. Cell. 2014;159(2):428–39.
64. Russ HA, Parent AV, Ringler JJ, Hennings TG, Nair GG, Shveygert M, et al. Controlled induction of human pancreatic progenitors produces functional beta-like cells in vitro. EMBO J. 2015;34(13):1759–72.
65. Kim Y, Kim H, Ko UH, Oh Y, Lim A, Sohn JW, et al. Islet-like organoids derived from human pluripotent stem cells efficiently function in the glucose responsiveness in vitro and in vivo. Sci Rep. 2016;6:35145.
66. Shim JH, Kim J, Han J, An SY, Jang YJ, Son J, et al. Pancreatic islet-like three-dimensional aggregates derived from human embryonic stem cells ameliorate hyperglycemia in Streptozotocin-induced diabetic mice. Cell Transplant. 2015;24(10):2155–68.
67. Banerjee I, Sharma N, Yarmush M. Impact of co-culture on pancreatic differentiation of embryonic stem cells. J Tissue Eng Regen Med. 2011;5(4):313–23.
68. Jaramillo M, Banerjee I. Endothelial cell co-culture mediates maturation of human embryonic stem cell to pancreatic insulin producing cells in a directed differentiation approach. JoVE. 2012;61:e3759.
69. Jaramillo M, Mathew S, Mamiya H, Goh SK, Banerjee I. Endothelial cells mediate islet-specific maturation of human embryonic stem cell-derived pancreatic progenitor cells. Tissue Eng Part A. 2015;21(1–2):14–25.
70. Sneddon JB, Borowiak M, Melton DA. Self-renewal of embryonic-stem-cell-derived progenitors by organ-matched mesenchyme. Nature. 2012;491(7426):765–8.
71. Oh BJ, Oh SH, Choi JM, Jin SM, Shim WY, Lee MS, et al. Co-culture with mature islet cells augments the differentiation of insulin-producing cells from pluripotent stem cells. Stem Cell Rev Rep. 2015;11(1):62–74.
72. Yilmaz I, Sariboyaci AE, Subasi C, Karaoz E. Differentiation potential of mouse embryonic stem cells into insulin producing cells in pancreatic islet microenvironment. Exp Clin Endocrinol Diabetes. 2016;124(2):120–9.
73. Yoshihara E, O'Connor C, Gasser E, Wei Z, Oh TG, Tseng TW, et al. Immune-evasive human islet-like organoids ameliorate diabetes. Nature. 2020;586(7830):606–11.
74. Jun Y, Kang AR, Lee JS, Jeong GS, Ju J, Lee DY, et al. 3D co-culturing model of primary pancreatic islets and hepatocytes in hybrid spheroid to overcome pancreatic cell shortage. Biomaterials. 2013;34(15):3784–94.
75. Takebe T, Enomura M, Yoshizawa E, Kimura M, Koike H, Ueno Y, et al. Vascularized and complex organ buds from diverse tissues via mesenchymal cell-driven condensation. Cell Stem Cell. 2015;16(5):556–65.
76. Soltanian A, Ghezelayagh Z, Mazidi Z, Halvaei M, Mardpour S, Ashtiani MK, et al. Generation of functional human pancreatic organoids by transplants of embryonic stem cell derivatives in a 3D-printed tissue trapper. J Cell Physiol. 2019;234(6):9564–76.
77. Ghezelayagh Z, Zabihi M, Zarkesh I, Gonçalves CAC, Larsen M, Hagh-Parast N, et al. Improved differentiation of hESC-derived pancreatic progenitors by using human fetal pancreatic mesenchymal cells in a micro-scalable three-dimensional co-culture system. Stem Cell Rev Rep. 2022;18(1):360–77.
78. Murrow LM, Weber RJ, Gartner ZJ. Dissecting the stem cell niche with organoid models: an engineering-based approach. Development. 2017;144(6):998–1007.

79. Hunckler MD, García AJ. Engineered biomaterials for enhanced function of insulin-secreting β-cell organoids. Adv Funct Mater. 2020;30(48):2000134.
80. Candiello J, Grandhi TSP, Goh SK, Vaidya V, Lemmon-Kishi M, Eliato KR, et al. 3D heterogeneous islet organoid generation from human embryonic stem cells using a novel engineered hydrogel platform. Biomaterials. 2018;177:27–39.
81. Hakobyan D, Médina C, Dusserre N, Stachowicz ML, Handschin C, Fricain JC, et al. Laser-assisted 3D bioprinting of exocrine pancreas spheroid models for cancer initiation study. Biofabrication. 2020;12(3):035001.
82. Lin M, Gao M, Pandalai PK, Cavnar MJ, Kim J. An Organotypic microcosm for the pancreatic tumor microenvironment. Cancer. 2020;12(4)
83. Abadpour S, Aizenshtadt A, Olsen PA, Shoji K, Wilson SR, Krauss S, et al. Pancreas-on-a-chip technology for transplantation applications. Curr Diab Rep. 2020;20(12):72.
84. Lai Benjamin FL, Lu Rick X, Hu Y, Davenport HL, Dou W, Wang EY, et al. Recapitulating pancreatic tumor microenvironment through synergistic use of patient organoids and organ-on-a-chip vasculature. Adv Funct Mater. 2020;30(48)
85. Shahryari A, Saghaeian Jazi M, Mohammadi S, Razavi Nikoo H, Nazari Z, Hosseini ES, et al. Development and clinical translation of approved gene therapy products for genetic disorders. Front Genet. 2019;10:868.
86. Uddin F, Rudin CM, Sen T. CRISPR gene therapy: applications, limitations, and implications for the future. Front Oncol. 2020;10:1387.
87. Shahryari A, Burtscher I, Nazari Z, Lickert H. Engineering gene therapy: advances and barriers. Adv Ther. 2021;4(9):2100040.
88. Romanelli SM, MacDougald OA. Viral and nonviral transfer of genetic materials to adipose tissues: toward a gold standard approach. Diabetes. 2020;69(12):2581–8.
89. Tan SY, Wong JLM, Sim YJ, Wong SS, Elhassan SAM, Tan SH, et al. Type 1 and 2 diabetes mellitus: a review on current treatment approach and gene therapy as potential intervention. Diabetes Metab Syndr Clin Res Rev. 2019;13(1):364–72.

Chapter 5
EBM in Endocrinology

Akbar Soltani, Azadeh Aletaha, and Bagher Larijani

5.1 Definition and Principles of EBM

Evidence-based medicine (EBM) is an approach to medical practice that integrates the best available evidence from systematic research with clinical expertise and patient values to make informed healthcare decisions. The following are the key principles of EBM [1–4]:

- Asking Focused Clinical Questions: EBM emphasizes the formulation of clear and specific clinical questions that guide the search for evidence. Well-defined questions typically involve aspects such as diagnosis, prognosis, treatment, or patient preferences.
- Searching for and Appraising Evidence: EBM involves conducting systematic literature searches to identify relevant research studies. Critical appraisal is then applied to assess the validity, reliability, and applicability of the evidence. This process helps determine the quality and relevance of the studies. It involves critically appraising and synthesizing the available evidence from well-designed studies, such as randomized controlled trials, systematic reviews, and meta-analyses.

A. Soltani (✉) · A. Aletaha
Evidence Based Medicine Research Center, Endocrinology and Metabolism Clinical Sciences Institute, Tehran University of Medical Sciences, Tehran, Iran

B. Larijani
Endocrinology and Metabolism Research Center, Endocrinology and Metabolism Clinical Sciences Institute, Tehran University of Medical Sciences, Tehran, Iran

H. Gharib et al. (eds.), *Interdisciplinary Advances in Endocrinology*, https://doi.org/10.1007/978-981-95-2286-6_5

- Applying Evidence to Patient Care: EBM recognizes that evidence alone is not sufficient for clinical decision-making. Clinical expertise and knowledge of the patient's unique values and preferences are essential factors in integrating evidence into individualized patient care.
- Continuous Learning and Improvement: EBM encourages healthcare professionals to engage in continuous learning and improvement. This involves staying updated with the latest research, critically evaluating new evidence, and adapting practice based on new information to provide the best possible care.

5.2 Importance of EBM in Endocrinology

Endocrinology is a complex and rapidly evolving field that encompasses the study of various hormonal disorders and their impact on the body. Evidence-based medicine (EBM) plays a crucial role in guiding clinical decision-making and improving patient outcomes in endocrinology.

EBM involves integrating the best available evidence from high-quality research with clinical expertise and patient values to make informed decisions about patient care [2]. In the context of endocrinology, EBM helps healthcare professionals stay up-to-date with the latest research findings and apply them to their practice. The use of EBM in endocrinology has several key benefits. First, it ensures that healthcare providers base their decisions on scientific evidence rather than personal opinions or anecdotal experiences. This approach promotes consistency and reduces the potential for bias, leading to more reliable and effective patient care [5].

Additionally, EBM helps identify and evaluate the quality of research studies in endocrinology. By critically appraising the literature, healthcare professionals can assess the validity and reliability of the evidence, considering factors such as study design, sample size, statistical analysis, and potential sources of bias. This critical appraisal allows for a more accurate interpretation of research findings and a better understanding of their clinical implications [6]. Furthermore, EBM in endocrinology helps bridge the gap between research and practice. By incorporating the best available evidence into clinical decision-making, healthcare professionals can optimize patient outcomes and ensure that their interventions are based on the most reliable and up-to-date information. This approach also encourages continuous learning and professional development, as healthcare providers strive to stay informed about the latest advancements in the field [7]. Evidence-based medicine (EBM) plays a crucial role in the field of endocrinology for several reasons:

- *Complexity of Endocrine Disorders:* Endocrine disorders, such as diabetes and thyroid disorders, involve intricate hormonal pathways and interactions with multiple organ systems. The application of EBM principles is crucial to navigate the complexities of these conditions. For example, in the management of type 2 diabetes, EBM has led to significant advancements in treatment strategies. The UK Prospective Diabetes Study (UKPDS) demonstrated the benefits of intensive glycemic control in reducing the risk of microvascular complications, providing strong evidence for individualized treatment targets based on patient characteristics and comorbidities [8, 9]. EBM has also guided the use of newer classes of antidiabetic medications, such as sodium-glucose co-transporter-2 inhibitors (SGLT2 inhibitors) and glucagon-like peptide-1 receptor agonists (GLP-1 RAs), by demonstrating their cardiovascular benefits and improved glycemic control [10]

- *Evolving Treatment Landscape:* The field of endocrinology is characterized by ongoing advancements in treatment options and diagnostic techniques. EBM ensures that healthcare professionals remain up-to-date with the evolving landscape. For instance, in the management of differentiated thyroid cancer, the American Thyroid Association (ATA) guidelines provide evidence-based recommendations on risk stratification, surgical approaches, and radioactive iodine therapy [11]. These guidelines are regularly updated based on emerging evidence, ensuring clinicians have access to the most current best practices. EBM also plays a vital role in evaluating emerging therapies, such as targeted therapies and immunotherapies, to guide their integration into treatment algorithms [11].
- *Patient-Centered Care:* EBM emphasizes the importance of considering individual patient preferences, values, and goals in decision-making. In the management of hypothyroidism, for example, EBM supports shared decision-making regarding the choice of levothyroxine formulations based on patient preferences and individual factors. The American Thyroid Association guidelines recommend considering patient preference for branded versus generic formulations, as some patients may perceive differences in symptom control or quality of life [12]. By incorporating patient values alongside evidence-based recommendations, EBM promotes patient-centered care and improves treatment adherence.
- *Enhanced Clinical Decision-Making:* EBM equips healthcare professionals with the tools to make evidence-based clinical decisions. In the diagnosis of adrenal incidentalomas, for instance, EBM guides the evaluation of hormonal functionality and the risk of malignancy. The European Society of Endocrinology guidelines provide evidence-based algorithms to aid in the selection of appropriate biochemical and radiological investigations, enabling clinicians to make accurate diagnoses and determine the need for surgical intervention [13]. By following evidence-based guidelines, clinicians can improve diagnostic accuracy and avoid unnecessary interventions.
- *Resource Optimization:* The prevalence of endocrine disorders places a significant burden on healthcare resources. EBM plays a vital role in optimizing resource allocation. In the management of gestational diabetes mellitus (GDM), for example, EBM has demonstrated that lifestyle interventions, including diet and exercise, are effective in controlling blood glucose levels and reducing adverse outcomes [14]. By promoting lifestyle interventions as the first-line approach, EBM helps minimize the need for pharmacological interventions and reduces healthcare costs.
- *Addressing Practice Variation:* EBM promotes standardized care by providing evidence-based guidelines that address practice variation among healthcare pro-

fessionals. For instance, in the management of acromegaly, the Endocrine Society guidelines offer evidence-based recommendations on the use of somatostatin analogs, growth hormone receptor antagonists, and other therapeutic modalities [15]. These guidelines help ensure consistent, high-quality care across different healthcare settings and reduce variability in practice. In summary, the importance of EBM in endocrinology is evident in the complex nature of endocrine disorders, the evolving treatment landscape, the focus on patient-centered care, enhanced clinical decision-making, resource optimization, and addressing practice variation. By incorporating EBM principles into clinical practice, healthcare professionals can provide evidence-based, personalized care that improves patient outcomes and optimizes the management of endocrine disorders.

Evidence-based medicine (EBM) plays a crucial role in assessing study quality and bias in the field of endocrinology. Here are some key points regarding this role:

5.2.1 Assessing Study Quality and Bias

- Assessing study quality and potential biases is crucial in evidence-based medicine to ensure reliable findings. Various tools and frameworks are available to evaluate study quality, such as the Cochrane Collaboration's tool for assessing risk of bias in randomized trials [16]. This tool assesses key domains of bias, including random sequence generation, allocation concealment, blinding of participants and personnel, incomplete outcome data, selective reporting, and other sources of bias. By systematically assessing these domains, researchers and clinicians can determine the reliability and internal validity of a study.

5.2.2 Understanding Statistical Measures and Interpretation

- Statistical measures play a vital role in quantifying the strength of evidence and interpreting study findings. It is essential to understand concepts such as p-values, confidence intervals, and effect sizes. For a comprehensive understanding of statistical concepts in the context of endocrine literature, "Medical Statistics at a Glance" by Petrie and Sabin provides a concise overview. This resource covers statistical tests commonly used in clinical research, including t-tests, chi-square tests, and regression analysis, enabling researchers to appropriately interpret the statistical results reported in endocrine studies [17].

5.2.3 Evaluating Clinical Relevance and Applicability

- Assessing the clinical relevance and applicability of study findings is crucial for translating evidence into practice. The GRADE (Grading of Recommendations Assessment, Development, and Evaluation) system provides a framework for evaluating the quality of evidence and making recommendations. The GRADE approach considers factors such as study design, risk of bias, consistency of results, precision, directness, and applicability to patient populations and settings. By applying the GRADE framework, clinicians can assess the certainty of evidence and determine the applicability of research findings in their clinical practice [18].

Evidence-based medicine (EBM) plays a crucial role in guiding the management of specific endocrine conditions. By integrating the best available evidence with clinical expertise and patient preferences, healthcare professionals can make informed decisions that optimize patient outcomes. Here are some EBM approaches in specific endocrine conditions:

5.3 EBM in Diabetes Management

Diabetes is a chronic metabolic disorder that requires ongoing management. EBM provides a foundation for evidence-based diabetes care, including diagnosis, glycemic control, and prevention of complications. Clinical practice guidelines, such as those from the American Diabetes Association (ADA) and the International Diabetes Federation (IDF), offer evidence-based recommendations for diabetes management [19]. These guidelines incorporate findings from large randomized controlled trials (RCTs) and systematic reviews on topics like glucose-lowering medications, lifestyle interventions, and cardiovascular risk reduction strategies. By following evidence-based guidelines, healthcare providers can optimize glycemic control, reduce the risk of complications, and improve the quality of life for individuals with diabetes.

5.4 EBM in Thyroid Disorders

Thyroid disorders, such as hypothyroidism and hyperthyroidism, require accurate diagnosis and appropriate treatment. EBM approaches in thyroid disorders involve utilizing evidence-based guidelines, such as those from the American Thyroid Association (ATA) and the European Thyroid Association (ETA), to guide clinical decision-making [11]. These guidelines provide recommendations based on systematic reviews, meta-analyses, and expert consensus, addressing topics such as thyroid function testing, management of thyroid nodules, and thyroid hormone replacement therapy. By following evidence-based guidelines, healthcare professionals can ensure accurate diagnosis, appropriate treatment, and optimal outcomes for patients with thyroid disorders.

5.5 EBM in Adrenal Disorders

Adrenal disorders, including adrenal insufficiency and Cushing's syndrome, require evidence-based approaches for diagnosis and management. EBM in adrenal disorders involves utilizing clinical practice guidelines, such as those from the Endocrine Society, to guide decision-making [20]. These guidelines are based on systematic reviews and meta-analyses of the available evidence and address topics such as diagnostic testing, pharmacological interventions, and surgical management. By incorporating evidence-based guidelines, healthcare professionals can optimize the diagnosis, treatment, and long-term management of patients with adrenal disorders.

5.6 EBM in Reproductive Endocrinology

Reproductive endocrinology encompasses conditions such as polycystic ovary syndrome (PCOS), infertility, and menopausal hormone therapy. EBM in reproductive endocrinology involves utilizing evidence-based guidelines, such as those from the American Society for Reproductive Medicine (ASRM) and the International Federation of Gynecology and Obstetrics (FIGO), to guide clinical practice [21, 22]. These guidelines are based on systematic reviews, RCTs, and expert consensus, providing recommendations for the diagnosis and management of reproductive endocrine conditions. By following evidence-based guidelines, healthcare professionals can optimize fertility treatments, hormonal therapies, and overall reproductive health outcomes.

It is important for healthcare professionals to regularly update their knowledge by staying informed about the latest evidence-based guidelines and research in these specific endocrine conditions. By incorporating EBM approaches, healthcare providers can ensure the highest quality of care for patients with diabetes, thyroid disorders, adrenal disorders, and reproductive endocrine conditions.

5.7 EBM and Treatment Guidelines

Evidence-based medicine (EBM) plays a critical role in the development, evaluation, and implementation of clinical practice guidelines. These guidelines provide healthcare professionals with evidence-based recommendations to guide clinical decision-making and improve patient care. Let's explore the key aspects of EBM in relation to treatment guidelines.

5.8 Development and Evaluation of Clinical Practice Guidelines

Clinical practice guidelines are developed through a rigorous process that involves synthesizing the best available evidence, expert consensus, and consideration of patient values and preferences. EBM is at the core of this process, ensuring that guidelines are based on high-quality evidence from systematic reviews, meta-analyses, and well-conducted clinical trials.

The development of guidelines typically involves multidisciplinary panels of experts who review and critically appraise the available evidence. They assess the quality and strength of the evidence, weigh the benefits and harms of different interventions, and formulate recommendations based on the balance of these factors. EBM methods, such as the GRADE (Grading of Recommendations Assessment, Development, and Evaluation) system, are often used to standardize the evaluation and grading of evidence.

Once developed, guidelines undergo a rigorous evaluation process to ensure their validity, reliability, and applicability. This evaluation may involve external review by other experts, public consultation, and pilot testing to assess the feasibility and impact of implementing the guidelines in real-world clinical settings [23, 24].

5.9 Incorporating EBM into Clinical Decision-Making

Clinical practice guidelines serve as a valuable tool for healthcare professionals to incorporate EBM into their clinical decision-making process. Guidelines provide evidence-based recommendations that are tailored to specific patient populations and clinical scenarios. By following these recommendations, healthcare providers can optimize patient outcomes and deliver consistent, high-quality care.

Incorporating EBM into clinical decision-making involves critically appraising the available evidence and considering the individual patient's values, preferences, and clinical characteristics. It requires a balance between the best available evidence, clinical expertise, and the unique context of each patient. Healthcare professionals should be knowledgeable about the guidelines relevant to their practice and regularly update their knowledge to stay informed about the latest evidence and recommendations [5, 25].

5.10 Challenges and Controversies in Guideline Development

The development of treatment guidelines is not without challenges and controversies. Some of the common challenges include [26, 27]:

- *Conflicting Evidence*: In certain areas of medicine, the evidence base may be limited, conflicting, or of low quality. This can pose challenges in formulating clear and definitive recommendations.
- *Bias and Conflicts of Interest*: Guideline development panels should strive to minimize bias and conflicts of interest among panel members to ensure the integrity and objectivity of the recommendations.
- *Contextual Factors*: Guidelines may not always address the full range of clinical scenarios and patient preferences. Healthcare professionals need to consider the specific context, patient characteristics, and local resources when applying guidelines to individual patient care.
- *Updating Guidelines*: The rapid pace of scientific advancements necessitates regular updates to guidelines. However, keeping guidelines up-to-date can be challenging and time-consuming, leading to potential delays in incorporating new evidence into practice.

Controversies can arise when different guideline organizations or expert panels have divergent recommendations due to variations in their interpretation of the evidence or differing perspectives on the benefits and risks of interventions. These controversies highlight the importance of critical appraisal and considering multiple sources of guidelines when making clinical decisions.

In conclusion, EBM is essential in the development, evaluation, and implementation of clinical practice guidelines. These guidelines provide evidence-based recommendations to guide clinical decision-making and improve patient care. Incorporating EBM into clinical practice requires healthcare professionals to stay informed about the latest evidence, critically appraise the available guidelines, and consider the unique context of each patient.

5.10.1 EBM and Emerging Technologies in Endocrinology

Emerging technologies are rapidly transforming the field of endocrinology, and evidence-based medicine (EBM) plays a crucial role in evaluating and integrating these technologies into clinical practice. Here, we will explore two areas where EBM intersects with emerging technologies in endocrinology: precision medicine and telemedicine/remote monitoring.

5.10.2 *Precision Medicine and EBM*

Precision medicine aims to tailor medical treatments and interventions to individual patients based on their unique characteristics, including genetic makeup, biomarkers, and clinical data. EBM provides the foundation for incorporating precision medicine into endocrinology practice, ensuring that interventions are supported by robust evidence.

EBM enables the evaluation of genetic and molecular markers to identify patients who are likely to respond to specific therapies or have an increased risk of certain endocrine conditions. Through the use of systematic reviews, meta-analyses, and clinical trials, EBM helps determine the clinical utility and validity of biomarkers and genetic tests in guiding treatment decisions and predicting outcomes [28, 29].

Furthermore, EBM is critical in assessing the effectiveness, safety, and cost-effectiveness of emerging targeted therapies and interventions. By systematically evaluating the available evidence, EBM helps clinicians make informed decisions about incorporating precision medicine technologies into routine practice, considering factors such as patient preferences, clinical benefits, and potential risks.

5.10.3 *Telemedicine and Remote Monitoring in Endocrine Care*

Telemedicine and remote monitoring technologies have gained significant attention in recent years, especially in endocrine care. These technologies enable healthcare providers to deliver care remotely, monitor patients' conditions, and provide ongoing support. EBM provides a framework for evaluating the effectiveness, safety, and feasibility of telemedicine and remote monitoring in endocrine practice. Evidence-based studies have assessed the use of telemedicine for various endocrine conditions, including diabetes management, thyroid disorders, and adrenal diseases. These studies have examined outcomes such as glycemic control, patient satisfaction, and healthcare resource utilization. EBM helps determine the efficacy of telemedicine interventions, identify patient populations that benefit the most, and define the appropriate scope and limitations of remote care.

Similarly, remote monitoring technologies, such as continuous glucose monitors (CGMs) and wearable devices, offer opportunities for real-time data collection and personalized management of endocrine conditions. EBM plays a crucial role in evaluating the accuracy, clinical utility, and impact of these technologies on patient outcomes and healthcare delivery.

By incorporating EBM principles, healthcare providers can make evidence-based decisions about the integration of telemedicine and remote monitoring technologies into endocrine care, ensuring that these technologies are applied appropriately, effectively, and safely [30, 31].

In conclusion, EBM is essential in the integration of emerging technologies, such as precision medicine and telemedicine/remote monitoring, into endocrinology practice. EBM provides the necessary evidence to evaluate the effectiveness, safety, and feasibility of these technologies, ultimately improving patient care and outcomes.

Formulating clinical questions and searching for evidence are essential steps in the practice of evidence-based medicine (EBM) in endocrinology. When practicing evidence-based medicine (EBM), it is important to formulate well-structured clinical questions and effectively search for reliable sources of evidence. In this context, the PICO framework is often used to formulate clinical questions, while identifying reliable sources of evidence and employing effective search strategies are crucial for finding the best available evidence [32]. Here's an overview of these processes:

5.10.4 PICO Framework for Clinical Questions

The PICO framework is a widely used approach for formulating clinical questions in a structured manner. It stands for:

- P: Patient, Problem, or Population—describing the characteristics of the patient or population of interest
- I: Intervention, Exposure, or Test—specifying the intervention, exposure, or test being considered
- C: Comparison—identifying the alternative or comparison intervention, exposure, or test
- O: Outcome—defining the desired outcome or outcomes of interest

By using the PICO framework, clinicians can clearly define their clinical question and focus their search for evidence on the relevant aspects. This structured approach improves the efficiency and effectiveness of the evidence search process.

5.10.5 Identifying Reliable Sources of Evidence

Identifying reliable sources of evidence is essential for practicing EBM [5, 24, 33]. Here are some key sources to consider:

- Systematic Reviews and Meta-analyses: These studies summarize and critically appraise existing evidence on a particular topic, providing a comprehensive overview of the available literature.
- Randomized Controlled Trials (RCTs): RCTs are considered the gold standard for evaluating the effectiveness of interventions. They involve randomly assigning participants to different treatment groups and comparing outcomes.

- Clinical Practice Guidelines: Guidelines developed by reputable organizations synthesize evidence and provide recommendations for clinical decision-making.
- High-Quality Journals: Peer-reviewed journals with rigorous editorial processes often publish original research studies and systematic reviews.

It is important to critically appraise the sources of evidence to ensure their reliability, validity, and relevance to the clinical question at hand. Tools like the GRADE approach can help evaluate the quality of evidence.

5.10.6 Effective Search Strategies

To conduct an effective search for evidence, consider the following strategies:

- Define the clinical question using the PICO framework.
- Identify appropriate keywords and synonyms related to the PICO elements.
- Utilize databases such as PubMed, Embase, or Cochrane Library to search for relevant articles.
- Refine the search using filters, such as study design or publication date, to focus on the most relevant evidence.
- Review reference lists of relevant articles to identify additional sources.
- Consider using advanced search techniques, such as Boolean operators (AND, OR), truncation, or proximity searching, to refine the search further.

Keeping track of the search strategy, including the keywords used and the databases searched, is crucial for reproducibility and documentation purposes. In summary, formulating clinical questions using the PICO framework, identifying reliable sources of evidence, and employing effective search strategies are essential components of EBM. By following these principles, clinicians can find the best available evidence to inform their clinical decision-making and provide optimal care to their patients.

5.11 Future Directions in Evidence-Based Medicine (EBM) and Endocrinology

Future directions in evidence-based medicine (EBM) and endocrinology research hold exciting prospects for advancing knowledge, improving patient care, and addressing emerging challenges. Here are some key areas that are shaping the future of EBM and endocrinology research:

- *Precision Medicine and Personalized Treatments*: The field of endocrinology is increasingly recognizing the importance of precision medicine, which involves tailoring treatments to individual patients based on their unique characteristics. Future research will focus on identifying specific biomarkers, genetic variations, and molecular pathways associated with endocrine disorders. This knowledge will enable the development of targeted therapies and personalized treatment approaches, leading to improved outcomes and reduced adverse effects [34].

- *Omics Technologies and Data Integration*: With advancements in genomics, proteomics, metabolomics, and other "-omics" technologies, there is a growing opportunity to understand the molecular mechanisms underlying endocrine disorders. Future research will leverage these technologies to identify novel disease biomarkers, unravel disease pathways, and discover potential therapeutic targets. Additionally, integrating data from various sources, such as electronic health records, wearable devices, and patient-reported outcomes, will provide a comprehensive view of patients' health status and aid in evidence synthesis [35].
- *Big Data Analytics and Artificial Intelligence*: The increasing availability of large-scale datasets in endocrinology presents both challenges and opportunities. Advanced analytics techniques, including machine learning and artificial intelligence, will play a crucial role in extracting meaningful insights from complex data. These technologies can assist in identifying patterns, predicting disease outcomes, and improving diagnostic accuracy. Moreover, AI-powered decision support systems can aid clinicians in making evidence-based treatment decisions by synthesizing vast amounts of data and providing personalized recommendations [36].
- *Real-World Evidence and Comparative Effectiveness Research*: While randomized controlled trials (RCTs) remain the gold standard for establishing causality, there is a growing recognition of the importance of real-world evidence (RWE) and comparative effectiveness research (CER). Future research will focus on harnessing RWE from observational studies, registries, and electronic health records to understand treatment effectiveness, safety, and long-term outcomes in real-world settings. This will provide valuable insights into the broader impact of interventions and help guide clinical decision-making [37].
- *Patient Engagement and Shared Decision-Making*: Patient engagement is increasingly recognized as a key component of EBM. Future research will explore strategies to actively involve patients in research design, knowledge translation, and shared decision-making processes. Patient-reported outcomes and patient preferences will be integrated into research design and clinical practice to ensure patient-centered care and improve treatment adherence and satisfaction [35].
- *Health Equity and Disparities*: Addressing health disparities and promoting health equity are crucial aspects of future EBM and endocrinology research. Research efforts will focus on understanding and mitigating disparities in the prevention, diagnosis, and treatment of endocrine disorders across diverse populations. This includes examining social determinants of health, cultural factors, and access to care to ensure equitable distribution of evidence-based interventions [38].

In conclusion, future directions in EBM and endocrinology research involve embracing precision medicine, leveraging omics technologies and data integration, harnessing big data analytics and AI, utilizing real-world evidence, promoting patient engagement, and addressing health equity. These advancements will contribute to a more personalized, effective, and equitable approach to endocrine care, ultimately improving patient outcomes and quality of life.

References

1. Freddi G, Romàn-Pumar JL. Evidence-based medicine: what it can and cannot do. Annali dell'Istituto superiore di sanita. 2011;47(1):22–5.
2. Sackett DL, Rosenberg WM, Gray JA, Haynes RB, Richardson WS. Evidence based medicine: what it is and what it isn't. BMJ. 1996;312(7023):71–2.
3. Djulbegovic B, Guyatt GH. Progress in evidence-based medicine: a quarter century on. Lancet (London, England). 2017;390(10092):415–23.
4. Richardson PE. David Sackett and the birth of evidence based medicine: how to practice and teach EBM. BMJ. 2015;350:h3089.
5. Straus SE. Evidence-based medicine: how to practice and teach it; 2011.
6. Guyatt GH, Rennie D. Users' guides to the medical literature. JAMA. 1993;270(17):2096–7.
7. Gartlehner G, Hansen RA, Nissman D, Lohr KN, Carey TS. Criteria for distinguishing effectiveness from efficacy trials in systematic reviews; 2010.
8. UK Prospective Diabetes Study (UKPDS) Group. Intensive blood-glucose control with sulphonylureas or insulin compared with conventional treatment and risk of complications in patients with type 2 diabetes (UKPDS 33). Lancet (London, England). 1998;352(9131):837–53.
9. Marso SP, Bain SC, Consoli A, Eliaschewitz FG, Jódar E, Leiter LA, et al. Semaglutide and cardiovascular outcomes in patients with type 2 diabetes. N Engl J Med. 2016;375(19):1834–44.
10. Wiviott SD, Raz I, Bonaca MP, Mosenzon O, Kato ET, Cahn A, et al. Dapagliflozin and cardiovascular outcomes in type 2 diabetes. N Engl J Med. 2019;380(4):347–57.
11. Haugen BR, Alexander EK, Bible KC, Doherty GM, Mandel SJ, Nikiforov YE, et al. 2015 American Thyroid Association management guidelines for adult patients with thyroid nodules and differentiated thyroid cancer: the American Thyroid Association guidelines task force on thyroid nodules and differentiated thyroid cancer. Thyroid. 2016;26(1):1–133.
12. Jonklaas J, Bianco AC, Bauer AJ, Burman KD, Cappola AR, Celi FS, et al. Guidelines for the treatment of hypothyroidism: prepared by the american thyroid association task force on thyroid hormone replacement. Thyroid. 2014;24(12):1670–751.
13. Fassnacht M, Arlt W, Bancos I, Dralle H, Newell-Price J, Sahdev A, et al. Management of adrenal incidentalomas: European Society of Endocrinology Clinical Practice Guideline in collaboration with the European network for the study of adrenal tumors. Eur J Endocrinol. 2016;175(2):G1–g34.
14. Schoenaker DA, Mishra GD, Callaway LK, Soedamah-Muthu SS. The role of energy, nutrients, foods, and dietary patterns in the development of gestational diabetes mellitus: a systematic review of observational studies. Diabetes Care. 2016;39(1):16–23.
15. Katznelson L, Laws ER Jr, Melmed S, Molitch ME, Murad MH, Utz A, et al. Acromegaly: an endocrine society clinical practice guideline. J Clin Endocrinol Metab. 2014;99(11):3933–51.
16. Higgins JP, Altman DG, Gøtzsche PC, Jüni P, Moher D, Oxman AD, et al. The Cochrane collaboration's tool for assessing risk of bias in randomised trials. BMJ. 2011;343:d5928.
17. Petrie ASC. Medical statistics at a glance. Wiley-Blackwell; 2009.

18. Schünemann HJ, Cuello C, Akl EA, Mustafa RA, Meerpohl JJ, Thayer K, et al. GRADE guidelines: 18. How ROBINS-I and other tools to assess risk of bias in nonrandomized studies should be used to rate the certainty of a body of evidence. J Clin Epidemiol. 2019;111:105–14.
19. Association AD. American Diabetes Association standards of medical care in diabetes–2017. Diabetes Care. 2017;40(Suppl. 1):S1.
20. Nieman LK, Biller BM, Findling JW, Murad MH, Newell-Price J, Savage MO, et al. Treatment of Cushing's syndrome: an endocrine society clinical practice guideline. J Clin Endocrinol Metab. 2015;100(8):2807–31.
21. Medicine PCotASfR. Diagnostic evaluation of the infertile female: a committee opinion. Fertil Steril. 2015;103(6):e44–50.
22. Lee SR, Cho MK, Cho YJ, Chun S, Hong S-H, Hwang KR, et al. The 2020 menopausal hormone therapy guidelines. J Menopausal Med. 2020;26(2):69.
23. Institute of Medicine Committee on Standards for Developing Trustworthy Clinical Practice G. In: Graham R, Mancher M, Miller Wolman D, Greenfield S, Steinberg E, editors. Clinical practice guidelines we can trust. Washington: National Academies Press (US) Copyright 2011 by the National Academy of Sciences. All rights reserved.; 2011.
24. Guyatt GH, Oxman AD, Vist GE, Kunz R, Falck-Ytter Y, Alonso-Coello P, et al. GRADE: an emerging consensus on rating quality of evidence and strength of recommendations. BMJ. 2008;336(7650):924–6.
25. Guyatt GH, Meade MO, Jaeschke RZ, Cook DJ, Haynes RB. Practitioners of evidence based care: not all clinicians need to appraise evidence from scratch but all need some skills. Br Med J. 2000;320:954–5.
26. Qaseem A, Forland F, Macbeth F, Ollenschläger G, Phillips S, van der Wees P. Guidelines international network: toward international standards for clinical practice guidelines. Ann Intern Med. 2012;156(7):525–31.
27. Armstrong JJ, Goldfarb AM, Instrum RS, MacDermid JC. Improvement evident but still necessary in clinical practice guideline quality: a systematic review. J Clin Epidemiol. 2017;81:13–21.
28. Klonoff DC, Florez JC, German M, Fleming A. The need for precision medicine to be applied to diabetes. J Diabetes Sci Technol. 2020;14(6):1122–8.
29. Scott IA, Hilmer SN, Reeve E, Potter K, Le Couteur D, Rigby D, et al. Reducing inappropriate polypharmacy: the process of deprescribing. JAMA Intern Med. 2015;175(5):827–34.
30. Fatehi F, Armfield NR, Dimitrijevic M, Gray LC. Clinical applications of videoconferencing: a scoping review of the literature for the period 2002-2012. J Telemed Telecare. 2014;20(7):377–83.
31. Lee SWH, Ooi L, Lai YK. Telemedicine for the management of glycemic control and clinical outcomes of type 1 diabetes mellitus: a systematic review and meta-analysis of randomized controlled studies. Front Pharmacol. 2017;8:330.
32. Richardson WS, Wilson MC, Nishikawa J, Hayward RS. The well-built clinical question: a key to evidence-based decisions. ACP J Club. 1995;123(3):A12–3.
33. Jpt H. Cochrane handbook for systematic reviews of interventions. http://www cochrane-handbook org (2008).
34. Collins FS, Varmus H. A new initiative on precision medicine. N Engl J Med. 2015;372(9):793–5.
35. Snyder CF, Jensen RE, Segal JB, Wu AW. Patient-reported outcomes (PROs): putting the patient perspective in patient-centered outcomes research. Med Care. 2013;51(8 Suppl 3):S73–9.
36. Topol EJ. High-performance medicine: the convergence of human and artificial intelligence. Nat Med. 2019;25(1):44–56.
37. Sherman RE, Anderson SA, Dal Pan GJ, Gray GW, Gross T, Hunter NL, et al. Real-world evidence – what is it and what can it tell us? N Engl J Med. 2016;375(23):2293–7.
38. Braveman PA, Kumanyika S, Fielding J, Laveist T, Borrell LN, Manderscheid R, et al. Health disparities and health equity: the issue is justice. Am J Public Health. 2011;101(Suppl 1):S149–55.

Chapter 6
Molecular Modeling in Endocrinology

Elaheh Kashani-Amin, Joulia Alizadeh-Rahrovi, Latifeh Navidpour, and Azadeh Ebrahim-Habibi

6.1 Introduction

In the recent years, there has been a growing interest in the use of computational methods in order to design new drugs or improve existing drugs for the treatment of various diseases, including endocrine-related diabetes and obesity.

These methods, often referred to as in silico strategies, involve the use of computer simulations and modeling to mimic and predict the behavior of molecules and their interactions with biological targets. When those targets have no known experimentally solved structures, they were usually modelled using homology modeling, which predicts the 3D structure of a protein based on its similarity to known protein structures [1]. Although these methods are still used, in the recent years (i.e., from 2021) [2], the artificial-intelligence-based structure prediction tool "AlphaFold" has become the first resource to look at when a protein structure is not known.

After obtaining or preparing the target structure, structure-based virtual screening (VS) could help to identify potential hits (ligands) that could interact with it, by

E. Kashani-Amin
Antimicrobial Resistance Research Center, Institute of Immunology and Infectious Diseases, Iran University of Medical Sciences, Tehran, Iran

J. Alizadeh-Rahrovi
Endocrinology and Metabolism Research Center, Endocrinology and Metabolism Clinical Sciences Institute, Tehran University of Medical Sciences, Tehran, Iran

L. Navidpour
Department of Medicinal Chemistry, Faculty of Pharmacy, Tehran University of Medical Sciences, Tehran, Iran

A. Ebrahim-Habibi (✉)
Biosensor Research Center, Endocrinology and Metabolism Molecular-Cellular Sciences Institute, Tehran University of Medical Sciences, Tehran, Iran
e-mail: aehabibi@tums.ac.ir

H. Gharib et al. (eds.), *Interdisciplinary Advances in Endocrinology*,
https://doi.org/10.1007/978-981-95-2286-6_6

computationally screening large collections of molecules [3]. Molecular docking is the method that predicts the orientation and strength of the binding of those hits, which are often small molecules [4]. In order to get a more precise insight into the interaction of those ligands and targets, molecular dynamics (MD) simulations can also be performed. MD simulations simulate atoms' motion over time, and may elucidate the dynamic behavior of biomolecular systems to some extent. They may also give details on how proteins and ligands interact with each other, how proteins change their shape and function, and how stable the ligand-protein complexes are [5].When quantum mechanics methods are used to provide more details into specific regions of a biological complex (usually in the binding cavity), and the rest of the complex is studied by MD simulations based on molecular mechanics (MM), the used method is designated as "QM/MM" [6].

Ligand-based methods can also provide novel alternatives to known drugs. In this context, pharmacophore modeling and computation of quantitative structure-activity relationship (QSAR) may come to aid. The first tool identifies the key features of a ligand that are essential for binding to a target protein. These features include atoms, groups, or regions that are involved in specific interactions, such as hydrogen bonds, electrostatic interactions, or hydrophobic contacts [7]. QSAR involves developing mathematical models that correlate the chemical structure of compounds with their biological activities. The activity of new compounds is then predicted based on their structural features such as size, shape, charge, or polarity [8]. Virtual screening of molecule databases could be performed by the ligand-based approach, using structural and chemical features of known active molecules [9] .

Finally, computational prediction of toxicity or pharmacokinetics properties (absorption, distribution, metabolism, excretion, and toxicity: ADMET) are also considered in the recent years when a suitable drug candidate has been obtained during a medicinal chemistry research [10].

In this chapter, we present an overview of selected recent investigations that have used at least one of the above-mentioned methods in order to obtain potential new therapeutic agents for diabetes as a major representative of endocrine disorders. This is by no mean an exhaustive review of all current drugs family or putative targets for diabetes; our focus has been on recent studies (mostly from 2017 onward) and approved or potential therapeutic targets, which have been most investigated by in silico methods, as found out by our search strategy.

6.2 Molecular Targeting of Diabetes

6.2.1 Glycosidase Inhibitors

Slowing down the digestion of carbohydrates by using inhibitors of intestinal digestive enzymes has been investigated since the 1980s as a new approach to treating diabetes. These inhibitors help in reducing high postprandial blood sugar levels as demonstrated with inhibitors of enzymes such as alpha-amylase and other glucosidases. An early example is a study conducted with trestatin, a carbohydrate-based compound extracted from *Streptomyces*, which was effective in reducing starch-meals increases in blood glucose levels in human subjects [11]. These compounds are relatively safe, and although effective on postprandial glucose levels, would not provoke hypoglycemic episodes [12]. Acarbose, miglitol, and voglibose are examples of approved glycosidase (alpha-glucosidase) inhibitors [13].

Use of computer-based rational methods can help to identify new inhibitors of these enzymes. For example, the development of novel α-amylase inhibitors involving the conversion of carbohydrates into drug-like fragments was presented by Mortier and Wolber [14].

On the other hand, flavonoids and similar structures are also known as inhibitors of this enzyme [15]. In a systematic in silico investigation published in 2020, polyphenols (flavonoids and phenolics acids) have been studied from various angles, including structural properties of the ligands (with quantum mechanics methods), their docking into glycoside enzymes followed by MD simulation, as well as an ADMET check. Furthermore, P450 site of metabolism was also studied. Finally, a pharmacophore was obtained for this type of compounds, showing Linarin to be a quite suitable potential glycosidase inhibitor [16]. Another polyphenol, namely, curcumin, is also an inhibitor of alpha-glucosidase [17]. The synthesis and evaluation of curcumin-based derivatives as potential antidiabetic agents has been described in a report by Khodarahmi et al. [18] . The study involved an in vitro and in silico analysis of the compounds' ability to inhibit the enzymes α-glucosidase and α-amylase.

The synthesis of another group of compounds with an aromatic heterocyclic scaffold, i.e., hydrazine containing piperazine or benzimidazole derivatives, and their potential as α-amylase inhibitors have been reported by Colak and his colleagues [19]. This study involved molecular docking, inhibition kinetics, and in vitro cytotoxicity activity studies to evaluate the potential of these compounds as α-amylase inhibitors.

An alternative to find suitable chemically synthesized compounds is a search in the large and diverse pool of natural compounds. As a recent example, phytochemical analysis, α-glucosidase and amylase inhibitory activity assessment as well as molecular docking studies have been performed on compounds extracted from *Persicaria hydropiper L.* leaves essential oils. The result of this study was the identification of β-caryophyllene epoxide as a potent alpha-glycosidase [20]. In a study that showed the in vivo potential of *Levisticum officinale* stem and leaf extract in diabetic rats, reduced serum glucose levels and amelioration of other related parameters (e.g., lipid profile and antioxidant enzyme levels) were observed. The most abundant natural compounds were also tested in vitro and in silico for their α-amylase inhibitory activity. The results revealed flavonoid compounds, as well as hexanoic acid as inhibitors of the enzyme [21].

Other recently reported structures with glycosidase inhibition activity include benzylidenebenzofuran (aurones) [22], 3,3-di(indolyl)indolin-2-ones [23], 5-amino-nicotinic acid derivatives [24], 1,2,4-triazole-bearing bis-hydrazones [25], bisindolylmethane sulfonamides [26], phthalimide-benzenesulfonamide hybrids [27], as well as caffeic acid derivatives (newboulaside B) obtained from natural sources [28] [29]. In most studies, at least a docking experiment has been performed, while MD simulations and affinity binding computations have been sometimes added to obtain details of interaction between ligands and enzymes at atomic level.

There has been an increased interest toward finding novel inhibitors of glycosidase enzymes (alpha-amylase and alpha-glucosidase) in recent years, and we have cited a limited number of those. While many of these reports include at least a docking experiment, it would be of interest to see an integrative study that would collect all structure types and extract pharmacophore(s) for them, as well as clarify (or predict) possible interaction sites of these compounds. So far, most of these studies have discussed polyphenols, and more specifically flavonoids.

6.2.2 PPARγ-Modulators

PPARγ (peroxisome proliferator-activated receptor gamma) is a nuclear receptor that regulates the expression of multiple genes including genes involved in glucose and lipid metabolism, inflammation, and cell differentiation. PPARγ-modulators affect its function and have been investigated as potential antidiabetic agents.

While antidiabetic thiazolidinediones (TZDs), such as rosiglitazone and pioglitazone, are agonists of PPARγ, an early 2000s study reported that modest antagonism of the receptor can also counteract insulin resistance and obesity (caused by a high-fat diet). These compounds act by influencing leptin and adiponectin. On the other hand, too much reduction of PPARγ can also lead to insulin resistance, since this will reduce white adipose tissue and increase triglyceride levels [30]. These results indicated the need to be cautious in modulating PPARγ function, but also suggested other possibilities such as designing partial agonists of the receptor with less side effects than full agonists (such as weight gain) [31]. Since PPARγ undergoes a number of posttranslational modification, targeting those would also be a way to modulate its activity. A recent review has highlighted an approach consisting of blocking PPARγ phosphorylation at a specific position (Ser 273). For now, the exact mechanism of action of phosphorylation blockers is not understood, and in silico experiments (including MD simulations) have suggested that these compounds may actually stabilize the ligand-binding domain of the receptor [32].

In a recent study, isobutyric acid derivatives have been shown to be interesting antihyperglycemics in a mice diabetes model, while also increasing the expression of PPARγ (and GLUT-4) mRNA in adipocytes cell lines. The nitro-compounds were especially effective, and a docking experiment showed their abilities to interact with the receptor in a similar way with previously co-crystallized ligands. With the use of MD simulation, the authors further clarify the interaction details of their best compound and the receptor. Finally, in an "in silico toxicology" computation, ADMET values of the best compounds were verified. The results were that while potential toxicity of these compounds could be of concern when the structures are considered, they would probably not show problematic characteristics in vivo, and that they could be classified as "toxicity cliffs." In conclusion, these compounds could be partial modulators of PPARγ [33].

Another set of compounds, namely, 1,2,4-oxadiazole-based trans-acrylic acid derivatives, were designed based on a pharmacophore with these characteristics: an acidic head group linked to a lipophilic tail with an aryl or methylene linker, which was suggested to be a dual agonist of PPARs (alpha and gamma). Designed compounds that had best docking scores were synthesized and tested in vitro on the receptors. ADMET properties were also predicted and the best compounds were indeed effective in an in vivo model [34]. Another study has used aryl propionic acid as scaffold and, in a combination of synthesizing compounds and docking them in PPARγ, reported active compounds as tested in a diabetic in vivo model [35].

As mentioned in the previous section, natural sources are also explored in order to find specific compounds that would act on therapeutic targets. It is possible to construct a compound library for VS experiments based on natural product libraries and literature that lists known modulators of PPARγ, it is possible to construct compounds library to perform VS experiments. By the use of VS, designing pharmacophores and anti-pharmacophores (in order to exclude full agonists of the receptor), and in some cases, validation of computational results by experimental methods, flavonoids, sesquiterpene lactone derivatives, neolignans (dieugenol, tetrahydrodieugenol and magnolol), and oleanolic acid have been identified as PPARγ (partial) agonists [36]. Based on the structure of scutellarin (a flavonoid), an extensive computational study has explored a phenol compounds database, in order to find other polyphenols with antidiabetic potential and fewer side effects. In this study, various conformations of the receptor and co-crystallized ligands have been used for a precise analysis of the binding cavity that accommodates itself to the bonded ligand. A high number of polyphenols was suggested to have therapeutic potential, and satisfied the ADMET criteria, as tested by predictive tools [37].

In a slightly different approach, isolated compounds from a traditional Indian medicinal plant were investigated, again by starting to dock the compounds into PPARγ structure, and choosing the best scoring compound, which was "nymphayol," for further in vitro and in vivo tests, in which it performed well [38].

In line with the recent interest toward "drug repositioning," which aims at finding other uses for approved drugs, an investigation was conducted on FDA-approved drugs with an extensive set of proteins structures, in order to find similar affinity fingerprints, with eight known PPARγ antagonists as a reference set. Between the ten found hits (which were also docked onto PPARγ structure), according to experimental validations, the best drug was nitazoxanide, which is originally used to treat parasitic infections [39].

Other PPARγ targeting structures that have been checked in silico (at least with a docking experiment) and tested in vitro and/or in vivo include novel thiazolidinedione derivatives [40], 1,3,4-oxadiazole and 2-4-thiazolidinedione based bisheterocycles [41], 1, 3, 4-thiadiazole derivatives [42], cinnamic acid derivatives [43], and indole derivatives [44].

6.2.3 Multitarget Approaches Involving PPARγ

In a "multitarget" approach toward antidiabetics design (i.e., targeting several receptors and enzymes involved in glucose metabolism), a unified pharmacophore has been used that possesses "an acid moiety, an aromatic ring, a flexible linker group, and a bulky hydrophobic group." This pharmacophore is proposed to be effective toward PPARγ but also PPARα and GPR-40 (G-protein-coupled receptor 40), PTP-1B (protein tyrosine phosphatase-1B), and aldose reductase (AR). Bioisosteres were designed based on this pharmacophore from which a phenylpropanoic acid derivative and a benzylidenethiazolidine-2,4-dione derivative were proven to be antihyperglycemic in an in vivo model. Docking of these compounds as well as MD simulations was performed on two of the targets, and a pharmacological consensus analysis was done with the use of multiple tools [45].

While inhibition of glycosidase enzymes is a mean to lessen postprandial glucose levels, aldose reductase inhibition would prevent potential complications arisen from polyols accumulation in various tissues [46]. A flavonoid named diosmin, which is obtained from citrus is effective against alpha-amylase, alpha-glucosidase, and aldol reductase, which makes it an interesting core structure for further optimization [47]. In this study, molecular docking, MD simulation, and pharmacokinetic prediction have been used.

Sulfonylurea receptors (SUR) and PPARs are considered as two essential molecular drug targets in the treatment of type 2 diabetes mellitus. Stimulation of sulfonylurea receptors existing in pancreatic β-cells increases insulin secretion [48]. Sulfonylureas are classified into three generations based on their antidiabetic efficiency, which interact with different binding sites in SUR [49]. Furthermore, some sulfonylureas have also demonstrated agonistic activity on PPARγ [48, 50], including pyrazoline containing benzenesulfonylureas for which docking experiments have been performed in addition to experimental studies [51]. Further efforts to design new analogs exerting their antidiabetic clinical efficacy by acting through both receptors resulted in a new pharmacophore model development. Therefore, quinoline-4(3*H*)-one [52] and phthalimide-sulfonylurea hybrids [53] bearing three lipophilic centers separated by amidic and anionic linkers were synthesized and showed in vivo activities against STZ-induced hyperglycemic rats, in vitro PPARγ-binding affinities, and insulin-secreting abilities. The binding mode of these analogs in the PPARγ and SUR was also examined by molecular docking experiments and the structural requirements were explored by QSAR models, while in silico ADMET tests were also performed.

6.2.4 Dipeptidyl Peptidase-4 (DPP-4) Inhibitors

Lowering blood glucose levels can be achieved by inhibiting the serine peptidase DPP-4, which degrades the incretin hormones glucagon-like peptide-1 (GLP-1) and glucose-dependent insulinotropic polypeptide (GIP). These hormones are released postprandial and stimulate insulin secretion while inhibiting glucagon secretion, slowing gastric emptying, and reducing appetite.

Approved DPP-4 inhibitors include sitagliptin, vildagliptin, saxagliptin, linagliptin, and alogliptin. They are interesting antidiabetic with regard to their low risk of hypoglycemia, being weight-neutral or slightly weight-reducing, and they have a potential to prevent or delay the progression of diabetic complications [54].

Triazolotriazine derivatives possess an effective scaffold as DPP-4 inhibitors. These compounds were designed based on 3D-QSAR results obtained on quinoline/isoquinoline and a generated pharmacophore that had been used in a VS study. The designed compounds efficacy was then demonstrated with an in vivo experiment on an animal diabetes model [55].

Another tested structure was thiosemicarbazones with pyrazole components. Both of these structures had shown antidiabetic properties, and designed compounds containing both were synthesized and tested in vitro. These tests were followed by docking experiments that further suggested the importance of some substitutions (e.g., bromo and trifluoromethyl substitutions), as well as ADMET predictions, which showed the suitability of the compounds [56]. With a similar reasoning (combination of different scaffolds with antidiabetic activities), hybrids of dihydropyrimidine phthalimide have been synthesized and tested in vitro and in an in vivo model, again followed by docking and a proposed structure-activity relationship pattern [57]. Other proposed DPP-4 inhibitor structures include uracil-based benzoic acid and ester derivatives [58], and Schiff's bases [59].

Based on the antidiabetic effect of *Ephedra* species extract, and an extensive computational study of 2012 that had performed VS, docking, and MD simulations to find DPP-4 inhibitors from natural sources, and that had predicted ephedrine and pseudoephedrine to have antidiabetic properties [60], an investigation on those and other derivatives of ephedrine showed their abilities to inhibit this enzyme in vitro [61]. The results showed norephedrine to be a promising candidate and a potential lead to develop other DPP-4 inhibitors. Computational experiments (docking, pharmacophore proposal) have then been performed to propose potentially more effective ligands. Other potential DPP-4 inhibitors from natural sources include compounds from *Amberboa ramosa*, which is a plant with antidiabetic activity. In a recent study, phytochemicals of the plant have been subjected to VS followed by detailed computation (MD simulation and QM/MM calculation for best hits) as well as ADME test. The study has suggested three compounds as probable enzyme inhibitors [62].

Peptides inhibitors are also an interesting alternative to classical small molecules. As an example, tripeptide analogs of Ile-Pro-Ile (diprotin A), a potent, food-derived DPP-4 inhibitor, have been designed by the use of a method called minimum analog peptide set (MAPS). This method enables the generation of smaller peptide libraries, by focusing on desired physicochemical characteristics of a peptide. In this case, a QSAR model was first generated to find these characteristics. An interesting result of the study was the generation of a particularly stable peptide (Ile-Pro-Ala), which is, however, less potent than the original tripeptide [63]. Interestingly, Ile-Pro-Ala has also been found in the protein hydrolysate of an Antarctic marine organism [64]. A subsequent study has used previously reported di- and tripeptides to generate a 3D QSAR model after which six tripeptides had been synthesized and it was found that they have moderate DPP-4 inhibitory activity. In this work, MD simulation and dockings were also performed and key residues involved in the inhibitors interactions were suggested [65]. In another study, screening of pea protein hydrolysates, which had antihyperglycemic effect, led to the identification of four peptides with 5 to 7 residues and DPP-4 inhibitory effect. Peptides of the hydrolysates had been first experimentally separated and sequenced, after which a VS and docking was performed to find probable inhibitors [66].

6.2.5 Sodium-Glucose Cotransporter 2 (SGLT2) Inhibitors

SGLT2 inhibitors are a relatively new class of antidiabetics that inhibit glucose reabsorption in kidneys. This results in lower blood glucose levels and an increased urinary glucose elimination (glucosuria). Marketed SGLT2 inhibitors include anagliflozin, dapagliflozin, empagliflozin, and ertugliflozin. Besides decreased blood glucose levels, they may also induce weight loss and show cardiovascular benefits. On the other hand, they may increase genitourinary infections, and they are associated with diabetic ketoacidosis and a higher risk of bone fractures [67]. Their adverse effects are especially a matter of concern in the elderly, who, incidentally, would constitute an increasingly large part of people with diabetes [68].

In studies by Wai-Lung Ng et al., new "carbasugars" were synthesized based on the structure of known SGLT2 inhibitors and their mode of interaction with SGLT2 was hypothesized by modeling the receptor and performing docking simulations. The in silico experiment helped to explain the unexpected structure-activity relationship that was obtained based on experimental tests [69]. Another studied scaffold has been C-glucosyl dihydrochalcones, derivatives of which were shown to be selective SGLT2 inhibitors. In this study, MD simulations were performed to verify whether the best suggested SGLT2 inhibitor (nothofagin) was a pan-assay interference compound (PAINS), that is, a compound that can interact with numerous targets, and in this case, membrane proteins. The result was that nothofagin was not likely to be PAINS [70]. Another new compound is the flavonoid C-glycoside swertisin, which has been checked experimentally, but also investigated by docking simulations [71].

Other theoretical studies on SGLT2 inhibitors, which are either found with VS on databases or designed new compounds, suggest these structure as potential effective hits: 1,2,4 triazoles and 1,2,4 oxadiazoles scaffold [72], and dioxabicyclo[3.2.1] octane [73]. There are also several in silico studies, which start at known SGLT2 inhibitors and suggest putative modifications but without going further into experimental tests (e.g., dapagliflozin [74]).

6.2.6 *Other Explored Targets*

6.2.6.1 Protein Tyrosine Phosphatase 1B

Protein tyrosine phosphatase 1B (PTP1B) negatively regulates insulin signaling by dephosphorylating the insulin receptor and its substrate. It is also involved in the regulation of leptin signaling, which affects energy balance and body weight. Inhibition of PTP1B could enhance insulin sensitivity and positively affect glucose metabolism, as well as reduce type 2 diabetes associated obesity and inflammation. Designing selective inhibitors of this enzyme is challenging due to its similarity with other phosphatases, and oral inhibitors may have shortages with regard to high cell permeability and bioavailability, due to the highly charged nature of PTP1B active site [75].

In examples of search for inhibitors involving in silico methods, natural compounds databases have been explored and isosilybin has been obtained as a putative PTP1B inhibitor [76], while another computational study suggests 1,6- dihydropyrimidine derivatives [77]. In another study, natural compounds that had been previously identified as PTP1B inhibitors and antidiabetics were more closely examined via MD simulations experiments. An allosteric binding mode, alongside with possible conformational changes in PTP1B upon ligands binding, was detected, and the authors conclude that Aloe emodin glycoside, 3β-taraxerol (3BT), chlorogenic acid (CGA) and cichoric acid (CHA) are effective allosteric inhibitors of the enzyme [78]. Other natural compounds include geranylated flavonoid analogs [79], furancoumarin [80], stilbene dimers [81], phloroglucinols [82], and unsaturated alkynyl phenols [83] to name a few. Recent reviews provides more insight into the current research situation with regard to PTP1B inhibitors from natural sources as well as synthetic ones [84, 85].

6.2.6.2 Glycogen Phosphorylase

Glycogen phosphorylase catalyzes the breakdown of glycogen to glucose in the liver and muscles. Inhibiting this enzyme will result in the decrease of liver glucose output, which may help to improve glycemic control. One limitation in developing selective and effective glycogen phosphorylase inhibitors (GPI) is related to adverse effects on muscle fatigue, which is important in terms of hindering exercising in people with diabetes [86].

N-acyl-β-d-glucopyranosylamines, and biphenyl-N-acyl-β-d--glucopyranosylamines are GPIs, which were designed based on the crystallographic information on the enzyme, and the characteristics of the ligand-binding pocket. Subsequent synthesis and testing the compounds showed their activity and their crystallization with the enzyme proved the reliability of the molecular modeling method [87]. 3-(β-d-glucopyranosyl)-5-substituted-1,2,4-triazole derivatives have also been reported as GPIs. The in silico approach used in this study was a VS experiment done with the help of QM/MM docking [88].

From the natural products pool, flavonoids have also been identified as GPIs with genistein, 8-prenylgenistein, apigenin, 8-prenylapigenin, 8-prenylnaringenin, galangin, and valoneic acid dilactone being effective inhibitors [89]. In this study, important residues in the interaction of flavonoids and GP have also been suggested by computational methods.

6.2.6.3 Glucokinase

Glucokinase (GK) catalyzes the first step of glycolysis, by facilitating the conversion of glucose to glucose-6-phosphate. It is a glucose sensor in the liver and pancreas and a target for diabetes treatment, since its activation would lead to lower levels of blood glucose, and may ultimately improve glucose metabolism and insulin secretion in people with type 2 diabetes. GK activators that have been so far developed have shown side effects such as hypoglycemia (as found in a meta-analysis) [90], weight gain [91], and liver toxicity [92].

Several structures have been designed as GK activators (GKA). A number of hetero-substituted sulfonamido-benzamide hybrids have been designed and tested for in vitro and in vivo activities; compounds were also docked into GK structure and checked for ADMET properties, and suggested to be safe for further development [93]. Quinazolin-4-one clubbed with thiazole acetates/acetamides was found to lower blood glucose to a desirable level in an animal OGTT (oral glucose tolerance test). In this study, docking was performed to find out details of compound-enzyme interaction [94]. Other synthetic GKA structures whose investigation includes at least one in silico method (usually docking) include new benzamides derivatives, such as thiazol-2-yl benzamide derivatives and the allosteric activators 3,5-disubstituted benzamide derivatives and N-pyridin-2-yl benzamide analogs or N-benzimidazol-2yl benzamide analogs [95], and pyridoxine derivatives (two pyridoxine rings connected with a sulfur-containing linker) [96]. In some cases, compounds have been first designed by an in silico method. Examples are amino phosphonate derivatives [97], which have been designed by joining fragments in the binding cavity, new benzamides including diazole-benzamide and benzamide-sulfonamide derivatives, which have been designed and then docked to find the best compound before in vitro experimentation [98], or mangiferin, a natural compound suggested by a preliminary VS study [99].

A theoretical approach (i.e., screening by in silico methods) has been applied to natural compounds and resulted in suggesting these molecules as potential GKAs: prenylated flavonoids [100], some compounds of the hydro-alcoholic extract of *Allium hirtifolium Boiss* (Persian shallot) including cinnamic acid and flavonoids [101], and swertiamarin and apigenin, from the traditional anti-diabetic plant *Enicostemma littorale* [102].

6.3 A Special Case: MD Simulations of Insulin

Insulin, the 51-residues double-chain, disulfide bridged molecule that has a central role in glucose homeostasis, is also one of the most thoroughly explored biological structures. Its 3D structure was reported in 1969, by Dorothy Hodgkin and her team, making it the sixth protein structure to be ever elucidated [103].

Insulin was used as a therapeutic from the early 1920s, though. Since then, variants of the peptide have been designed that are either short acting, regular, or long acting [13].

Among various issues with insulin, its conformational changes needed for exerting its physiological function, its propensity to form amyloid fibrils, and its stability as a therapeutic protein are subjects that can be explored via MD simulation. The small size of insulin makes it also an excellent model protein for such studies that are usually computationally expensive.

The active form of insulin, i.e., the one that binds to its receptor, is a monomeric form that should be obtained by the dissociation of its oligomeric and finally dimeric forms. A recent MD simulation has shown that this process can take place via more than one path, and essentially by either dissociation of alpha-helices or beta-strands [104]. In order to give details about insulin binding to its receptor, a study by Papaioannou et al. showed that the C-terminal part of the insulin's B chain (BC-CT), which is crucial in this process, acquires random open and close conformations, as well as a rare and active conformation (the wide-open conformation). Mutating chain B's Y26 could affect the propensity of insulin to take the active conformation, and the mutants (in particular Y26N) were suggested to make suitable insulin analogs [105]. In a subsequent study, the authors suggested mutations Y26S and Y26E as potential choice to make analogs with higher probability for the active conformation, leading to better effectiveness [106]. Other studies have shown interesting details about specific segments of insulin that are particularly important in insulin binding, such as the relatively flexible intrachain disulfide of chain A (C6-C11), which is influencing the B-chain conformation [107]. Small molecules can also affect the active conformation of insulin, as demonstrated by an MD simulation study on vitamin E, which has an activator effect not seen for vitamin D, even though both molecules have shown suitable binding affinity toward insulin [108].

Pathogenic mutations can affect the normal folding of proteins or cause important conformational changes in its structure. One such pathogenic mutation occurs in a type of neonatal diabetes named mutant INS-gene-induced diabetes of youth (MIDY). A MD simulation study has shown that the A chain C7Y mutation will affect the secondary structure at residues 2 to 8, causes an extended alpha-helix formation downward (residues 9 to 19), and increases N-terminal flexibility of the A-chain. The result is a structure that may go toward a partially folded state [109].

As a biopharmaceutical, the stability of insulin is of particular importance. Use of additives or modifications such as PEGylation is a common means of stabilizing proteins. In the case of insulin, MD simulations have shown how trehalose can protect insulin during desiccation (lyophilization) by maintaining the H-bond content of insulin and acting as water surrogate [110]. Amino acids are another class of additives used to stabilize various proteins. A study on Arg, Lys, and His showed the individual stabilizing properties of each amino acid. For example, Arg had a more pronounced effect on generating a hydration shell over the protein, while Lys formed salt bridges with insulin [111]. Ionic liquids are another class of stabilizers that are also acting by protecting insulin from water's interactions [112] and preserve insulin native conformation [113]. PEGylation was found to decrease the solvent accessible area of insulin and prevent water to disrupt the hydrophobic regions [114, 115]. Another tested modification was O-glycosylation, that is also a stabilizing modification, which occurs via glycan H-bonds [116].

Formation of amyloid fibrils, that is, a particular ordered form of aggregation from monomers of insulin, may affect its therapeutic effectiveness, when occurring both in vitro (over storage) and in vivo (e.g., after multiple injections at the same site) [117]. Studying various aspects of insulin aggregation can help to gather more information on its mechanism and lead to proposals of appropriate measures to prevent it.

Pressure-induced conformational change in insulin was studied by crystallography and MD simulations as a mean to explore nonnative structures of insulin, which may appear in the initial stages of aggregation. The results showed the propensity of the B-chain, and especially its terminal fragments to undergo deleterious conformational changes [118]. Temperature-induced initial changes of insulin structure have been related to several residues of the B-chain C-terminus, and other environmental conditions such as acidic pH were found to be important, in accordance with experimental results [119]. Stabilizing methods mentioned previously such as use of additives, ionic liquids, and modifications or mutations may all have a role in preventing aggregates or amyloid formation of insulin, as, for example, demonstrated in an experimental and MD simulation study of chemically modified insulins [120].

In summary, MD simulations have been used to investigate insulin structure, function, and stability, providing additional validation (or explanation) for experimental data, or giving new hints about an overlooked issue. Given the importance of this therapeutic molecule, and its many unexplored aspects, it is likely that we will still witness more investigations in this regard.

6.4 Conclusion

In silico methods are now routinely used in the process of drug discovery, repositioning or optimization. We have briefly presented a limited number of examples concerning diabetes therapeutics. There is at least one major development that is perceptible in recent researches that aim to discover new molecules: the wide use of ADMET tools, which are an invaluable aid in predicting the developability of a molecule, in addition to its druggability, which is covered by other in silico tools. The use of artificial intelligence, and especially machine learning, is very likely to expand to a great extent in the use of all in silico methods, which could become an integrated and essential tool to assess new drugs and even new biological targets.

References

1. Cavasotto CN, Phatak SS. Homology modeling in drug discovery: current trends and applications. Drug Discov Today. 2009;14(13–14):676–83.
2. Callaway E. Deepmind's AI for protein structure is coming to the masses. Nature. 2021;
3. Reddy AS, Pati SP, Kumar PP, Pradeep H, Sastry GN. Virtual screening in drug discovery-a computational perspective. Curr Protein Peptide Sci. 2007;8(4):329–51.
4. Meng X-Y, Zhang H-X, Mezei M, Cui M. Molecular docking: a powerful approach for structure-based drug discovery. Curr Comput Aided Drug Des. 2011;7(2):146–57.
5. Kerrigan JE. Molecular dynamics simulations in drug design. In: In silico models for drug discovery; 2013. p. 95–113.
6. Kulkarni PU, Shah H, Vyas VK. Hybrid quantum mechanics/molecular mechanics (QM/MM) simulation: A tool for structure-based drug design and discovery. Mini Rev Med Chem. 2022;22(8):1096–107.
7. Yang S-Y. Pharmacophore modeling and applications in drug discovery: challenges and recent advances. Drug Discov Today. 2010;15(11–12):444–50.
8. Cherkasov A, Muratov EN, Fourches D, Varnek A, Baskin II, Cronin M, et al. QSAR modeling: where have you been? Where are you going to? J Med Chem. 2014;57(12):4977–5010.
9. Ripphausen P, Nisius B, Bajorath J. State-of-the-art in ligand-based virtual screening. Drug Discov Today. 2011;16(9–10):372–6.
10. Pawar G, Madden JC, Ebbrell D, Firman JW, Cronin MT. In silico toxicology data resources to support read-across and (Q) SAR. Front Pharmacol. 2019;10:561.
11. Eichler H, Korn A, Gasic S, Pirson W, Businger J. The effect of a new specific α-amylase inhibitor on post-prandial glucose and insulin excursions in normal subjects and type 2 (non-insulin-dependent) diabetic patients. Diabetologia. 1984;26:278–81.
12. Hedrington MS, Davis SN. Considerations when using alpha-glucosidase inhibitors in the treatment of type 2 diabetes. Expert Opin Pharmacother. 2019;20(18):2229–35.
13. Brunton LL, Knollmann BC. Goodman & Gilman's the pharmacological basis of therapeutics. New York: McGraw Hill; 2023.
14. Al-Asri J, Fazekas E, Lehoczki G, Perdih A, Görick C, Melzig MF, et al. From carbohydrates to drug-like fragments: rational development of novel α-amylase inhibitors. Bioorg Med Chem. 2015;23(20):6725–32.
15. Ćorković I, Gašo-Sokač D, Pichler A, Šimunović J, Kopjar M. Dietary polyphenols as natural inhibitors of α-amylase and α-glucosidase. Life. 2022;12(11):1692.
16. Chenafa H, Mesli F, Daoud I, Achiri R, Ghalem S, Neghra A. In silico design of enzyme α-amylase and α-glucosidase inhibitors using molecular docking, molecular dynamic, conceptual DFT investigation and pharmacophore modelling. J Biomol Struct Dyn. 2022;40(14):6308–29.
17. Tshiyoyo KS, Bester MJ, Serem JC, Apostolides Z. In-silico reverse docking and in-vitro studies identified curcumin, 18α-glycyrrhetinic acid, rosmarinic acid, and quercetin as inhibitors of α-glucosidase and pancreatic α-amylase and lipid accumulation in HepG2 cells, important type 2 diabetes targets. J Mol Struct. 2022;1266:133492.
18. Ezati M, Ghavamipour F, Khosravi N, Sajedi RH, Chalabi M, Farokhi A, et al. Synthesis and potential antidiabetic properties of curcumin-based derivatives: an in vitro and in silico study of α-glucosidase and α-amylase inhibition. Med Chem. 2023;19(1):99–117.
19. Cakmak U, Oz-Tuncay F, Basoglu-Ozdemir S, Ayazoglu-Demir E, Demir İ, Colak A, et al. Synthesis of hydrazine containing piperazine or benzimidazole derivatives and their potential

as α-amylase inhibitors by molecular docking, inhibition kinetics and in vitro cytotoxicity activity studies. Med Chem Res. 2021;30(10):1886–904.

20. Mahnashi MH, Alqahtani YS, Alyami BA, Alqarni AO, Ayaz M, Ghufran M, et al. Phytochemical analysis, α-glucosidase and amylase inhibitory, and molecular docking studies on Persicaria hydropiper L. leaves essential oils. Evid Based Complement Alternat Med. 2022;2022:1–11.
21. Ghaedi N, Pouraboli I, Askari N. Antidiabetic properties of Hydroalcoholic leaf and stem extract of Levisticum officinale: an implication for α-amylase inhibitory activity of extract ingredients through molecular docking. Iran J Pharm Res. 2020;19(1):231–50.
22. Roshanzamir K, Kashani-Amin E, Ebrahim-Habibi A, Navidpour L. Aurones as new porcine pancreatic α-amylase inhibitors. Letters Drug Design Discov. 2019;16(3):333–40.
23. Santoso M, Ong LL, Aijijiyah NP, Wati FA, Azminah A, Annuur RM, et al. Synthesis, α-glucosidase inhibition, α-amylase inhibition, and molecular docking studies of 3, 3-di (indolyl) indolin-2-ones. Heliyon. 2022;8(3):e09045.
24. Nawaz M, Taha M, Qureshi F, Ullah N, Selvaraj M, Shahzad S, et al. Structural elucidation, molecular docking, α-amylase and α-glucosidase inhibition studies of 5-amino-nicotinic acid derivatives. BMC chemistry. 2020;14(1):1–11.
25. Khan I, Rehman W, Rahim F, Hussain R, Khan S, Rasheed L, et al. Synthesis and in vitro α-amylase and α-glucosidase dual inhibitory activities of 1, 2, 4-Triazole-bearing bis-Hydrazone derivatives and their molecular docking study. ACS Omega. 2023;8:22508.
26. Taha M, Noreen T, Imran S, Nawaz F, Chigurupati S, Selvaraj M, et al. Synthesis, α-amylase inhibition and molecular docking study of bisindolylmethane sulfonamide derivatives. Med Chem Res. 2019;28:2010–22.
27. Askarzadeh M, Azizian H, Adib M, Mohammadi-Khanaposhtani M, Mojtabavi S, Faramarzi MA, et al. Design, synthesis, in vitro α-glucosidase inhibition, docking, and molecular dynamics of new phthalimide-benzenesulfonamide hybrids for targeting type 2 diabetes. Sci Rep. 2022;12(1):10569.
28. Basnet S, Ghimire MP, Lamichhane TR, Adhikari R, Adhikari A. Identification of potential human pancreatic α-amylase inhibitors from natural products by molecular docking, MM/GBSA calculations, MD simulations, and ADMET analysis. PLoS One. 2023;18(3):e0275765.
29. Mbagwu IS, Akah PA, Ajaghaku DL, Ike JC, Okoye FBC. Newboulasides A and B, two new caffeic acid glycosides from Newbouldia laevis with α-amylase inhibitory activity. Nat Prod Res. 2022;36(3):726–34.
30. Kadowaki T. PPAR gamma agonist and antagonist. Nihon Yakurigaku zasshi Folia Pharmacologica Japonica. 2001;118(5):321–6.
31. Burgermeister E, Schnoebelen A, et al. A novel partial agonist of peroxisome proliferator-activated receptor-γ (PPARγ) recruits PPARγ-coactivator-1α, prevents triglyceride accumulation, and potentiates insulin signaling in vitro. Mol Endocrinol. 2006;20(4):809–30.
32. Frkic RL, Richter K, Bruning JB. The therapeutic potential of inhibiting PPARγ phosphorylation to treat type 2 diabetes. J Biol Chem. 2021;297(3):101030.
33. Colin-Lozano B, Torres-Gomez H, Hidalgo-Figueroa S, Chávez-Silva F, Estrada-Soto S, Almanza-Pérez JC, et al. Synthesis, in vitro, in vivo and in silico antidiabetic bioassays of 4-nitro(thio)phenoxyisobutyric acids acting as unexpected PPARγ modulators: an in combo study. Pharmaceuticals. 2022;15(1):102.
34. Kaur P, Bhat ZR, Bhat S, Kumar R, Kumar R, Tikoo K, et al. Synthesis and evaluation of new 1,2,4-oxadiazole based trans- acrylic acid derivatives as potential PPAR-alpha/gamma dual agonist. Bioorg Chem. 2020;100:103867.
35. Kharbanda C, Alam MS, Hamid H, Ali Y, Nazreen S, Dhulap A, et al. In silico designing, in vitro and in vivo evaluation of potential PPAR-γ agonists derived from aryl propionic acid scaffold. Bioorg Chem. 2021;106:104458.
36. El-Houri R, Mortier J, Murgueitio M, Wolber G, Christensen L. Identification of PPARγ agonists from natural sources using different in silico approaches. Planta Med. 2014;81(06):488–94.

37. Encinar JA, Fernández-Ballester GJ, Galiano-Ibarra V, Micol-Molina V. In silico approach for the discovery of new PPARγ modulators among plant-derived polyphenols. In: Drug design, development and therapy; 2015. p. 5877.
38. Stalin A, Stephen Irudayaraj S, Ramesh Kumar D, Balakrishna K, Ignacimuthu S, Al-Dhabi NA, et al. Identifying potential PPARγ agonist/partial agonist from plant molecules to control type 2 diabetes using in silico and in vivo models. Med Chem Res. 2016;25(9):1980–92.
39. Kovács D, Simon Z, Hári P, Málnási-Csizmadia A, Hegedűs C, Drimba L, et al. Identification of PPARγ ligands with one-dimensional drug profile matching. In: Drug design, development and therapy; 2013. p. 917–28.
40. Li Y, Ks N, Byran G, Krishnamurthy PT. Identification of selective PPAR-γ modulators by combining pharmacophore modeling, molecular docking, and Adipogenesis assay. Appl Biochem Biotechnol. 2023;195(2):1014–41.
41. Nazreen S, Alam MS, Hamid H, Yar MS, Shafi S, Dhulap A, et al. Design, synthesis, in silico molecular docking and biological evaluation of novel oxadiazole based thiazolidine-2,4-diones bis-heterocycles as PPAR-γ agonists. Eur J Med Chem. 2014;87:175–85.
42. Vaishnav Y, Dewangan D, Verma S, Mishra A, Thakur AS, Kashyap P, et al. PPAR gamma targeted molecular docking and synthesis of some new amide and urea substituted 1, 3, 4-thiadiazole derivative as antidiabetic compound. J Heterocyclic Chem. 2020;57(5):2213–24.
43. Chauhan A, Grewal AS, Pandita D, Lather V. Novel Cinnamic acid derivatives as potential PPARδ agonists for metabolic syndrome: design, synthesis, evaluation and docking studies. Curr Drug Discov Technol. 2020;17(3):338–47.
44. Eeda V, Wu D, Lim H-Y, Wang W. Design, synthesis, and evaluation of potent novel peroxisome proliferator-activated receptor γ indole partial agonists. Bioorg Med Chem Lett. 2019;29(22):126664.
45. Domínguez-Mendoza EA, Galván-Ciprés Y, Martínez-Miranda J, Miranda-González C, Colín-Lozano B, Hernández-Núñez E, et al. Design, synthesis, and in silico multitarget pharmacological simulations of acid bioisosteres with a validated in vivo antihyperglycemic effect. Molecules. 2021;26(4):799.
46. Thakur S, Gupta SK, Ali V, Singh P, Verma M. Aldose reductase: a cause and a potential target for the treatment of diabetic complications. Arch Pharm Res. 2021;44:655–67.
47. Dubey K, Dubey R, Gupta R, Gupta A. Exploration of Diosmin to control diabetes and its complications-an in vitro and in silico approach. Curr Comput Aided Drug Des. 2021;17(2):307–13.
48. Fukuen S, Iwaki M, Yasui A, Makishima M, Matsuda M, Shimomura I. Sulfonylurea agents exhibit peroxisome proliferator-activated receptor γ agonistic activity. J Biol Chem. 2005;280(25):23653–9.
49. Vila-Carriles WH, Zhao G, Bryan J. Defining a binding pocket for sulfonylureas in ATP-sensitive potassium channels. FASEB J. 2007;21(1):18–25.
50. Arrault A, Rocchi S, Picard F, Maurois P, Pirotte B, Vamecq J. A short series of antidiabetic sulfonylureas exhibit multiple ligand PPARγ-binding patterns. Biomed Pharmacother. 2009;63(1):56–62.
51. Kharbanda C, Alam MS, Hamid H, Javed K, Dhulap A, Bano S, et al. Antidiabetic effect of novel benzenesulfonylureas as PPAR-γ agonists and their anticancer effect. Bioorg Med Chem Lett. 2015;25(20):4601–5.
52. Ibrahim MK, Eissa IH, Alesawy MS, Metwaly AM, Radwan MM, ElSohly MA. Design, synthesis, molecular modeling and anti-hyperglycemic evaluation of quinazolin-4 (3H)-one derivatives as potential PPARγ and SUR agonists. Bioorg Med Chem. 2017;25(17):4723–44.
53. El-Zahabi MA, Elbendary ER, Bamanie FH, Radwan MF, Ghareib SA, Eissa IH. Design, synthesis, molecular modeling and anti-hyperglycemic evaluation of phthalimide-sulfonylurea hybrids as PPARγ and SUR agonists. Bioorg Chem. 2019;91:103115.
54. Capuano A, Sportiello L, Maiorino MI, Rossi F, Giugliano D, Esposito K. Dipeptidyl peptidase-4 inhibitors in type 2 diabetes therapy–focus on alogliptin. Drug Des Devel Ther. 2013:989–1001.

55. Patel BD, Bhadada SV, Ghate MD. Design, synthesis and anti-diabetic activity of triazolotriazine derivatives as dipeptidyl peptidase-4 (DPP-4) inhibitors. Bioorg Chem. 2017;72:345–58.
56. Sever B, Soybir H, Görgülü Ş, Cantürk Z, Altıntop MD. Pyrazole incorporated new Thiosemicarbazones: design, synthesis and investigation of DPP-4 inhibitory effects. Molecules. 2020;25(21):5003.
57. Mourad AA, Khodir AE, Saber S, Mourad MA. Novel potent and selective DPP-4 inhibitors: design, synthesis and molecular docking study of dihydropyrimidine phthalimide hybrids. Pharmaceuticals. 2021;14(2):144.
58. Li Q, Deng X, Jiang N, Meng L, Xing J, Jiang W, et al. Identification and structure–activity relationship exploration of uracil-based benzoic acid and ester derivatives as novel dipeptidyl Peptidase-4 inhibitors for the treatment of type 2 diabetes mellitus. Eur J Med Chem. 2021;225:113765.
59. Abu Khalaf R, Awad M, Al-Essa L, Mefleh S, Sabbah D, Al-Shalabi E, et al. Discovery, synthesis and in combo studies of Schiff's bases as promising dipeptidyl peptidase-IV inhibitors. Mol Divers. 2021;26:1–13.
60. Guasch L, Sala E, Ojeda MJ, Valls C, Blade C, Mulero M, et al. Identification of novel human dipeptidyl peptidase-IV inhibitors of natural origin (part II): in silico prediction in antidiabetic extracts. PLoS One. 2012;7
61. Ojeda-Montes MJ, Ardid-Ruiz A, Tomás-Hernández S, Gimeno A, Cereto-Massagué A, Beltrán-Debón R, et al. Ephedrine as a lead compound for the development of new DPP-IV inhibitors. Future Med Chem. 2017;9(18):2129–46.
62. Paul RK, Ahmad I, Patel H, Kumar V, Raza K. Phytochemicals from Amberboa ramosa as potential DPP-IV inhibitors for the management of type-II diabetes mellitus: inferences from in-silico investigations. J Mol Struct. 2023;1271:134045.
63. Nongonierma AB, Dellafiora L, Paolella S, Galaverna G, Cozzini P, FitzGerald RJ. In silico approaches applied to the study of peptide analogs of Ile-pro-Ile in relation to their dipeptidyl peptidase IV inhibitory properties. Front Endocrinol. 2018;9:329.
64. Ji W, Zhang C, Ji H. Purification, identification and molecular mechanism of two dipeptidyl peptidase IV (DPP-IV) inhibitory peptides from Antarctic krill (Euphausia superba) protein hydrolysate. J Chromatogr B. 2017;1064:56–61.
65. Liang Z, Li H, Lu X, Lin G, Li Y, Zhang R. 3D-QSAR, in vitro assay and MD simulations studies on the design, bioactivities and different inhibitory modes of the novel DPP-IV inhibitory peptides. J Mol Struct. 2023;1283:135271.
66. Zhang M, Zhu L, Wu G, Liu T, Qi X, Zhang H. Rapid screening of novel dipeptidyl peptidase-4 inhibitory peptides from pea (Pisum sativum L.) protein using peptidomics and molecular docking. J Agric Food Chem. 2022;70(33):10221–8.
67. Lupsa BC, Inzucchi SE. Use of SGLT2 inhibitors in type 2 diabetes: weighing the risks and benefits. Diabetologia. 2018;61(10):2118–25.
68. Ferrannini E, Solini A. SGLT2 inhibition in diabetes mellitus: rationale and clinical prospects. Nat Rev Endocrinol. 2012;8(8):495–502.
69. Ng W-L, Li H-C, Lau K-M, Chan AK, Lau CB-S, Shing TK. Concise and stereodivergent synthesis of carbasugars reveals unexpected structure-activity relationship (SAR) of SGLT2 inhibition. Sci Rep. 2017;7(1):5581.
70. Jesus AR, Vila-Viçosa D, Machuqueiro M, Marques AP, Dore TM, Rauter AP. Targeting type 2 diabetes with C-glucosyl dihydrochalcones as selective sodium glucose co-transporter 2 (SGLT2) inhibitors: synthesis and biological evaluation. J Med Chem. 2017;60(2):568–79.
71. Bhardwaj G, Vakani M, Srivastava A, Patel D, Pappachan A, Murumkar P, et al. Swertisin, a novel SGLT2 inhibitor, with improved glucose homeostasis for effective diabetes therapy. Arch Biochem Biophys. 2021;710:108995.
72. Sharma S, Mittal A. 1, 2, 4 Triazoles and 1, 2, 4 Oxadiazoles scaffold as SGLT2 inhibitors: molecular docking and ADMET studies. Lett Drug Design Discov. 2023;20(11):1799–811.

73. Kumar S, Khatik GL, Mittal A. In silico molecular docking study to search new SGLT2 inhibitor based on Dioxabicyclo[3.2.1] octane scaffold. Curr Comput Aided Drug Des. 2020;16(2):145–54.
74. Feng R, Dong L, Wang L, Xu Y, Lu H, Zhang J. Development of sodium glucose co-transporter 2 (SGLT2) inhibitors with novel structure by molecular docking and dynamics simulation. J Mol Model. 2019;25:1–11.
75. Teimouri M, Hosseini H, ArabSadeghabadi Z, Babaei-Khorzoughi R, Gorgani-Firuzjaee S, Meshkani R. The role of protein tyrosine phosphatase 1B (PTP1B) in the pathogenesis of type 2 diabetes mellitus and its complications. J Physiol Biochem. 2022;78:1–16.
76. Bibi S, Sakata K. An integrated computational approach for plant-based protein tyrosine phosphatase non-receptor type 1 inhibitors. Curr Comput Aided Drug Des. 2017;13(4)
77. Patel AD, Barot R, Parmar I, Panchal I, Shah U, Patel M, et al. Molecular docking, in-silico ADMET study and development of 1,6- Dihydropyrimidine derivative as protein tyrosine phosphatase inhibitor: an approach to design and develop antidiabetic agents. Curr Comput Aided Drug Des. 2018;14(4):349–62.
78. SarathKumar B, Lakshmi BS. In silico investigations on the binding efficacy and allosteric mechanism of six different natural product compounds towards PTP1B inhibition through docking and molecular dynamics simulations. J Mol Model. 2019;25(9)
79. Niu S-L, Tong Z-F, Zhang Y, Liu T-L, Tian C-L, Zhang D-X, et al. Novel protein tyrosine phosphatase 1B inhibitor-geranylated flavonoid from mulberry leaves ameliorates insulin resistance. J Agric Food Chem. 2020;68(31):8223–31.
80. Yang Y, Tian J-Y, Ye F, Xiao Z. Identification of natural products as selective PTP1B inhibitors via virtual screening. Bioorg Chem. 2020;98:103706.
81. Yang J-B, Ye F, Tian J-Y, Song Y-F, Gao H-Y, Liu Y, et al. Multiflorumisides HK, stilbene glucosides isolated from Polygonum multiflorum and their in vitro PTP1B inhibitory activities. Fitoterapia. 2020;146:104703.
82. Phong NV, Oanh VT, Yang SY, Choi JS, Min BS, Kim JA. PTP1B inhibition studies of biological active phloroglucinols from the rhizomes of Dryopteris crassirhizoma: kinetic properties and molecular docking simulation. Int J Biol Macromol. 2021;188:719–28.
83. Le DD, Nguyen DH, Zhao BT, Seong SH, Choi JS, Kim SK, et al. PTP1B inhibitors from Selaginella tamariscina (Beauv.) spring and their kinetic properties and molecular docking simulation. Bioorg Chem. 2017;72:273–81.
84. Liu Z, Gao H, Zhao Z, Huang M, Wang S, Zhan J. Status of research on natural protein tyrosine phosphatase 1B inhibitors as potential antidiabetic agents: update. Biomed Pharmacother. 2023;157:113990.
85. Hussain H, Green IR, Abbas G, Adekenov SM, Hussain W, Ali I. Protein tyrosine phosphatase 1B (PTP1B) inhibitors as potential anti-diabetes agents: patent review (2015-2018). Expert Opin Ther Pat. 2019;29(9):689–702.
86. Baker DJ, Greenhaff PL, MacInnes A, Timmons JA. The experimental type 2 diabetes therapy glycogen phosphorylase inhibition can impair aerobic muscle function during prolonged contraction. Diabetes. 2006;55(6):1855–61.
87. Parmenopoulou V, Kantsadi AL, Tsirkone VG, Chatzileontiadou DSM, Manta S, Zographos SE, et al. Structure based inhibitor design targeting glycogen phosphorylase b. virtual screening, synthesis, biochemical and biological assessment of novel N-acyl-β-d-glucopyranosylamines. Bioorganic Med Chem. 2014;22(17):4810–25.
88. Kun S, Begum J, Kyriakis E, Stamati EC, Barkas TA, Szennyes E, et al. A multidisciplinary study of 3-(β-d-glucopyranosyl)-5-substituted-1, 2, 4-triazole derivatives as glycogen phosphorylase inhibitors: computation, synthesis, crystallography and kinetics reveal new potent inhibitors. Eur J Med Chem. 2018;147:266–78.
89. Brás NF, Neves RP, Lopes FA, Correia MA, Palma AS, Sousa SF, et al. Combined in silico and in vitro studies to identify novel antidiabetic flavonoids targeting glycogen phosphorylase. Bioorg Chem. 2021;108:104552.

90. Gao Q, Zhang W, Li T, Yang G, Zhu W, Chen N, et al. The efficacy and safety of glucokinase activators for the treatment of type-2 diabetes mellitus: a meta-analysis. Medicine. 2021;100(40):e27476.
91. Toulis KA, Nirantharakumar K, Pourzitaki C, Barnett AH, Tahrani AA. Glucokinase activators for type 2 diabetes: challenges and future developments. Drugs. 2020;80:467–75.
92. Sharma P, Singh S, Sharma N, Singla D, Guarve K, Grewal AS. Targeting human Glucokinase for the treatment of type 2 diabetes: an overview of allosteric Glucokinase activators. J Diabetes Metab Disord. 2022;21(1):1129–37.
93. Khadse SC, Amnerkar ND, Dighole KS, Dhote AM, Patil VR, Lokwani DK, et al. Hetero-substituted sulfonamido-benzamide hybrids as glucokinase activators: design, synthesis, molecular docking and in-silico ADME evaluation. J Mol Struct. 2020;1222:128916.
94. Khadse SC, Amnerkar ND, Dave MU, Lokwani DK, Patil RR, Ugale VG, et al. Quinazolin-4-one derivatives lacking toxicity-producing attributes as glucokinase activators: design, synthesis, molecular docking, and in-silico ADMET prediction. Fut J Pharm Sci. 2019;5:1–14.
95. Singh R, Lather V, Pandita D, Judge V, Arumugam N, K, Singh Grewal A. Synthesis, docking and antidiabetic activity of some newer benzamide derivatives as potential glucokinase activators. Lett Drug Design Discov. 2017;14(5):540–53.
96. Dzyurkevich MS, Babkov DA, Shtyrlin NV, Mayka OY, Iksanova AG, Vassiliev PM, et al. Pyridoxine dipharmacophore derivatives as potent glucokinase activators for the treatment of type 2 diabetes mellitus. Sci Rep. 2017;7(1):16072.
97. Yellapu NK, Kilaru RB, Chamarthi N, Sarma P, Matcha B. Structure based design, synthesis and biological evaluation of amino phosphonate derivatives as human glucokinase activators. Comput Biol Chem. 2017;68:118–30.
98. Hamid AA, Abdul-Rasheed OF, Mahdi MF, Atia A-J. Design, synthesis, characterization, and biological evaluation of new diazole-benzamide derivatives as glucokinase activators with antihyperglycemic activity. Egypt J Chem. 2022;65(8):451–69.
99. Min Q, Cai X, Sun W, Gao F, Li Z, Zhang Q, et al. Identification of mangiferin as a potential glucokinase activator by structure-based virtual ligand screening. Sci Rep. 2017;7(1):44681.
100. Faloye KO, Bekono BD, Fakola EG, Ayoola MD, Bello OI, Olajubutu OG, et al. Elucidating the glucokinase activating potentials of naturally occurring prenylated flavonoids: an explicit computational approach. Molecules. 2021;26(23):7211.
101. Kaur A, Thakur S, Deswal G, Chopra B, Dhingra AK, Guarve K, et al. In silico docking based screening of constituents from Persian shallot as modulators of human glucokinase. J Diabetes Metab Disord. 2023;22(1):547–70.
102. Khan A, Unnisa A, Sohel M, Date M, Panpaliya N, Saboo SG, et al. Investigation of phytoconstituents of Enicostemma littorale as potential glucokinase activators through molecular docking for the treatment of type 2 diabetes mellitus. In Silico Pharmacol. 2022;10:1–16.
103. Lawrence MC. Understanding insulin and its receptor from their three-dimensional structures. Mol Metab. 2021;52:101255.
104. Antoszewski A, Feng CJ, Vani BP, Thiede EH, Hong L, Weare J, et al. Insulin dissociates by diverse mechanisms of coupled unfolding and unbinding. J Phys Chem B. 2020;124(27):5571–87.
105. Papaioannou A, Kuyucak S, Kuncic ZJPO. Molecular dynamics simulations of insulin: elucidating the conformational changes that enable its binding. PLoS One. 2015;10(12):e0144058.
106. Papaioannou A, Kuyucak S, Kuncic Z. Computational study of the activity, dynamics, energetics and conformations of insulin analogues using molecular dynamics simulations: application to hyperinsulinemia and the critical residue B26. Biochem Biophys Rep. 2017;11:182–90.
107. Ong SC, Belgi A, Van Lierop B, Delaine C, Andrikopoulos S, MacRaild CA, et al. Probing the correlation between insulin activity and structural stability through introduction of the rigid A6–A11 bond. J Biol Chem. 2018;293(30):11928–43.

108. Soleymani H, Ghorbani M, Allahverdi A, Shojaeilangari S, Naderi-Manesh H. Activation of human insulin by vitamin E: a molecular dynamics simulation study. J Mol Graph Model. 2019;91:194–203.
109. Kim YH, Kastner K, Abdul-Wahid B, Izaguirre JA. Evaluation of conformational changes in diabetes-associated mutation in insulin a chain: a molecular dynamics study. Proteins Struct Funct Bioinf. 2015;83(4):662–9.
110. Li D, Liu L, Yu H, Zhai Z, Zhang Y, Guo B, et al. A molecular simulation study of the protection of insulin bioactive structure by trehalose. J Mol Model. 2014;20(11):2496.
111. Santra S, Dhurua S, Jana M. Analyzing the driving forces of insulin stability in the basic amino acid solutions: a perspective from hydration dynamics. J Chem Phys. 2021;154(8):084901.
112. Palanisamy K, Prakash M. The molecular mechanism behind the stabilization of insulin by choline and geranate (CAGE) ionic liquids – computational insights into oral insulin drug formulation. Phys Chem Chem Phys. 2021;23(44):25298–307.
113. Sundaram V, Ramanan RN, Selvaraj M, Vijayaraghavan R, MacFarlane DR, Ooi CW. Structural stability of insulin aspart in aqueous cholinium aminoate ionic liquids based on molecular dynamics simulation studies. J Mol Liq. 2021;322:114501.
114. Yang C, Lu D, Liu ZJB. How PEGylation enhances the stability and potency of insulin: a molecular dynamics simulation. Biochemistry. 2011;50(13):2585–93.
115. Jia Y, Fernandez A, Sampath J. PEGylation of insulin and lysozyme to stabilize against thermal denaturation: a molecular dynamics simulation study. J Phys Chem B. 2023;127(31):6856–66.
116. Hsu WT, Ramirez DA, Sammakia T, Tan Z, Shirts MR. Identifying signatures of proteolytic stability and monomeric propensity in O-glycosylated insulin using molecular simulation. J Comput Aided Mol Des. 2022;36(4):313–28.
117. Das A, Shah M, Saraogi I. Molecular aspects of insulin aggregation and various therapeutic interventions. ACS Bio Med Chem Au. 2022;2(3):205–21.
118. Kurpiewska K, Miłaczewska A, Lewiński K. Insulin conformational changes under high pressure in structural studies and molecular dynamics simulations. J Mol Struct. 2020;1202:127251.
119. Chinisaz M, Larijani B, Ebrahim-Habibi A. A molecular modeling study on full-length insulin: insight into initial events of amyloid formation. Struct Chem. 2014;25:1175–85.
120. Chinisaz M, Ebrahim-Habibi A, Dehpour A-R, Yaghmaei P, Parivar K, Moosavi-Movahedi AA. Structure and function of anhydride-modified forms of human insulin: in silico, in vitro and in vivo studies. Eur J Pharm Sci. 2017;96:342–50.

Chapter 7
Metabolomics and Genomics in Endocrinology

Fatemeh Bandarian, Hojat Dehghanbanadaki, Patricia Khashayar, Mostafa Rezaei-Tavirani, Mahsa M.Amoli, Nekoo Panahi, Mahin Bandarian, and Farideh Razi

7.1 Introduction

The complicated fabric of endocrinology, characterized by its interplay of hormonal signaling, metabolic regulation, and genetic determinants, remains a focal point of keen interest for the researchers and clinicians alike. Recent scientific advancements have introduced a paradigm-shifting approach that combines two powerful disciplines—metabolomics and genomics—to unravel the complexities of the endocrine system. This integration has the potential to redefine our understanding of the

F. Bandarian · F. Razi (✉)
Metabolomics and Genomics Research Center, Endocrinology and Metabolism Molecular-Cellular Sciences Institute, Tehran University of Medical Sciences, Tehran, Iran
e-mail: fbandarian@tums.ac.ir; f-razi@tums.ac.ir

H. Dehghanbanadaki
Endocrinology and Metabolism Research Center, Endocrinology and Metabolism Clinical Sciences Institute, Tehran University of Medical Sciences, Tehran, Iran

P. Khashayar
Department of Chemistry, Ghent University, Ghent, Belgium
e-mail: patricia.khashayar@ugent.be

M. Rezaei-Tavirani
Proteomics Research Center, Shahid Beheshti University of Medical Sciences, Tehran, Iran

M. M.Amoli · N. Panahi
Metabolic Disorders Research Center, Endocrinology and Metabolism Molecular-Cellular Sciences Institute, Tehran University of Medical Sciences, Tehran, Iran
e-mail: amolimm@tums.ac.ir

M. Bandarian
Department of Obstetrics and Gynecology, Ziaean Hospital, Tehran University of Medical Sciences, Tehran, Iran

H. Gharib et al. (eds.), *Interdisciplinary Advances in Endocrinology*,
https://doi.org/10.1007/978-981-95-2286-6_7

endocrine disorders, revolutionizing the diagnostic processes, and tailoring the therapeutic strategies with unprecedented precision.

Genomics, the study of an organism's genetic profile and their interactions, has provided a foundation for our understanding of the endocrine disorders. Genetic variations influence the susceptibility to as well as the onset and the severity of these disorders, underscoring the need to unravel the genetic underpinnings. By identifying the genetic variants associated with specific endocrine conditions, genomics has unveiled hidden clues to the etiology and the progression of certain disorders.

The human genome, comprised of over 20,000 genes, harbors valuable information about the genetic basis of endocrine disorders. Genomic technology has promoted significant developments in the field of medicine and endocrinology, transforming the way we understand and treat diseases. The advent of advanced sequencing and genotyping techniques, such as next-generation sequencing (NGS) and Microchip technology, has enabled scientists to perform whole genome (WGS) and exome (WES) sequencing as well as genome-wide association studies (GWASs) to decode the human genome more rapidly and at a lower cost. The WGS provides a comprehensive view of an individual's genome, facilitating the identification of novel disease-associated genetic variants. This is while the WES shifts the focus toward the protein-coding regions, pinpointing the functionally of the relevant mutations. With the help of large-scale genomic studies, researchers are now able to identify genetic variants associated with increased susceptibility to or protection against certain conditions. Today, the growing knowledge on the genetic reasons behind various syndromes affecting organs is not limited to the pituitary, thyroid, parathyroid, pancreas, adrenal, and the gonads as well as on the genomic loci harboring risk alleles for common traits, and certain endocrine conditions make the application of precision medicine in everyday clinical practice imperative [1].

Metabolomics, an evolution of the traditional biochemical analysis, entails the systematic measurement and investigation of small metabolites, ranging from amino acids and organic acids to nucleic acids and lipids, within biological samples like plasma, urine, saliva, and tissues. This comprehensive approach illustrates a panoramic portrayal of the metabolic state while revealing the pathophysiological changes in the body. It, thereby, furnishes a holistic understanding of the cellular or biological systems. The use of metabolomics to explore various diseases has witnessed a notable increase in recent years, particularly in the quest for new biomarkers. Biomarkers encompass a spectrum of small molecules, including metabolites, capable of elucidating the metabolic pathways and their deviations as a result of the pathological conditions. Technological advancements in metabolomics, including mass-spectrometry-based techniques and nuclear magnetic resonance (NMR) spectroscopy alongside sophisticated statistical methodologies, have propelled the field forward. High-resolution and high-throughput platforms enable the simultaneous detection and quantification of extensive metabolite arrays, permitting the construction of intricate metabolic maps to highlight the altered pathways of the endocrine disorders [2].

The application of genomics and metabolomics in endocrinology has been a transformative force in the exploration of disorders such as diabetes mellitus and obesity, which is the focus of this chapter. The synergistic fusion of metabolomics and genomics in endocrinology marks a paradigm shift with far-reaching implications. This interdisciplinary approach not only unravels the complex mosaic of molecular interactions governing endocrine disorders but also lays the foundation for precision medicine tailored to an individual's metabolic and genetic profile.

Similar to other fields of medicine, various omics are poised to alter the process of prevention, diagnosis, and treatment of endocrine conditions. We now have the opportunity to not only understand the cellular processes, the glandular development, and the pathophysiology of the diseases but also apply the molecularly targeted therapies. The evolution is fast and presents us with new challenges ranging from the protection of personal data to the interpretation, implementation, and overall use of genomic information [3].

In recent years and with the expansion of omics science, there has been a concerted effort to leverage bioinformatics and molecular modeling. The goal is to integrate the rapidly expanding data from various omics disciplines—such as genomics, epigenomics, transcriptomics, metabolomics, and proteomics—with phenotypic information, providing valuable insights.

The chapter navigates through the landscape of genetic variations, unveiling the molecular signatures that predispose individuals to conditions such as diabetes, obesity, metabolic syndrome, poly cystic ovary, and thyroid and adrenal disorders.

7.2 Type 1 Diabetes

Type 1 diabetes (T1D), a metabolic disorder and the second most common type of diabetes, is caused by a complex interplay between genetic susceptibility and environmental risk factors [4]. It imposes a heavy burden on global health systems. This multifactorial disorder has a strong genetic component, caused by the autoimmune destruction of pancreatic β cells [5] responsible for insulin deficiency. Pancreas in the sufferers, therefore, does not produce sufficient insulin, leading to patients being dependent on insulin use. Elucidating the genomic and metabolomics landscape of T1D, thus, has been a major goal in the past decade to help revolutionize our understanding of the underlying mechanisms involved in this complex disorder.

7.2.1 Genomics of Type 1 Diabetes

Recent advancements in genomic research have significantly contributed to our knowledge of the genetic architecture of T1D susceptibility and pathogenesis. GWAS, and high-throughput sequencing endeavors have identified numerous genetic loci, including the major histocompatibility complex (MHC) regions, associated with T1D risk [6]. From among these regions, the HLA class II gene is particularly considered as the pivotal locus implicated in disease susceptibility and onset. The involvement of other immune-related genes like PTPN22, INS, and CTLA4 has also been well known. The profound impact of specific HLA alleles, such as *HLA-DR* and *HLA-DQ* variants, on T1D risk has been extensively documented [7, 8].

HLA class II alleles account for up to 30–50% of genetic risk for T1D, whereas *HLA-DRB1* and *HLA-DQB1* on chromosome 6p21 are considered as the major susceptibility loci [7, 9]. Beyond the HLA regions, the genomic canvas of T1D encompasses a spectrum of genes involved in immune regulation, antigen presentation, and beta cell function. Variants such as INS, PTPN22, and CTLA4 intricately intertwine with certain immune pathways, modulating the balance between immune tolerance and autoimmunity in T1D pathogenesis (Table 7.1) [5, 10]. Latest bioinformatics and GWAS studies have identified over 50 susceptible regions for T1D on all 23 human chromosomes except for chromosome 8 and y (Table 7.2) [11, 12].

Furthermore, the clinical heterogeneity of T1D, spanning diverse age-of-onset spectra and disease progression trajectories, reflects the nuanced genetic predispositions and environmental interactions shaping the disease phenotypes [8]. The integration of these genetic insights into clinical practice heralds promising prospects for tailored therapeutic interventions and precision medicine in T1D [13]. Leveraging genomic information exploits the potential to refine risk prediction, stratify patient cohorts for targeted therapies, and advances the efforts toward disease interception or prevention.

Despite such strides, comprehending the intricate genetic underpinnings of T1D remains an ongoing endeavor. Unraveling the complex interplay of genetic variants, epigenetic modifications, and environmental triggers necessitates a continued synergy between cutting-edge genomic technologies and translational research efforts.

Genomic research in T1D has made significant progress in recent years. Biomarkers have been established to assess the risk of developing certain disease, monitor its progression, and evaluate the response to treatments. Genetic screening, particularly for the human leukocyte antigens (HLA) genes, has been effective in identifying individuals at risk of T1D. Personalized medicine, including patient-specific targeted interventions based on genetic mutations, shows promise for improving the clinical management of diabetes. GWAS has uncovered novel genetic factors involved in T1D, while further research using whole genome sequencing approaches is needed to uncover additional loci.

Table 7.1 Main genetic factors associated with type 1 diabetes and related pathways

Gene	Chromosome	Function
HLA	6	Antigen presentation
INS	11	Encodes insulin
PTPN22	1	Regulates T-cell activation
CTLA4	2	Regulates T-cell activation
IL-2RA	10	Suppressing T-cell immune responses

Table 7.2 Genetic loci associated with type 1 diabetes

Chromosome	Region	Gene	Variant	Coding protein
Chr 1	1p13.2	*PTPN22*	rs2476601	Protein tyrosine phosphatase, nonreceptor type 22 putative homeodomain transcription factor1
		PHTF1	rs6679677	
	1q32.1	*CAMSAP2*	rs6691977	Calmodulin regulated spectrin-associated protein family member 2
	1q32.1	*IL-10*	rs3024505	Interleukin 10
Chr 2	2q24.2	*IFIH1*	rs2111485	Interferon induced with helicase C domain 1
	2q32.3	*STAT4*	rs7574865	Signal transducer and activator of transcription 4 (STAT4)
	2q33.2	*CTLA4*	rs11571316 rs3087243	Cytotoxic T-lymphocyte-associated protein 4 (CTLA4)
	2q13	*ACOXL*	rs4849135	Acyl-CoA oxidase like
	2p23.3	*EFR3B*	rs478222	EFR3 homolog B
	2q11.2	*AFF3*	rs9653442	AF4/FMR2 family member 3
Chr 3	3p21.31	*CCR5*	rs113010081	C-C chemokine receptor 5 (CCR5)
Chr4	4q32.3	*AC080079.1* or *NOL8P1*	rs2611215	Tripartite motif-containing 38 (TRIM38) pseudogenes or Nucleolar protein 8 pseudogene 1
	4q27	*ADAD1* *IL21* *IL2*	rs6827756 rs4505848 rs17388568	Adenosine deaminase domain containing 1 interleukin 21 Interleukin 2
	4p15.2	*LINC02357*	rs10517086	Long intergenic nonprotein coding RNA 2357
Chr 5	5p13.2	*IL7R*	rs11954020	Interleukin 7 receptor
Chr 6	6q22.32	*CENPW*	rs9388489	Centromere protein W
	6q15	*BACH2*	rs11755527	BTB domain and CNC homolog 2
	6q27	*AL596442.1* or *AL049612.1*	rs924043	Novel transcript
	6q23.3	*TNFAIP3*	rs6920220 rs10499194	TNF-α induced protein 3
	6p21.3	*HLA class II*	rs6927022 rs2157051 rs9275184 rs7744001	Major histocompatibility complex
Chr 7	7p15.2	*SKAP2*	rs7804356	Src kinase-associated phosphoprotein 2
	7p12.1	*COBL*	rs4948088	Cordon-Bleu WH2 repeat protein
	7P12.2	*IKZF1*	rs10272724 rs62447205	IKAROS family zinc finger 1
Chr 9	9p24.2	*GLIS3*	rs7020673 rs10758593	GLIS family zinc finger 3

(continued)

Table 7.2 (continued)

Chromosome	Region	Gene	Variant	Coding protein
Chr 10	10p11.22	*NRP1*	rs722988	Neuropilin 1
	10p15.1	*IL2RA*	rs41295061 rs2104285 rs706778	Interleukin 2 receptor subunit α
	10q23.31	*RNLS*	rs10509540	Renalase FAD-dependent amine oxidase
Chr 11	11p15.5	*INS*	rs7111341	Insulin
	11q13.1	*BAD*	rs694739	BCL2-associated agonist of cell death
Chr 12	12q13.13	*ITGB7*	rs11170466	Integrin subunit β7
	12q13.2	*ERBB3* *DGKA*	rs2292239 rs11171710	Erb-B2 receptor tyrosine kinase 3 Diacylglycerol kinase α
	12q21.2	*ZDHHC17*	rs2632214	Zinc finger DHHC-type containing 17
	12q24.13	*SH2B3*	rs3184504	SH2B adaptor protein 3
	12p13.31	*CD69*	rs4763879	CD69 molecule
Chr 13	13q22.2	*LMO7*	rs539514	LIM domain 7
	13q32.3	*GPR183*	rs9585056	G-protein-coupled receptor 183
Chr 14	14q32.2	*AL163932.1* *or* *LINC01550*	rs4900384	Novel transcript or long intergenic nonprotein coding RNA 1550
	14q24.1	*ZFP36L1* or *MAGOH3P*	rs1465788	ZFP36 ring finger protein-like 1 or mago homolog 3, pseudogene
	14q32.2	*DLK1*	rs941576	Delta-like noncanonical notch ligand 1
Chr 15	15q25.1	*CTSH*	rs3825932	Cathepsin H
	15q14	*RASGPR1*	rs72727394	RAS guanyl-releasing protein1
Chr 16	16p11.2	*IL27*	rs151234	Interleukin 27
	16p13.13	*CLEC16A* *DEXI*	rs12708716 rs12927355 rs193778	C-type lectin domain containing 16A dexamethasone-induced protein
	16q23.1	*BCAR1*	rs8056814	Breast cancer antiestrogen resistance 1
Chr 17	17q21.2	*SMARCE1*	rs7221109	SWI/SNF-related, matrix-associated, actin-dependent regulator of chromatin, subfamily e, member 1 or TEC
	17q12	*ORMDL3*	rs2290400	ORMDL sphingolipid biosynthesis regulator 3
Chr 18	18q22.2	*CD226*	rs763361	CD226 molecule
	18p11.21	*PTPN2*	rs1893217	Protein tyrosine phosphatase, nonreceptor type 2

(continued)

Table 7.2 (continued)

Chromosome	Region	Gene	Variant	Coding protein
Chr 19	19q13.33	*FUT2*	rs601338	Fucosyltransferase 2
	19q13.32	*PRKD2*	rs425105	Protein kinase D2
	19p13.2	*TYK2*	rs34536443	Tyrosine kinase 2
	19p13.3	*CDC34* *MADCAM1*	rs12982646	Ubiquitin-conjugating MaDcaM1 enzyme E2 R1 Mucosal vascular addressin Cell adhesion molecule 1
Chr 20	20p13	*SIRPG*	rs2281808	Signal regulatory protein gamma
Chr 21	21q22.3	*UBASH3A*	rs11203203	Ubiquitin associated and SH3 domain containing A
Chr 22	22q12.2	*AC002378*	rs5753037	Novel transcript
	22q12.3	*C1QTNF6* *RAC2*	rs229533	C1q- and TNF-related 6 Ras-related C3 botulinum toxin substrate 2
Chr X	Xp22.2	*TLR7/8*	rs5979785	Toll-like receptor 7/8
	Xq28	*GAB3*	rs2664170	GRB2-associated binding protein 3

The integration of genomic data with other -omics disciplines, including transcriptomics, epigenomics, and proteomics using bioinformatics analysis, machine learning and system biology, has facilitated the identification of key novel biological pathways and networks involved in T1D pathogenesis [14].

7.2.2 Metabolomics of Type 1 Diabetes

Metabolomics studies in T1D explore the metabolites linked to the disease. As mentioned earlier, this chronic autoimmune disorder manifests when the body fails to produce sufficient insulin due to the destruction of insulin-producing pancreatic cells [15]. Two distinct patterns involved in the development of autoimmunity contributing to the disease have been proposed: younger children who first exhibit insulin autoantibodies (IAAs) generally experience a swifter progression toward multiple autoantibody positivity and T1D. This pattern is correlated with the *HLA-DR4* haplotypes. The second pattern consists of older children who initially have positive test for glutamic acid decarboxylase autoantibodies (GADA). This pattern typically demonstrates a slower progression toward additional autoantibodies, and is associated with the *HLA-DR3* haplotypes. Beyond genetic influences, the environmental factors are likely to play a role in determining the occurrence and sequence of autoantibody appearance [16]. The metabolomic profile is also intricately influenced by genetic predispositions, environmental factors, dietary patterns, and health conditions [17].

Metabolomic profiling of samples from the BABYDIAB study revealed that children seroconverting early in life (≤2 years) had significantly lower levels of methionine and hydroxyproline compared to those developing autoantibodies at an older age or autoantibody-negative controls [17]. This pattern was consistent with findings from the MIDIA cohort, which studied the Norwegian genetically high-risk infants. Despite the statistically nonsignificant difference in methionine levels, the MIDIA study suggested potential associations influenced by factors like age and breastfeeding duration [18]. These findings indicate that methionine deficits in early childhood may have multifaceted consequences, potentially impacting lymphocyte proliferation and the regulation of T-helper17 cell differentiation, thereby suggesting a potential connection with the T1D pathogenesis. The role of methionine as a key intermediate in choline catabolism, a component of phospholipids, aligns with studies identifying lower levels of phospholipids in cord blood of T1D children [16].

In the type 1 Diabetes Prediction and Prevention (DIPP) cohort, Oresic et al. conducted studies on 129 genetically high-risk children who later developed early childhood diabetes (<3.6 years). Their findings indicated reduced total content of phosphatidylcholine in cord blood and a general decrease in triglycerides (TGs), various phospholipids, including ether phosphatidylcholines and sphingomyelins, before seroconversion. The study highlighted a 1.5-fold increase in the pro-inflammatory lysophosphatidylcholine (LPC) 18:0/0:0 approximately 9–18 months prior to the seroconversion [19]. This association was corroborated in the Diabetes Prediction in Skåne (DiPiS) cohort, where the cord blood samples from children diagnosed with T1D before 8 years of age were prospectively analyzed alongside healthy controls. The predictive model for T1D in children under the age of 2 consisted of phosphatidylcholines, phosphatidylethanolamines, and triglyceride levels, that made a distinct lipid patterns between the cases and the controls [20]. Conflicting results surfaced from the investigations within the BABYDIAB cohort on a group of 1650 children with familial T1D which sowed that autoantibody-positive children exhibited elevated levels of certain lipids, such as odd-chain TGs and polyunsaturated fatty acid-containing phospholipids [17]. The discrepancies between the DIPP and BABYDIAB cohorts likely stem from variations in the timing of lipid profiling, with the DIPP cohort assessing samples before seroconversion and at birth, while the BABYDIAB cohort conducted profiling at the time of seroconversion [17].

Overall, the observations suggest the potential of cord blood phospholipids to predict the development of autoimmunity, possibly reflecting the intrauterine environment and maternal factors such as nutrition, infections, and microbiome composition. While the association between the phospholipids' levels at birth and the development of autoimmunity has been demonstrated in very young age groups, no study has yet established any links between these phospholipids and the specific autoantibody profiles linked with T1D in early childhood [16].

Certain alterations in the circulating amino acids (AA) were found in both diabetes types, impaired glucose tolerance, and obesity [21]. Galderisi et al. showed an excess of tryptophan metabolites (including kynurenine) along with an increase in certain types of small urinary peptides in T1D children [15]. Some studies suggest elevated levels of these aromatic amino acids to be associated with an increased risk of developing T1D. Additionally, contradictory findings regarding branched-chain amino acids have been reported, with some studies suggesting their positive impact on the insulin action and signaling processes, while others indicate a worsening of insulin resistance in T1D patients. It is possible that association of branched-chain amino acids level and T1D is attributed to their increased concentrations in obese individuals [22].

7.3 Type 2 Diabetes, Insulin Resistance, and Metabolic Syndrome

Type 2 diabetes (T2D) is the most common diabetes that affects millions of people worldwide. It is projected that more than 784 million people globally would be suffering from the condition by 2045, showing a 46% increase in its prevalence [23].

7.3.1 Genomics of Type 2 Diabetes, Metabolic Syndrome, and Insulin Resistance

Recent large-scale genome-wide research, such as GWAS, NGS, and high-throughput technologies, has identified several genetic factors contributing to the development of the disease. As insulin resistance and beta-cell failure are the main known pathogenesis of T2D, genetic factors related to these pathways contribute in T2D. Decoding the genetic landscape for personalized management offers an in-depth assessment of how genomics is transforming our understanding of T2D. Here, we will explore the genetic factors contributing to the disease as well as the latest research on the topic.

GWAS has revealed 65 different loci and genes associated with T2D [24]. Figure 7.1 shows the main genetic factors contributing to T2D and the related pathways based on the most recent large studies [25, 26]. A recent large-scale meta-analysis of GWAS on 228,499 cases and 1,178,783 controls identified 568 associations, including 286 autosomal and 7 X-chromosomal genes, 25 others (identified in the ancestry-specific analyses), that were unreported previously [27]. Moreover, the transcriptome-wide association analysis identified 3568 T2D associations with genetically predicted gene expressions in 687 novel genes; of these, 54 were known to interact with the FDA-approved drugs [27].

Different rare and common genetic variants contribute to T2D. Rare variants have greater effect size, while common ones have small effect size [28].

Metabolic Syndrome Metabolic syndrome (MetS) is a cluster of interconnected risk factors including obesity, hyperlipidemia, insulin resistance, and hypertension (Fig. 7.2). It is therefore linked with cardiovascular diseases and T2D. Genomic investigations unveiling the intricate genetic underpinnings of metabolic syndrome are revolutionizing our comprehension of its origins and manifestations.

Genes Associated with Type 2 Diabetes: Pathway	Detection Method	Gene		
Insulin Resistance	Candidate Gene Studies	IRS1		PPARG
	GWAS and GWAS meta-analysis	FTO	HMGA2	RBMS1
		GRB14	KLF14	PEPD
	GWAS and GWAS meta-analysis of both imputed and genotyped SNPs	ARL15	LEP	SLC16A11
	GWAS and GWAS meta-analysis for T2D related quantitative traits	GCKR		
	GWAS based on Metabochip custom beadchip	ANKRD55		ANK1
		MC4R		BCAR
		TBC1D4		
Insulin Secretion/ Beta Cell or Islet Function	Linkage Studies	HNF4A		TCF7L2
	Candidate Gene Studies	GCK		KCNJ11
		HNF1B		WES1
	GWAS and GWAS meta-analysis	ARAP1	CDKAL1	IGF2BP2
		BCL11A	CDKN2A/B	KCNQ1
		C2CD4A/C2CD4B	DUSP9	MAEA
		CDC123/CAMK1D	GLIS3	PAX4
		HHEX/IDE	UBE2E2	SLC30A8
		HNF1A	UPS26A	THADA
		ZFAND3	ZBED3	
	GWAS and GWAS meta-analysis of both imputed and genotyped SNPs	GPSM1		SSR1/RREB1
		LPP		
	GWAS and GWAS meta-analysis for T2D related quantitative traits	ADCY5		MTNR1B
		DGKB		PROX1
	GWAS based on Metabochip custom beadchip	GIRP		
Unknown Pathway	GWAS and GWAS meta-analysis	ADAMTS9	KCNK16	SGCG
		AP3S2	LAMA1	SPRY2
		CHCHD2P9	MOB2	SRR
		DNER	NOTCH2	ST6GAL1
		FITM2/R3HDML	PRC1	TLE4
		GCC1	PSMD6	TMEM163
		CRK5	PTPRD	TP53INP1
		HIMG20A	RASGRP1	TSPAN8/LGR6
		JAZF1	RND/RBM43	ZFAND6
	GWAS and GWAS meta-analysis of both imputed and genotyped SNPs	FAF1	IGF2	SLC16A13
		HLA-B	POU5F1/TCF19	TMEM154
		MPHOSPH9		
	GWAS based on Metabochip custom beadchip	CCND2	KLHDC5	ZMIZ1
		CILP2	TLE1	BCAR1
		ANK1		
	WES	COBLL1		MACF1

Fig. 7.1 Genes associated with T2D and related pathways with their identification method

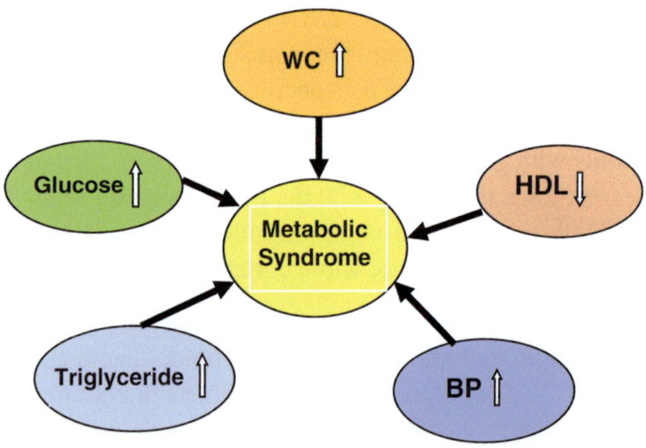

Fig. 7.2 Criteria for clinical diagnosis of the metabolic syndrome. *WC* waist circumference, *BP* blood pressure

The amalgamation of genetic predisposition and environmental factors contributes to MetS. Through GWAS, various genetic loci, such as IRS1, APOA5, TNF, FTO, Leptin, and SERPINA12, associated with MetS components were identified.

Cutting-edge genomic techniques are powering the MetS research. High-throughput sequencing, epigenomics, and transcriptomics provide insights into the genetic variants, epigenetic modifications, and gene expression patterns contributing to the complexity of the syndrome.

Genetic variants affect key metabolic pathways. Genes linked to insulin resistance (IRS1, IRS2), lipid metabolism (APOA5, LPL), inflammation (TNF, IL6), and obesity (FTO) take center stage in these alterations. Dissecting these pathways elucidates the genetic foundation of the metabolic syndrome. Moreover, the genetic variants that contribute to each component of MetS (obesity, hypertension and hyperglycemia) are involved in MetS genomics as well as these contribute in the pathogenesis of MetS (Table 7.3).

Genomic approaches provide risk prediction models for metabolic syndrome. Polygenic risk scores combine the genetic information to quantify individual risk of MetS. Incorporating the genomic data with clinical parameters enhances the risk prediction accuracy, facilitating early intervention.

Genetic variants also influence drug response and adverse effects. Tailoring therapies based on the genetic makeup maximizes treatment efficacy while minimizing the risks.

Insulin Resistance Insulin resistance (IR) is the central pathogenesis of MetS and other metabolic disorders like diabetes and obesity. Different common and rare genetic variants also contribute to IR and its outcomes such as diabetes and MetS (Table 7.3) [29, 30].

Table 7.3 Variants associated with insulin resistance

Variant	Chromosome	Gene
rs4311394 rs702634	Chr 12	*ARL15*
rs7077836	Chr 10	*TCERGIL*
rs17046216	Chr 4	*SC4MOL*
rs12970134	Chr 18	*MC4R*
rs35767	Chr 12	*IGF1*
rs6723108 rs998451	Chr 2	*TMEM163*
rs1208	Chr 8	*NAT2*
rs7903146	Chr 10	*TCF7L2*
rs8050136	Chr 16	*FTO*
rs780094	Chr 2	*GCKR*
rs2943641	Chr 2	*IRS1*
rs972283	Chr 7	*KLF14*
rs13081389	Chr 3	*PPARG*

7.3.2 Metabolomics in Type 2 Diabetes and Insulin Resistance

In recent decades, researchers have devoted efforts to unravel the metabolic profile of the diabetic individuals [21, 31]. Initially, the focus was on the identification of individual metabolites, leveraging from high-throughput technologies that subsequently made the comprehensive metabolite profiling feasible. The majority of researchers have observed a distinct correlation between the amino acids and lipids metabolites and the risk of prediabetes and diabetes [32–34]. The precise role of these metabolites in diabetes, however, is not precisely defined.

7.3.2.1 Amino Acids

Nearly 50 metabolites have emerged as potential indicators of T2D and insulin resistance, underscoring the complexity of the metabolic dysregulation linked with this disorder. Among them, amino acids, specifically branched-chain amino acids (BCAAs) and aromatic amino acids (AAAs), are more extensively studied [35–38].

Branched-Chain Amino Acids Elevated BCAA levels have consistently been linked with hyperglycemia, suggesting their promising potential as early biomarkers for T2D risk assessment. This association has rigorously been examined in numerous cross-sectional studies, and its reliability has been further substantiated by robust evidence from large prospective studies [39, 40]. A seminal contribution to our understanding originates from the Framingham Heart Study [41], which highlighted a significant association between three BCAAs (isoleucine, leucine, and valine) and two AAAs (tyrosine and phenylalanine) and an increased risk of T2D development over a comprehensive 12-year follow-up period. Notably, these associations retained their significance even after meticulous adjustments for key variables such as age, sex, body mass index, and fasting glucose levels. The cumulative impact of three specific amino acids, namely isoleucine, tyrosine, and phenylalanine, was demonstrated as a predictive tool for T2D, with an odds ratio of 2.42 (95% confidence interval: 1.66–3.54) [41].

BCAAs can be produced in various tissues through the breakdown of the skeletal muscle, adipose tissue, and liver. Changes in the metabolism of BCAAs, such as reduced activity of the branched-chain α-keto acid dehydrogenase (BCKD), have been linked to insulin resistance [42]. The catabolism of BCAAs occurs through the branched-chain aminotransferase (BCAT), which converts them into branched-chain α-keto acids (BCKAs). Subsequently, the BCKD oxidizes BCKAs into acetyl- or succinyl-CoA, which act as intermediates in the citric acid cycle, also known as the Krebs cycle [42]. BCKD deficiency leads to the accumulation of BCKAs, resulting in increased levels of BCAAs. Excess BCKAs, on the other hand, activates an alternative pathway, converting them into C3- and C5-acylcarnitines, which are then degraded through beta-oxidation. If the beta-oxidation capacity is surpassed, diacylglycerol (DAG) and ceramides are generated, contributing to insulin resistance [42, 43].

This implies that reduced BCAA degradation is not only associated with insulin resistance but also probably contributes to elevated BCAA levels during hyperglycemia. Another potential mechanism for escalated BCAA levels during hyperglycemia could involve a diminished uptake of as well as an augmented release of BCAAs from the skeletal muscle, possibly due to increased protein catabolism during insulin resistance. These evidences suggest a two-way relationship, in which insulin resistance could contribute to elevated BCAA levels [44]. Regardless of the primary cause, BCAA can impact T2D in various and sometimes opposing ways. They can act as substrates for processes such as gluconeogenesis and mitochondrial oxidation, or as signaling molecules to induce either insulin resistance or secretion [45]. Additionally, infusing amino acids reduce insulin-stimulated glucose uptake in the skeletal muscle. This is associated with the overactivation of the mTOR-S6K1 signaling pathway, increased phosphorylation of insulin receptor substrate 1 (IRS1) at specific sites, and reduced insulin-induced phosphoinositide 3-kinase (PI3K) activity [46]. The inhibition of mTOR-S6K1 with rapamycin counteracts with the hyperphosphorylation of IRS1 and restores the insulin-stimulated glucose disposal [33, 46, 47].

Despite the above-mentioned findings, the causal relationship between BCAAs and diabetes remains unclear. This is mainly because residual confounding and reverse causation often impede the establishment of causation in observational studies linking biomarkers to outcomes. The Mendelian randomization (MR) studies have helped address this by using genetic variants as instrumental variables to mimic the lifelong environmental exposure effects secured at conception. In one MR study, a genetic risk score (GRS) for insulin resistance was found to causally increase BCAAs levels, while no associations were documented between genetically increased BCAAs and insulin resistance [48]. Another MR study demonstrated the causal relationship between BCAAs levels and the risk of T2D development, suggesting a potential causal role for isoleucine, leucine, and valine in the pathogenesis of T2D [49]. These findings insinuate BCAAs as a possible segment of the causal pathway from insulin resistance to diabetes. In other words, it is implied that insulin resistance can cause diabetes through increasing BCAAs levels, mainly due to its effects on obese microbiomes and decreased oxidation in adipose tissue and liver. Consequently, BCAAs could potentially serve as a predictive biomarker in this regard, as their levels may rise as early as a decade before the onset of overt diabetes [2].

Aromatic Amino Acids The elevated levels of two circulating AAAs, phenylalanine and tyrosine, are frequently observed in individuals with conditions such as obesity, insulin resistance, or T2D [50, 51]. Notably, the changes in these metabolites often occur simultaneously. Cross-sectional studies of blood metabolite levels and insulin sensitivity, as well as those predicting T2D development, have consistently revealed strong associations with elevated phenylalanine and tyrosine [50, 51]. In rodent studies, the plasma phenylalanine concentration is notably higher in young, insulin-resistant rats compared to nonobese ones, indicating disturbed phenylalanine and tyrosine metabolisms in insulin-resistant conditions [52]. Beyond their association with insulin resistance, these two AAAs were linked to an increased risk of diabetes. The MR analyses of individuals with normal fasting glucose levels have shown a positive association between the phenylalanine levels and future risk of diabetes, which supports the potential causal role of phenylalanine in T2D [53]. Additionally, 3-(4-hydroxyphenyl) lactate, a breakdown product of phenylalanine, is associated with decreased insulin secretion/insulin sensitivity and subsequently an increased risk of T2D [54]. Results from the Southall And Brent REvisited (SABRE) study demonstrated a stronger link between tyrosine levels and diabetes in the South Asians compared to the Europeans, indicating the ethnic difference in the metabolic profile of the individuals and the importance of exploring the ethnic disparities in the metabolite levels, which could potentially lead to differences in the incidence of diabetes among various ethnic groups [55].

As for the AAAs, some suggest the elevated levels of tyrosine and phenylalanine may result from the reduced activity of tyrosine aminotransferase as a consequence of insulin resistance. Moreover, the increased breakdown of methionine into cysteine/cystine and ultimately into alpha-hydroxybutyrate may result in increased T2D risk, which potentially inhibits tyrosine aminotransferase [56, 57].

Other Amino Acids The constant observation of diminished plasma glycine levels in obese and diabetic individuals compared with their healthy counterparts suggests a potential correlation between the glycine metabolism and the pathogenesis of these conditions [58]. Several studies have indicated that interventions to reduce insulin resistance, including weight loss, exercise, or insulin-sensitizing drugs, can lead to augmented plasma concentrations of glycine in individuals suffering from obesity or T2D [58, 59]. In line with these findings, the offspring of T2D parents have been demonstrated to have lower plasma glycine concentrations compared to those with healthy parental backgrounds [60]. Notably, a communal defective human glycine metabolism is observed among individuals with obesity and diabetes, potentially contributing to the increased risk of cardiovascular diseases associated with these conditions [60–62]. Prospective studies have provided additional support for the predictive value of diminished plasma glycine levels in identifying individuals at risk of impaired glucose tolerance and T2D. Lower glycine levels, even years before the clinical onset of the disease, are associated with an elevated risk of these conditions [51, 63]. Conversely, elevated serum glycine levels are linked with a decreased risk of T2D [64]. The association of glycine derivatives, such as betaine, with insulin resistance and the risk of T2D further emphasizes on the intricate nature of the glycine-related pathways involved in the metabolic health. Reduced plasma levels of betaine serve as a predictor of diabetes risk; interventions to promote betaine levels are, therefore, associated with a lower incidence of diabetes [65].

The amino acids involved in gluconeogenesis, primarily alanine and glutamine, are reported to be capable of promoting the production of hepatic glucose, resulting in hyperglycemia [66]. Glutamate exhibits a positive association with T2D, independent of other clinical risk factors [67]. Elevated plasma levels of glutamate are documented in various diseases, characterized by chronic oxidative stress and inflammation. Moreover, persistent high extracellular glutamate levels may directly or indirectly contribute to the progressive loss of beta cells in both T1D and T2D. Platelet activation, on the other hand, is prevalent in obesity, metabolic syndrome, T1D, and T2D, has the potential to induce hyperglutamatemia in these respective conditions [67, 68].

Alanine, a nonessential amino acid synthesized from pyruvate and other amino acids and the primary source being BCAAs, is predominantly generated in the skeletal muscle and gut. It is considered as a crucial substrate for gluconeogenesis in the liver, significantly contributing to fasting hyperglycemia by promoting the gluconeogenic process. Moreover, alanine serves as the stimulator of glucagon secretion, exerting additional influence on glucose metabolism. Studies have highlighted elevated alanine levels during hyperglycemia, regardless of the obesity status, to be associated with insulin resistance. This relationship supports a notable positive correlation between insulin sensitivity and the mRNA levels of alanine aminotransferase, a pivotal enzyme in alanine metabolism. Alanine exhibits both cross-sectional and prospective correlations with impaired insulin sensitivity. Two separate prospective studies on the Finnish and the South Asian males in the UK as well as another two large, independent cohort research in China have observed a correlation between elevated alanine levels and an increased risk of developing T2D [55, 66, 69].

Lipids Most studies have identified significant links between certain lipid metabolites and prediabetes/T2D [70, 71]. On average, targeted approaches focused on 40 to 50 lipid metabolites, with triglycerides, phosphatidylcholines, and sphingomyelins being the most frequently analyzed lipid classes. For instance, the Framingham cohort, with a 12-year follow-up, indicated that 15 of the over 100 analyzed lipid metabolites were associated with diabetes. Notably, lipids with lower carbon numbers and double-bond content, particularly triacylglycerols (TAGs), were linked with a higher risk of prediabetes and T2D. Conversely, those with higher carbon numbers and more double bonds were associated with a lower risk of the condition [72].

In the same cohort, individuals in the upper quartile of the combination of strongest positive predictor (TAG 50:0) and negative predictor (TAG 58:0), exhibited a 4.30-fold higher risk of T2D independent of fasting insulin and glucose levels [72]. Additionally, lower levels of lysophosphatidylcholine (LPC) 18:2 at baseline predicted impaired glucose tolerance and T2D after a 7-year follow-up in the KORA study. This study also highlighted the combination of higher acetylcarnitine (C2) with lower LPC 18:2 and glycine as the predictor of diabetes [73]. Ferrannini et al. observed that α-hydroxybutyrate was positively linked whereas linoleoyl-glycerophosphocholine (L-GPC) was inversely associated with the risk of dysglycemia in the Relationship between Insulin Sensitivity and Cardiovascular disease (RISC) study and T2D [74]. A case-cohort study within the framework of the European Prospective Investigation into Cancer and Nutrition (EPIC)-Potsdam research, replicating the KORA study, concluded that diacyl-phosphatidylcholines

(C32:1, C36:1, C38:3, and C40:5) were associated with a higher risk of T2D, whereas sphingomyelin and acyl-alkyl-phosphatidylcholine (C18:2) were linked with a lower risk of the condition [73].

With respect to acylcarnitines, from among five targeted and two untargeted analyses on acylcarnitines, three studies identified significant associations between these esters and prediabetes/ T2D [75]. The Insulin Resistance Atherosclerosis Study (IRAS) revealed greater concentrations of carnitine C4-OH and C10:3 and lower levels of carnitine C5:1 and C20 were associated with insulin resistance [64].

The metabolism of free fatty acids (FFAs) is also dysregulated in T2D. FFAs are the by-products of triglyceride hydrolysis. Moreover, they can derive from dietary triglycerides and phospholipids. In insulin-resistant conditions, however, heightened lipolysis of triglycerides can result in the excessive production of glycerol and FFAs. Furthermore, the METabolic Syndrome in Men (METSIM) study highlighted the association between saturated FAs and an increased risk of T2D, while an inverse correlation was observed between unsaturated FAs and T2D. This population-based study demonstrated that fasting serum levels of glycerol, FFAs, monounsaturated FAs (MUFAs), saturated FAs, n-7 FAs, and n-9 FAs can predict the worsening of hyperglycemia and the development of T2D over a 4.5-year follow-up. Importantly, these associations remained independent of known T2D risk factors. Conversely, elevated levels of serum n-6 FAs, indicative of dietary linoleic acid intake, were associated with a reduced risk of hyperglycemia and T2D [76]. Furthermore, a prospective study spanning four Finnish cohorts over an 8–15 year follow-up revealed the association between MUFAs and the risk of diabetes, while n-6 FAs, were linked with a diminished risk of T2D [77]. A two-sample MR study suggested the potential causal link between FAs and fasting glucose levels, beta cell function, and T2D. Individuals with a genetic predisposition to elevate certain fatty acids, including α-linolenic acid, linoleic acid, palmitoleic acid, and oleic acid, exhibit a reduced risk of diabetes. Conversely, a genetic inclination toward increased levels of arachidonic acid, stearic acid, and eicosapentaenoic acid is associated with a higher risk of diabetes [78].

7.4 Obesity

Obesity is a complex multifactorial disease, in which accumulated excess body fat has negative effects on health. Overall, 39% of adults aged 18 years and over were overweight in 2016, and another 13% were obese [79]. Obesity, a global health concern, results from intricate interactions between genetics and environmental factors. Genomic research has revolutionized our understanding of obesity, shedding light on the genetic variations that influence susceptibility to, pathogenesis of, and treatment response in this condition.

7.4.1 *Genomics in Obesity*

Familial clustering and twin studies have long indicated a hereditary component in obesity. Recent advancements in genomics have highlighted the contributions of monogenic and polygenic factors, demonstrating the complexity of obesity inheritance. Various genes have been identified to contribute to monogenic obesity (Table 7.4) [80]. Different genes with rare and common variants contribute to polygenic obesity through various metabolic pathways [81] (Table 7.5). The genes involved in appetite regulation (FTO), energy homeostasis (MC4R), lipid metabolism (PPARG), and insulin sensitivity (INSR) are the centerpiece of these studies. Genomic variants that disrupt these pathways, therefore, contribute to obesity development.

The GWAS and next-generation sequencing have unveiled genetic variants associated with increased obesity risk. Cutting-edge techniques like single-cell genomics provide insight into the cellular heterogeneity within the adipose tissue. Different obesity predisposing genes detected in GWAS and related adiposity traits are shown in Fig. 7.3 [82, 83].

DNA methylation, histone modification, and noncoding RNAs are the link between the genetics and the environmental factors. Epigenetic alterations in adipose tissue impact adipogenesis, inflammation, and metabolic dysregulation, perpetuating obesity (Fig. 7.4) [84].

The outcome of bariatric surgeries, similarly, is influenced by genetic factors, pointing out the importance of personalized treatment strategies based on the genetic profile of the individual that can optimize the long-term success.

Table 7.4 Genetic variants associated with monogenic obesity

Gene	Inheritance	Protein	Clinical phenotype
MC4R	AD	Melanocortin receptor 4	Obesity, hyperphagia, accelerated growth
LEP	AR	Leptin	Obesity, hyperphagia, frequent infection, neuroendocrine dysfunction
LEPR	AR	Leptin receptor	Obesity, hyperphagia, neuroendocrine dysfunction, hypogonadism
PCSK1	AR	Proprotein canvertase subilisin/Kexin	Obesity, enteropathy, defect in prohormones, postprandial hypoglycemia
POMC	AR	Proopiomelanocortin	Obesity, red hair, pale skin, ACTH deficiency
SH2B1	AR	SH2B adaptor protein1	Obesity
SIM1	AR	Single-minded homologue1	Obesity, developmental delay
ADCY3	AR	Adenylate cyclase type3	Obesity
BDNF	AR	Brain-derived neurotrophic factor	Obesity, hyperphagia, impaired memory, impaired pain sensation, hyperactivity, developmental delay
SEMA3A-G	AR	Semaphorin 3A-G	Obesity, hypogonadotropic hypogonadism with or without anosemia

Table 7.5 Genetic variants associated with polygenic obesity

Genetic variant	Implicated gene	Role in obesity
FTO rs9939609	FTO	Appetite regulation
MC4R mutations	MC4R	Energy homeostasis
PPARG mutations	PPARG	Adipogenesis
POMC mutations	POMC	Regulation of the HPA axis and adrenal development
LEP mutations	Leptin	Regulation of body weight

Post-GWAS studies, which combine new omics technologies with bioinformatics analysis and system biology approaches, have facilitated the translation of genetic loci into meaningful biological statements and thus new avenues for treatment modalities [85]. Tailoring the dietary, lifestyle, and pharmacological interventions based on individual genetic profiles, therefore, enhances treatment efficacy and reduces adverse effects.

7.4.2 Metabolomics in Obesity

In the past 10 years, various reports and reviews have delved into the metabolic alterations linked to human obesity. Amino acids, specifically BCAAs and AAAs, are among the significant categories of metabolites causing dysregulations linked with obesity. The research conducted on obese children and young Chinese men indicated that elevated concentrations of BCAAs and, consequently, higher levels of the by-products resulted from their breakdown among obese individuals. Also, recent studies believe the heightened levels of serum BCAAs are correlated with metabolic disorders irrespective of the body weight [86].

Phenylalanine concentrations are found to be elevated in obese individuals [87]. In a separate study conducted in Finland, the authors concluded that BCAAs, AAAs, and orosomucoids serve as significant risk factors for obesity [88]. The heightened plasma levels of BCAAs in obese subjects reflect altered metabolic signatures and the deregulations associated with obesity [89].

Obese individuals are found to exhibit elevated concentrations of tryptophan and its metabolites, namely, kynurenine and kynurenic acid, which are correlated with BMI. Similarly, changes in the kynurenine pathway are documented in individuals with both obesity and insulin resistance (IR). The heightened levels of these compounds may indicate immune activation or low-grade systemic inflammation, potentially attributed to increased activity of the indoleamine 2,3-dioxygenase (IDO) enzyme [90].

Another category of metabolites that has been the focus of several investigations is lipids. Various studies have reported alterations in the concentration of fatty acids (FAs), including polyunsaturated (PUFAs) and saturated fatty acids (SFAs) as well as more complex lipids such as sentinel lysophospholipids and sphingomyelins in

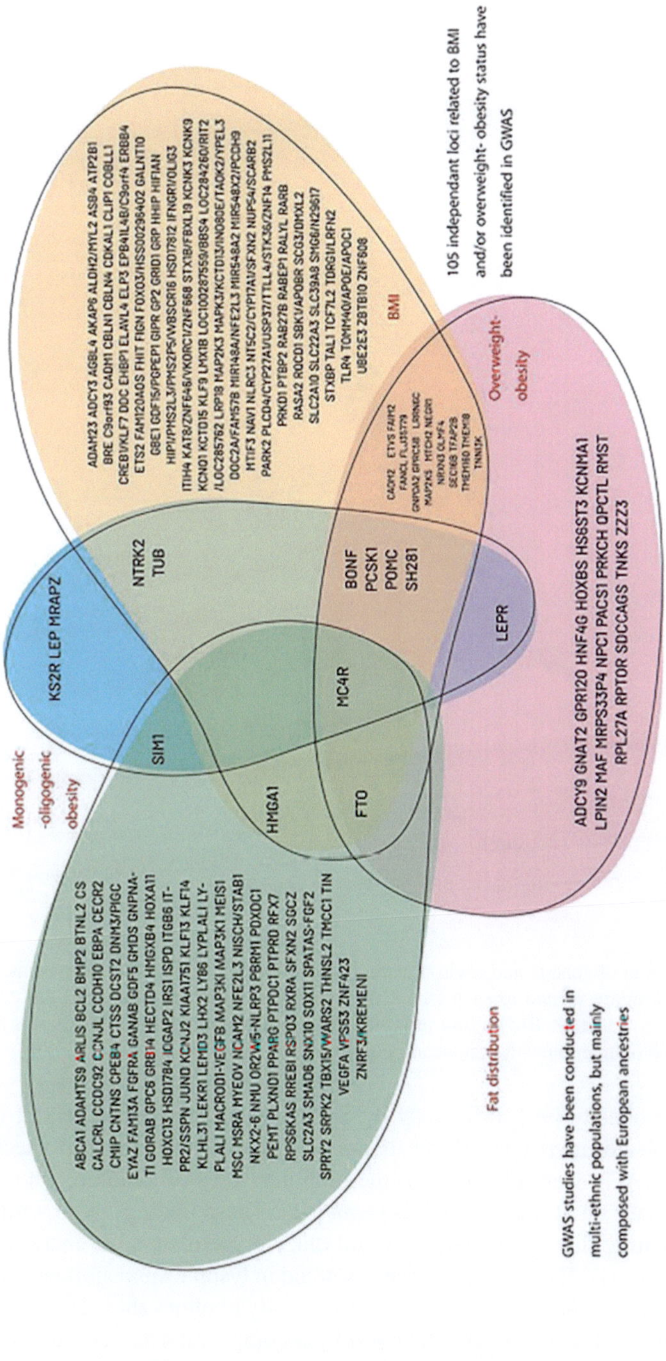

Fig. 7.3 Obesity-predisposing gene and related adiposity traits

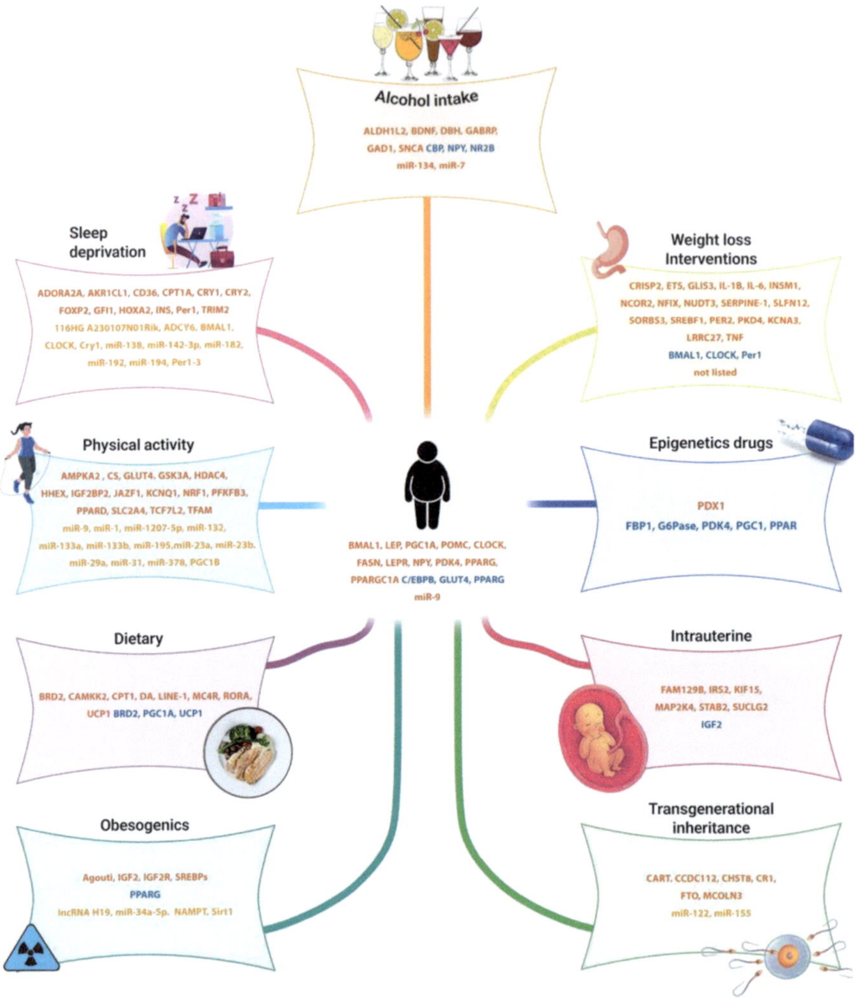

Fig. 7.4 Interaction of genetic and environmental factors through epigenetic mechanisms. Genes within each section are related to each factor, and genes placed in the core space are common between at least two factors. Brown font indicates DNA methylation, blue font indicates histone modification, and orange font shows noncoding RNAs

the context of obesity [90]. In a study by Sorrow et al., elevated levels of lipids, including linoleate, myristate, oleate, palmitate, stearate, caprate, and species of acylcarnitines (AC), were identified in the umbilical cord of children, who developed obesity later on at the age of 3–5 years [91]. These findings align with prior research indicating that sphingomyelins and diacylglycerols tend to increase with Body Mass Index (BMI), while a decrease is noted in lysophosphocholines levels in the same condition. Additionally, various phosphatidylcholines show effects in both directions, contributing to the complexity of lipid composition associated with BMI

[87, 92]. Metabolically healthy obese individuals are found to have elevated levels of nonessential fatty acids, including oleic acid, palmitic acid, palmitoleic acid, stearic acid, stearoyl carnitine, 2 hydroxybutanoic acid, and 3 hydroxybutanoic acid. These compounds are linked with dyslipidemia, an imbalance in lipids levels [86].

Furthermore, a significant and specific increase in C3 and C5 acylcarnitine levels is reported in these individuals. The elevated concentration of branched-chain amino acids (BCAAs) in obese individuals is associated with increased catabolism of these products in the liver and the skeletal muscles. This elevation in BCAAs is hypothetically linked to higher concentrations of short-chain acylcarnitines (C3 and C5), where C3 reflects the propionyl CoA pool, a by-product of isoleucine and valine catabolism, and C5 is comprised of α-methylbutyryl and isovalerylcarnitine species, intermediates in mitochondrial isoleucine and leucine catabolism, respectively [93].

Kang et al. observed significant increases in plasma levels of both medium- (MCACs) and long-chain acylcarnitines (LCACs) in overweight adults following a low-calorie diet. These changes showed a negative correlation with altered visceral fat areas. These findings could be interpreted as a result of intensified oxidation of the FFA released from visceral fat during weight loss, leading to the generation of MCAC and LCAC. Moreover, elevated MCAC and LCAC levels may be attributed to enhanced acetyltransferase activity, suggesting an improvement in the mitochondrial fatty acid oxidation rather than an imbalance in the process [94].

Future similar studies are essential to predict the emergence of metabolic and cardiovascular risks among the metabolically healthy obese (MHO) individuals. Furthermore, precise identification of such individuals is crucial, as it can help with tailored and targeted treatments with optimal outcomes.

7.5 Polycystic Ovary Syndrome (PCOS)

Polycystic ovary syndrome (PCOS) is a common endocrine disorder that affects women of reproductive age and is characterized by menstrual dysfunction, anovulation, and signs of hyperandrogenism, such as hirsutism, acne, infertility, and irregular periods, often presenting during late teens or early 20 s. It is one of the most common causes of infertility in women. Insulin resistance and hyperinsulinemia have the main role in the pathogenesis of PCOS. Lifestyle and environmental factors also play a role in the development of PCOS.

7.5.1 Genomics of PCOS

Advancements in genomics have unearthed the intricate genetic factors contributing to the PCOS pathogenesis, transforming our understanding of this multifaceted condition. Considering both genetic and environmental components, PCOS is considered as an inherently complex disorder. Recent genomic studies have identified susceptibility genes, shedding light on the hereditary factors influencing the PCOS risk. Although the exact cause of PCOS is yet to be known, a change or mutation in one or more genes is believed to be responsible for the disorder. GWAS, transcriptomics, and epigenomics have uncovered genetic variants, gene expression patterns, and epigenetic modifications contributing to the PCOS phenotypes.

Based on the primary characteristics of the disease, early PCOS candidate genes were those involved in steroidogenesis (e.g., *CYP11A1, CYP17A1, STAR*), steroid hormone effects including those involved in androgen and gonadotropin action (e.g., FSHR, LHCGR, *SHBG, AR*), and insulin resistance (e.g., *INSR*, *INS*-VNTR, *IGF1, IGF1R, IRS1, PPARG*) [95]. The genes involved in the production of the ovarian and adrenal hormone, such as CYP11a, CYP21, CYP17, and CYP19, are logical targets for study, and their variants are associated with PCOS (Table 7.6). Variants in the androgen receptor (AR) gene located on the X chromosome have also been reported in PCOS (Fig. 7.5) [96].

Altered DNA methylation and histone modifications influence the hormonal signaling pathways, contributing to androgen excess, ovulatory dysfunction, and metabolic disturbances.

Hyperandrogenic, anovulatory, and metabolic subtypes exhibit distinct genetic profiles. Integrating genomic data with clinical features enhances subtyping and personalized management. Genetic variations influence response to treatment and possible side effects. Genomic data can therefore help with tailored treatment plans, optimizing the therapeutic outcomes and therefore patient satisfaction.

Table 7.6 PCOS GWAS susceptibility loci

Locus	Related gene	Locus	Related gene
15q24.1	*CYP11a*	**9q22.32**	*C9orf3*
6p21. 3	*CYP21*	**9q33.3**	*DENND1A*
10q24-q25	*CYP17*	**11p14.1**	*FSHB*
15q21.2	*CYP19*	**11q22.1**	*YAP1*
2q36.3	*IRS-1*	11q23.1	*ZBTB16*
13q34	*IRS-2*	**12q13.2**	*RAB5B/SUOX/ERBB3*
2p16.3	*LHCGR*	12q14.3	*HMGA2*
2p16.3	*FSHR*	**12q21.2**	*KRR1*
2p21	*THADA*	2p16.3	***FSHR***
2q34	*ERBB4*	**16q12.1**	*TOX3*
5q13.1	*IRF1/RAD50*	19q13.3	*INSR*
6q25.3	*SOD2*	20q11.21	*SUMO1P1*
8p32.1	*GATA4/NEIL2*	20q13.2	*MAPRE1*
9p24.1	*PLGRKT*	2q37.3	*CAPN10*
16q12.2	*FTO*		

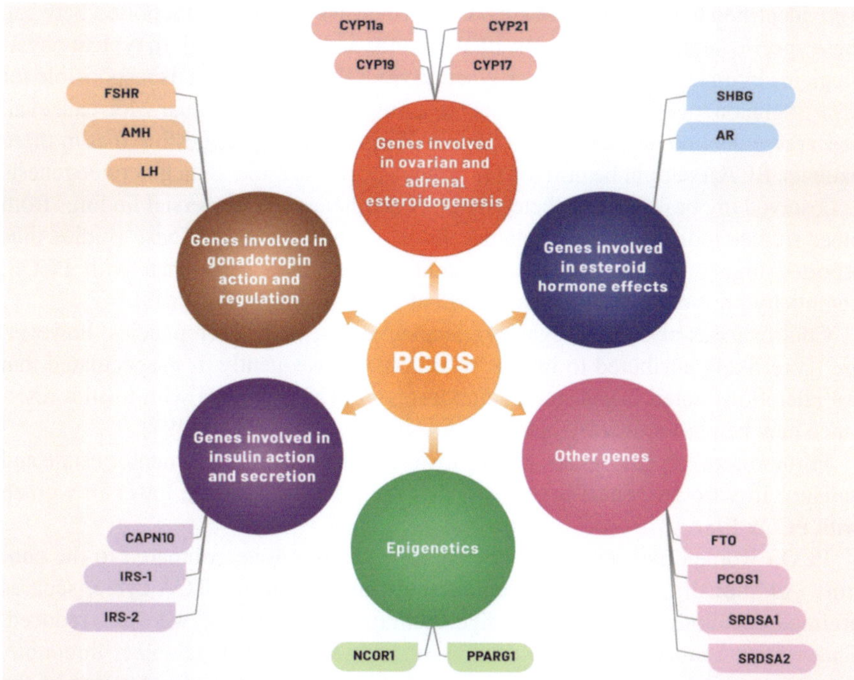

Fig. 7.5 Genes involved in PCOS and related pathways

7.5.2 *Metabolomics in PCOS*

Lipid metabolism is significantly disrupted in women with PCOS. These lipids are integral to diverse metabolic pathways, including steroid hormone biosynthesis, sphingolipid metabolism, and various facets of fatty acids metabolism, encompassing oxidation and amide metabolism [97].

A comprehensive study conducted by Zhao et al. revealed the upregulation of fatty acids, such as palmitic, stearic, and linoleic acid, in PCOS women. This observation implies escalated lipolysis, indicative of concurrent insulin resistance in adipose tissue. Particularly, the increase in linoleic acid levels can inhibit oocyte maturation and disrupt ovulation in PCOS. Additionally, the pro-inflammatory attributes of linoleic acid are implicated in the chronic low-grade inflammation characteristic of PCOS [98].

In contrast, phospholipids, integral to multifaceted biological pathways, are found to be downregulated in PCOS. The main phospholipids in this regard are phosphatidylcholine (PC), phosphatidylethanolamine (PE), lysophosphatidylcholine (LPC), and lysophosphatidylethanolamine (LPE) [97].

Amino acids (AAs) are the subsequent category of endogenous compounds scrutinized in samples obtained from women with PCOS. Elevated concentrations of various BCAA and AAA, including valine, tyrosine, tryptophan, and phenylalanine, were identified in the PCOS patients. Established associations are reported between these specific amino acids and insulin resistance and diabetes [93]. In typical physiological circumstances, alanine, originating from BCAA nitrogen, is responsible for 25% of gluconeogenesis derived from the amino acids [99]. Escobar-Morreale et al. observed a decline in the alanine concentrations in PCOS, suggesting that in these patients, BCAAs might be utilized for protein synthesis rather than gluconeogenesis as observed in obesity and diabetes [100]. Nevertheless, controversial findings from other studies indicate elevated alanine levels in these patients. These studies thus reported higher serum alanine aminotransferase (ALT) in women with PCOS, potentially promoting the transamination of pyruvate into alanine [98].

Controversies also exist regarding leucine levels; such discrepancies, however, are more likely attributed to insulin resistance. Consequently, it is speculated that the alterations noted in plasma leucine levels in PCOS patients with insulin resistance may be predominantly linked to impaired insulin signaling [97].

Furthermore, glycine levels, known to ameliorate the pro-inflammatory state and enhance in vitro adiponectin gene expression, were found to be lower in women with PCOS [98].

PCOS women have exhibited decreased levels of citrate compared to the controls. Additionally, the levels of amino acids involved in the TCA cycle, such as arginine, citrulline, glutamine, histidine, methionine, and proline, were also reduced. This was accompanied by an elevation in the levels of phenylalanine, threonine, tyrosine, and valine, potentially inducing fluctuations in the concentrations of the TCA cycle components. These findings suggest impaired TCA cycle in women with PCOS, which is indicative of insulin resistance. Hyperandrogenism, another characteristic of PCOS, has been noted to influence the TCA cycle by diminishing citrate levels. Moreover, the TCA cycle is recognized for its crucial role in oocyte maturation, whereas lower citrate levels may signify reduce their competence [99].

7.6 Thyroid Disorders

Thyroid disorders are one of the common endocrine disorders. Hypothyroidism affects up to 5% of the population that increases in elderly [101]. Here, we highlight the importance of genomics and metabolomics in understanding thyroid diseases, highlighting the role of genetic factors in disease development, diagnosis, treatment, and prognosis and present the latest research on the genomics of thyroid disorders.

7.6.1 Genomics of Thyroid Disorders

Recent research has identified several genetic factors that influence the thyroid function (Fig. 7.6) [102]. The most recent GWAS identified 260 independent sentinel variants at 156 unique genomic loci that can affect TSH levels: 158 sentinel variants at 78 genomic loci were newly diagnosed [103].

Genes associated with serum TSH/ FT4							
Identification Method	Whole Genome Sequencing	Candidate Gene Studies	Small GWAS (N<5000)	Large GWAS (N>15000)		Very large GWAS (N>50000)	
Gene	GNAS SYN2 B4GALT6	FOXE1 OATP1B1 MCT8 TSHR DIO1	XKR4 CAPZB NR3C2 PDE8B LOC440389	FOXA2 VAV3 GLIS3 LHX3 SASH1 ELK3 AADAT IGFBP5 SIVA1 NICX23 MBIP DIRC3 INSR FGF7	VEGFA NFIA SOX9 ITPK1 TPO MAF MIR1179 NRG1 NETO1 PRDM11 PDE10A ABO LPCAT2	GATA3 BCAS3 TG DIO2 DIO3OS NSF SLCO1B1 SULF1 MIR365A ADCY9 FNBP4 HES1 EK6 IGF2BP2 GNAS GLIS3	ACMSD SNX29 SLC17A4 CADM1 CA9 PTEN SPATA13 LOC728012 TM4SF4 ID4 MC4R NCOR1 SOX2-OT PSORS1C1 PRKX USP3

Fig. 7.6 Genetic factors contribute to thyroid function identified by various methods

The first group includes sentinel variants associated with hypothyroidism but not hyperthyroidism (including AKT1, IGFBP5, INSR, GLIS3, SPATA13, CADM1, BCAS3, SASH1, PDE4D, VEGFC, SPPL3, BNC2, PDE10A, PDE8B, NR3C2, VAV3, SOX9, B4GALNT3, CGA, C9orf92, NEK6, NSF, CCBE1, GNG7, TPPP, WNT4, SNX8, C1orf116, RBM47, KCTD5, PPP2R1B, PTPRJ, OCLN, C9orf156, GATA3, WWTR1, MAL2, ZBTB17, ARNT, CDC16). The second group is associated with hyperthyroidism but not hypothyroidism (including TSHR, NRG1, SDCCAG8, HMGA2, APOH, BMP2, SMAD6). The third group is associated with both hypothyroidism and hyperthyroidism with an opposite direction of effect (including TPO, PTEN, CAPZB, VEGFA, NFIA, MBIP, HLA-C, SLC25A37, SLC25A37, NKX2-1, NKX2-3, FOXA2). This is while tolerated SH2B3 missense variant, rs3184504 (allele T), is associated with increased TSH levels and at the same time high risk of both hypothyroidism and hyperthyroidism [103].

7.6.2 Metabolomics in Thyroid Disorders

Metabolomics has emerged as a powerful tool for a better understanding of metabolic alterations observed in thyroid diseases, such as hypothyroidism, hyperthyroidism, and thyroid cancer. Previous studies demonstrated the impact of thyroid hormones on lipid metabolism and amino acid turnover, resulting in the systemic effects of thyroid dysfunction. Therefore, researchers have found specific metabolic signatures associated with various diseases through analyzing the metabolite profiles.

Metabolomics analysis has revealed that both subclinical and clinical hypothyroidism are characterized by disrupted lipid metabolism, corroborated by elevated plasma levels of lysophosphatidylcholine (LPC), lysophosphatidylethanolamine (LPE), phosphatidylcholine (PC), phosphatidylglycerol (PG), phosphatidylethanolamine (PE), phosphatidylserine (PS), phosphatidylinositol (PI), and lysobisphosphatidic acid (LPA). In addition, hypothyroidism has been linked with altered amino acid metabolism, manifested by elevated plasma levels of glycine and L-arginine, and reduced L-tyrosine, L-lysine, and L-histidine concentrations. The disturbed metabolic pathways identified in hypothyroidism encompass the biosynthesis of *steroid hormone and primary bile acid*, *tryptophan metabolism*, *lysine degradation*, and *thiamine metabolism* [104]. Moreover, 65 metabolites are correlated with the parameters of thyroid function, namely, serum TSH, Free T4, Tg Ab (anti thyroglobulin antibody), and TPO Ab (Thyroid peroxidase antibody) levels. For instance, the metabolites involved in lysine degradation and tryptophan metabolism, including 5-phosphonoxy-L-lysine, glycine, 3-hydroxyanthranilic acid, 5-hydroxytryptamine, and 2-aminomuconate, are correlated positively with TSH levels and negatively with that of free T4.

In Hashimoto's thyroiditis (HT), metabolomics analysis has shown disrupted lipid metabolism, including increased levels of sphingomyelin (SM) 34:1, SM 34:2, SM 36:2, LPC 18:0 sn-1, LPC 18:1 sn-1, LPC 18:2 sn-1, PC 34:3, PC 36:5, PC 38:6, and L-acetylcarnitine. Additionally, SM 34:1, LPC 18:1 sn-1, PC 38:6, and SM34:2 were identified as potentially efficient biomarkers in discriminating euthyroid patients with HT from healthy controls. It has been found that *Fatty acid degradation* along with the *arginine and proline metabolism* are two key metabolic pathways involved in the HT development [105].

Hyperthyroidism is characterized by increased metabolic activity, resulting in altered metabolism of amino acids and lipids and the tricarboxylic acid cycle. The metabolomic investigation has revealed elevated levels of 33 metabolites and reduced concentrations of 15 others, mainly involved in aminoacyl-tRNA biosynthesis as well as alanine, aspartate, glutamate, and phenylalanine metabolism in individuals with hyperthyroidism [106].

Additionally, the metabolomics profile of patients with hyperthyroidism is reported to change following treatment [107, 108]. The elevated levels of fatty acids such as stearic acid, palmitic acid, and oleic acid, as well as carnitine and amino acids such as cysteine, valine, and dimethylglycine in these patients are shown to reduce after treatment. Concurrently, an increase is noted in the levels of nervonic acid, LPC 16:0, LPC 18:0, LPC 18:1, and glycine after treatment [107]. Similarly, the medium-chain acylcarnitines, such as octanoylcarnitine and decanoylcarnitine, which are increased in individuals with hyperthyroidism, are reported to be reduced after becoming euthyroid thanks to treatment. This suggests their potential to act as a promising biomarker to monitor the restoration of the euthyroid status. Hyperthyroidism treatment is also associated with the downregulation of kynurenine, a metabolite of tryptophan. The kynurenine 3-hydroxylase enzyme, which is suppressed due to hyperthyroidism, therefore, is believed to be upregulated following treatment. Additionally, the levels of L-cystine, a dimer of cysteine formed through cysteine oxidation, are decreased after treatment that suggests reduced oxidative stress in these patients. As a result, monitoring the plasma levels of L-cystine could offer insights into the progress of euthyroid state restoration in hyperthyroid patients [108].

The metabolomic profiling of thyroid cancer has identified distinct alterations in various metabolites, such as tyrosine, leucine, phenylalanine, lysine, alanine, taurine, valine, glutamine, glutamate, glycine, and fatty acids. These metabolic changes not only reflect the heterogeneous nature of thyroid cancer subtypes but also offer potential diagnostic biomarkers and therapeutic targets [109].

The amino acid metabolism is one of the prominent targets of the metabolic reprogramming in thyroid cancer. Metabolomics analysis of papillary thyroid carcinoma has elucidated changes in the levels of amino acids and their derivatives, mainly those involved in the biosynthesis of valine, leucine, and isoleucine, phenylalanine, tyrosine, and tryptophan, and arginine as well as the metabolism glycine, serine, and threonine, alanine, aspartate, and glutamate, glutamate and glutamine, and arginine and proline. These metabolic alterations play pivotal roles in the cellular proliferation and signaling pathways involved in tumor growth and progression [110].

Moreover, lipid metabolism is changed in thyroid cancer, with studies revealing aberrant lipid profiles and altered metabolites metabolism, including elevated levels of triacylglyceride (TAG), SM, phosphatidic acid (PA), phosphatidyl ethanolamine (PE), lysophosphatidic ethanolamine (LPE), diacylglycerol (DAG), ceramide (CER), cholesteryl ester (CE), and reduced concentrations of fatty acids, PC, and acylcarnitine. These changes indicate higher lipid metabolism and lower fatty acids synthesis and β-oxidation in individuals with thyroid tumor [110]. These metabolic signatures may present opportunities for targeted interventions aimed at disrupting lipid metabolism as a therapeutic strategy for thyroid cancer.

Interestingly, metabolomics analysis has the potential to help with the early diagnosis of thyroid diseases, such as thyroid cancer. The metabolite panel consisting of glutamine, sebacic acid, and indole-3-carboxaldehyde has been identified as a promising diagnostic tool for papillary thyroid carcinoma. This panel has 93.8% sensitivity, 97.1% specificity, and 99.4% diagnostic accuracy for the detection of PTC compared to histologic diagnosis [110].

7.7 Adrenal Disorders

Adrenal disorders are a group of diseases that affect the adrenal glands, which are responsible for producing hormones that regulate various bodily functions.

7.7.1 Genomics of Adrenal Disorders

Recent research has identified several genetic factors contributing to the development of adrenal disorders (Table 7.7) [111].

7.7.2 Metabolomics in Adrenal Disorders

Distinct alterations in various metabolites are reported in biological samples diagnosed with adrenal diseases such as Cushing's syndrome and adrenal tumors. These alterations are detectable in blood, urine, and tissue samples, and provide valuable insights into the metabolic signatures associated with these conditions.

Table 7.7 Genes involved in adrenal gland disorders

Region	Gene	Inheritance	disease
9q33.3	*SF1/NR5A1*	AD	Steroidogenic factor 1 deficiency
7p14.1	*GLI3*	AD	Pallister-Hall syndrome
7q21.2	*SAMD9*	AD	MIRAGE syndrome
11p15.4	*CDKN1C*	AD/ imprinting	IMAGE syndrome
1p36.12	*WNT4*	AR	SERKAL syndrome
1q24.2	*TPIT*	AR	Isolated ACTH deficiency
12q13.13	*AAAS*	AR	Triple A syndrome
8q11.21	*MCM4*	AR	FGD DNA repair defect
18p1.21	*MC2R*	AR	Familial glucocorticoid deficiency type 1 (FGD1)
21q22.11	*MRAP*	AR	Familial glucocorticoid deficiency type 2 (FGD2)
5p12	*NNT*	AR	FGD deficiency of mitochondrial ROS detoxification
22q11.21	*TXNRD2*	AR	FGD deficiency of mitochondrial ROS detoxification
17q22	*MKS1*	AR	Meckel-Gruber syndrome
15q25.2	*WDR73*	AR	Galloway-Mowat syndrome
9q31.3 11p.11.2 4p.16.3	*MUSK (FADS1)* *RAPSN (FADS2)* *DOK7 (FADS3)*	AR	Fetal akinesia deformation sequence (FADS)
11q24.2	*HYLS1*	AR?	Hydrolethalus syndrome
xp21.2	*DAX1/NROB1*	XLR	X-linked adrenal hypoplasia congenital (AHC)

As for Cushing's syndrome, characterized by excessive cortisol production, metabolomic studies have demonstrated perturbations in steroid hormone metabolites, such as increased levels of glucocorticoid and mineralocorticoid precursor metabolites. ACTH-independent Cushing's syndrome is depicted with decreased urine excretion of androgen metabolites, whereas a totally contrary condition is reported in the ACTH-dependent version of the syndrome [112]. Additionally, excess levels of cortisol inhibit 11β-hydroxysteroid dehydrogenase type 2, an enzyme responsible for converting cortisol to cortisone, leading to an elevated ratio of urinary tetrahydrocortisol + 5α-tetrahydrocortisol/tetrahydrocortisone [112]. The understanding of the metabolomics dysregulation in Cushing's syndrome can therefore help in both diagnosis and treatment monitoring. This includes the use of specific metabolite profiles as diagnostic markers and for the assessment of treatment efficacy.

Metabolomic studies have also revealed unique metabolic signatures in adrenal tumors, shedding light on the dysregulated metabolic pathways associated with these conditions [113, 114]. These altered metabolite profiles could be used as potential biomarkers for diagnostic and prognostic applications.

Elevated levels of 11-deoxycortisol metabolites, particularly tetrahydro-11-deoxycortisol, are the most consistent urinary markers for distinguishing adrenocortical carcinoma (ACC) from other adrenal cortical adenomas (ACAs). Additionally, elevated levels of intermediate-pathway steroid metabolites, such as 17-hydroxypregnenolone and 17-hydroxyprogesterone, were confirmed in the urine of ACC patients [114]. Further metabolomics studies also found significantly increased plasma levels of progesterone, 17-hydroxyprogesterone, 11-deoxycorticosterone, 11-deoxycortisol, dehydroepiandrosterone, dehydroepiandrosterone sulfate, and estradiol in ACC patients compared to the ACA sufferers. These metabolites can thus help to discriminate ACC from ACAs with an accuracy of 95% in males and 94% in females, suggesting their potential as an accurate diagnostic biomarkers for ACC [115].

Compared to normal adrenal cortical tissue, metabolomic investigation of tissue samples from the adrenal cortex of ACC patients has revealed higher abundance of glycine, glutathione, myo-inositol, lactate, total choline-containing compounds, glutamine, glutamate, and scyllo-inositol along with lower levels of isoleucine, N-acetyl aspartate, and fatty acids. In comparison between ACC and ACA, higher levels of glycine, glutathione, myo-inositol, lactate, total choline-containing compounds, glutamine, glutamate, valine, lysine, ethanolamine, γ-aminobutyric acid (GABA), acetate, alanine, N-acetyl aspartate, isoleucine, and fatty acid were identified as distinguishing factors for ACCs [116].

The identification of such specific metabolite signatures not only contributes to our better understanding of the underlying dysregulated metabolic pathways in adrenal diseases but also holds potential for promising clinical applications. This also guides researchers to determine metabolite-based biomarkers for early disease detection, disease subtyping, monitoring treatment responses as well as development of targeted therapies.

7.8 Conclusion

In recent years, the study of metabolomics and genomics has revolutionized our understanding of various endocrine disorders, such as type 1 diabetes, type 2 diabetes, obesity, thyroid disease, and adrenal disease. Additionally, the metabolomics and genomics investigations hold the potential for various clinical applications, including early detection, prognosis assessment, risk stratification, treatment monitoring, and targeted therapy for these endocrine disorders. The metabolomics and genomics have enabled the identification and characterization of the specific metabolic profile and genetic variants observed in endocrine disorders. Advanced analytical techniques, such as mass spectrometry and next-generation sequencing, allow for identifying specific biomarkers and genetic markers with high diagnostic accuracy for these endocrine conditions, facilitating their early detection.

Additionally, the identification of specific metabolic and genetic patterns linked to endocrine diseases has contributed to more precise risk stratification for individuals predisposed to these conditions, enabling proactive preventive strategies and early intervention in high-risk populations.

The specific metabolic patterns and genetic variants can also be utilized as potential prognostic tools for predicting the progression and outcomes of endocrine diseases. Moreover, metabolic profiles can be utilized as potential markers for treatment monitoring. The metabolic changes following treatment have promise in the understanding of the metabolic pathways upregulated/downregulated with treatment, providing the therapeutic targets for intervention.

By elucidating the metabolic and genetic signatures associated with endocrine disorders, precision medicine has been tailored to target specific pathways and molecular targets. The integration of multi-omics data has shown promise in the identification of biomarker-driven therapeutic targets and the development of personalized intervention strategies with optimized efficacy and minimize adverse effects.

Challenges in metabolomics and genomics studies encompass the necessity for large-scale validation studies, standardization of analytical techniques, and data interpretation. Additionally, the complexity of the metabolome and genome contributes to more complexity in the analysis of metabolomics data. However, advancements in analytical methods, data processing, and bioinformatics tools are continuously enhancing the reproducibility and reliability of metabolomics and genomics studies.

As the field of metabolomics and genomics continues to advance, ongoing research holds promise for revolutionizing our understanding of the complex metabolic and genetic aspects of endocrine diseases, ultimately leading to better patient care and outcomes.

References

1. Stratakis CA. Genomics and precision medicine and their impact on endocrinology. Endocr Connect. 2023;12(7)
2. Jin Q, Ma RCW. Metabolomics in diabetes and diabetic complications: insights from epidemiological studies. Cells. 2021;10(11):2832.
3. Abul-Husn NSKE. Personalized medicine and the power of electronic health records. Cell. 2019;177(1):58–69.
4. Jerram ST, Leslie RD. The genetic architecture of type1 diabetes mellitus. Genes (Basel). 2017;8:209.
5. Todd JA. Etiology of type 1 diabetes. Immunity. 2010;32(4):457–67.
6. Pociot F. Type 1 diabetes genome-wide association studies: not to be lost in translation. Clin Transl Immunol. 2017;6(12):e162.
7. Robertson CC, Rich SS. Genetics of type 1 diabetes. Curr Opin Genet Dev. 2018;50:7–16.
8. Redondo MJ, Steck AK, Pugliese A. Genetics of type 1 diabetes. Pediatr Diabetes. 2018;19(3):346–53.
9. Steck AK, Rewers MJ. Genetics of type 1 diabetes. Clin Chem. 2011;57(2):176–85.

10. Onengut-Gumuscu S, et al. Fine mapping of type 1 diabetes susceptibility loci and evidence for colocalization of causal variants with lymphoid gene enhancers. Nat Genet. 2015;47(4):381–6.
11. Klak M, et al. Type 1 diabetes: genes associated with disease development. Cent Eur J Immunol. 2020;45(4):439–53.
12. Barrett JC, Concannon P, et al. Genome wide association study and meta-analysis find that over 40 loci affect risk of type 1 diabetes. Nat Genet. 2009;41:703–7.
13. Carr ALJ, Evans-Molina C, Oram RA. Precision medicine in type 1 diabetes. Diabetologia. 2022;65(11):1854–66.
14. Nyaga DM, Vickers MH, Jefferies C, Perry JK, O'Sullivan JM. Type 1 diabetes mellitus-associated genetic variants contribute to overlapping immune regulatory networks. Front Genet. 2018;9:535.
15. Galderisi A, Pirillo P, Moret V, Stocchero M, Gucciardi A, Perilongo G, et al. Metabolomics reveals new metabolic perturbations in children with type 1 diabetes. Pediatr Diabetes. 2018;19(1):59–67.
16. Overgaard AJ, Kaur S, Pociot F. Metabolomic biomarkers in the progression to type 1 diabetes. Curr Diab Rep. 2016;16:1–5.
17. Pflueger M, Seppänen-Laakso T, Suortti T, Hyötyläinen T, Achenbach P, Bonifacio E, et al. Age- and islet autoimmunity–associated differences in amino acid and lipid metabolites in children at risk for type 1 diabetes. Diabetes. 2011;60(11):2740–7.
18. Jørgenrud B, Stene LC, Tapia G, Bøås H, Pepaj M, Berg JP, et al. Longitudinal plasma metabolic profiles, infant feeding, and islet autoimmunity in the MIDIA study. Pediatr Diabetes. 2017;18(2):111–9.
19. Oresic M, Simell S, Sysi-Aho M, Nanto-Salonen K, Seppänen-Laakso T, Parikka V, et al. Dysregulation of lipid and amino acid metabolism precedes islet autoimmunity in children who later progress to type 1 diabetes. J Exp Med. 2008;205(13):2975–84.
20. La Torre D, Seppänen-Laakso T, Larsson HE, Hyötyläinen T, Ivarsson SA, Lernmark Å, et al. Decreased cord-blood phospholipids in young age–at–onset type 1 diabetes. Diabetes. 2013;62(11):3951–6.
21. Knebel B, Strassburger K, Szendroedi J, Kotzka J, Scheer M, Nowotny B, et al. Specific metabolic profiles and their relationship to insulin resistance in recent-onset type 1 and type 2 diabetes. J Clin Endocrinol Metabol. 2016;101(5):2130–40.
22. Arneth B, Arneth R, Shams M. Metabolomics of type 1 and type 2 diabetes. Int J Mol Sci. 2019;20(10):2467.
23. Federation ID. IDF Diabetes Atlas. Brussels, 2021.
24. Ayub Q, Chen Y, Panoutsopoulou K, Colonna V, Pagani L, et al. Revisiting the thrifty gene hypothesis via 65 loci associated with susceptibility to type 2 diabetes. Am Hum Genet. 2014;94(2):176–85.
25. Flannick J, Beer NL, Jacobs SB, Grarup N, Burtt NP, et al. Loss-of-function mutations in SLC30A8 protect against type 2 diabetes. Nat Genet. 2014;46(4):357–63.
26. Ebrahimi Fana S, Esmaeili S, Bandarian F, Nasli-Esfahani E, Amoli MM, Razi F. Knowledge discovery in genetics of diabetes in Iran, a roadmap for future researches. J Diabetes Metab Disord. 2021;20:1785–91.
27. Vujkovic M, Lynch JA, Miller DR, Zhou J, Tcheandjieu C, et al. Discovery of 318 new risk loci for type 2 diabetes and related vascular outcomes among 1.4 million participants in a multi-ancestry meta-analysis. Nat Genet. 2020;52:680–91.
28. Bonnefond A, Froguel P. Rare and common genetic events in type 2 diabetes: what should biologists know? Cell Metab. 2015;21(3):357–68.
29. Brown AE, Walker M. Genetics of insulin resistance and the metabolic Syndrom. Curr Cardiol Rep. 2016;18:75.
30. Gharipour M, Sadeghian L, Eftekhari A, Rothenberg I, Jahanfar S. Precision medicine and metabolic syndrome. ARYA Atheroscler. 2022;18(4)
31. Skinner SC, Nemkov T, Diaw M, Mbaye MN, Diedhiou D, Sow D, et al. Metabolic profile of individuals with and without type 2 diabetes from sub-Saharan Africa. J Proteome Res. 2023;22:2319.

32. Hosseinkhani S, Aazami H, Hashemi E, Dehghanbanadaki H, Adibi-Motlagh B, Razi F. The trend in application of omics in type 2 diabetes researches; a bibliometric study. Diabetes Metab Syndr Clin Res Rev. 2021;15(5):102250.
33. Xourafa G, Korbmacher M, Roden M. Inter-organ crosstalk during development and progression of type 2 diabetes mellitus. Nat Rev Endocrinol. 2023;20:1–23.
34. Arjmand B, Ebrahimi Fana S, Ghasemi E, Kazemi A, Ghodssi-Ghassemabadi R, Dehghanbanadaki H, et al. Metabolic signatures of insulin resistance in non-diabetic individuals. BMC Endocr Disord. 2022;22(1):1–11.
35. Ramzan I, Ardavani A, Vanweert F, Mellett A, Atherton PJ, Idris I. The association between circulating branched chain amino acids and the temporal risk of developing type 2 diabetes mellitus: a systematic review & meta-analysis. Nutrients. 2022;14(20):4411.
36. Chen T, Ni Y, Ma X, Bao Y, Liu J, Huang F, et al. Branched-chain and aromatic amino acid profiles and diabetes risk in Chinese populations. Sci Rep. 2016;6(1):20594.
37. Hosseinkhani S, Arjmand B, Dilmaghani-Marand A, Mohammadi Fateh S, Dehghanbanadaki H, Najjar N, et al. Targeted metabolomics analysis of amino acids and acylcarnitines as risk markers for diabetes by LC–MS/MS technique. Sci Rep. 2022;12(1):8418.
38. Taghizadeh H, Emamgholipour S, Hosseinkhani S, Arjmand B, Rezaei N, Dilmaghani-Marand A, et al. The association between acylcarnitine and amino acids profile and metabolic syndrome and its components in Iranian adults: data from STEPs 2016. Front Endocrinol. 2023;14:1058952.
39. Savolainen O, Fagerberg B, Vendelbo Lind M, Sandberg A-S, Ross AB, Bergström G. Biomarkers for predicting type 2 diabetes development—can metabolomics improve on existing biomarkers? PLoS One. 2017;12(7):e0177738.
40. Suhre K. Metabolic profiling in diabetes. J Endocrinol. 2014;221(3):R75–85.
41. Wang TJ, Larson MG, Vasan RS, Cheng S, Rhee EP, McCabe E, et al. Metabolite profiles and the risk of developing diabetes. Nat Med. 2011;17(4):448–53.
42. Tanase DM, Gosav EM, Botoc T, Floria M, Tarniceriu CC, Maranduca MA, et al. Depiction of branched-chain amino acids (BCAAs) in diabetes with a focus on diabetic microvascular complications. J Clin Med. 2023;12(18):6053.
43. Gar C, Rottenkolber M, Prehn C, Adamski J, Seissler J, Lechner A. Serum and plasma amino acids as markers of prediabetes, insulin resistance, and incident diabetes. Crit Rev Clin Lab Sci. 2018;55(1):21–32.
44. White PJ, McGarrah RW, Herman MA, Bain JR, Shah SH, Newgard CB. Insulin action, type 2 diabetes, and branched-chain amino acids: a two-way street. Mol Metab. 2021;52:101261.
45. Yoon M-S. The emerging role of branched-chain amino acids in insulin resistance and metabolism. Nutrients. 2016;8(7):405.
46. Ardestani A, Lupse B, Kido Y, Leibowitz G, Maedler K. mTORC1 signaling: a double-edged sword in diabetic β cells. Cell Metab. 2018;27(2):314–31.
47. Mao Z, Zhang W. Role of mTOR in glucose and lipid metabolism. Int J Mol Sci. 2018;19(7):2043.
48. Mahendran Y, Jonsson A, Have CT, Allin KH, Witte DR, Jørgensen ME, et al. Genetic evidence of a causal effect of insulin resistance on branched-chain amino acid levels. Diabetologia. 2017;60(5):873–8.
49. Lotta LA, Scott RA, Sharp SJ, Burgess S, et al. Genetic predisposition to an impaired metabolism of the branched-chain amino acids and risk of type 2 diabetes: a Mendelian randomisation analysis. PLoS Med. 2016;13(11):e1002179.
50. Yamada C, Kondo M, Kishimoto N, Shibata T, Nagai Y, Imanishi T, et al. Association between insulin resistance and plasma amino acid profile in non-diabetic J apanese subjects. J Diabetes Investigat. 2015;6(4):408–15.
51. Ding Y, Wang S, Lu J. Unlocking the potential: amino acids' role in predicting and exploring therapeutic avenues for type 2 diabetes mellitus. Meta. 2023;13(9):1017.
52. Adams SH. Emerging perspectives on essential amino acid metabolism in obesity and the insulin-resistant state. Adv Nutr. 2011;2(6):445–56.

53. Merino J, Leong A, Liu C-T, Porneala B, Walford GA, von Grotthuss M, et al. Metabolomics insights into early type 2 diabetes pathogenesis and detection in individuals with normal fasting glucose. Diabetologia. 2018;61:1315–24.
54. Vangipurapu J, Fernandes Silva L, Kuulasmaa T, Smith U, Laakso M. Microbiota-related metabolites and the risk of type 2 diabetes. Diabetes Care. 2020;43(6):1319–25.
55. Tillin T, Hughes AD, Wang Q, Würtz P, Ala-Korpela M, Sattar N, et al. Diabetes risk and amino acid profiles: cross-sectional and prospective analyses of ethnicity, amino acids and diabetes in a south Asian and European cohort from the SABRE (Southall and Brent REvisited) study. Diabetologia. 2015;58:968–79.
56. Kawanaka M, Nishino K, Oka T, Urata N, Nakamura J, Suehiro M, et al. Tyrosine levels are associated with insulin resistance in patients with nonalcoholic fatty liver disease. Hepatic Med Evidence Res. 2015;7:29–35.
57. Hellmuth C, Kirchberg FF, Lass N, Harder U, Peissner W, Koletzko B, et al. Tyrosine is associated with insulin resistance in longitudinal metabolomic profiling of obese children. J Diabetes Res. 2016;2016:1.
58. Alves A, Bassot A, Bulteau A-L, Pirola L, Morio B. Glycine metabolism and its alterations in obesity and metabolic diseases. Nutrients. 2019;11(6):1356.
59. Glynn EL, Piner LW, Huffman KM, Slentz CA, Elliot-Penry L, AbouAssi H, et al. Impact of combined resistance and aerobic exercise training on branched-chain amino acid turnover, glycine metabolism and insulin sensitivity in overweight humans. Diabetologia. 2015;58:2324–35.
60. Adeva-Andany M, Souto-Adeva G, Ameneiros-Rodríguez E, Fernández-Fernández C, Donapetry-García C, Domínguez-Montero A. Insulin resistance and glycine metabolism in humans. Amino Acids. 2018;50:11–27.
61. Dehghanbanadaki H, Dodangeh S, Parhizkar Roudsari P, Hosseinkhani S, Khashayar P, Noorchenarboo M, et al. Metabolomics profile and 10-year atherosclerotic cardiovascular disease (ASCVD) risk score. Front Cardiovasc Med. 2023;10:1161761.
62. Dodangeh S, Taghizadeh H, Hosseinkhani S, Khashayar P, Pasalar P, Meybodi HRA, et al. Metabolomics signature of cardiovascular disease in patients with diabetes, a narrative review. J Diabetes Metab Disord. 2023;22(2):985–94.
63. Yan-Do R, MacDonald PE. Impaired "glycine"-mia in type 2 diabetes and potential mechanisms contributing to glucose homeostasis. Endocrinology. 2017;158(5):1064–73.
64. Palmer ND, Stevens RD, Antinozzi PA, Anderson A, Bergman RN, Wagenknecht LE, et al. Metabolomic profile associated with insulin resistance and conversion to diabetes in the insulin resistance atherosclerosis study. J Clin Endocrinol Metabol. 2015;100(3):E463–E8.
65. Walford GA, Ma Y, Clish C, Florez JC, Wang TJ, Gerszten RE, et al. Metabolite profiles of diabetes incidence and intervention response in the diabetes prevention program. Diabetes. 2016;65(5):1424–33.
66. Stančáková A, Civelek M, Saleem NK, Soininen P, Kangas AJ, Cederberg H, et al. Hyperglycemia and a common variant of GCKR are associated with the levels of eight amino acids in 9,369 Finnish men. Diabetes. 2012;61(7):1895–902.
67. Peddinti G, Cobb J, Yengo L, Froguel P, Kravić J, Balkau B, et al. Early metabolic markers identify potential targets for the prevention of type 2 diabetes. Diabetologia. 2017;60(9):1740–50.
68. Davalli AM, Perego C, Folli FB. The potential role of glutamate in the current diabetes epidemic. Acta Diabetol. 2012;49:167–83.
69. Qiu G, Zheng Y, Wang H, Sun J, Ma H, Xiao Y, et al. Plasma metabolomics identified novel metabolites associated with risk of type 2 diabetes in two prospective cohorts of Chinese adults. Int J Epidemiol. 2016;45(5):1507–16.
70. Xuan Q, Hu C, Zhang Y, Wang Q, Zhao X, Liu X, et al. Serum lipidomics profiles reveal potential lipid markers for prediabetes and type 2 diabetes in patients from multiple communities. Front Endocrinol. 2022;13:966823.
71. Yang J, Wang M, Yang D, Yan H, Wang Z, Yan D, et al. Integrated lipids biomarker of the prediabetes and type 2 diabetes mellitus Chinese patients. Front Endocrinol. 2023;13:1065665.

72. Rhee EP, Cheng S, Larson MG, Walford GA, Lewis GD, McCabe E, et al. Lipid profiling identifies a triacylglycerol signature of insulin resistance and improves diabetes prediction in humans. J Clin Invest. 2011;121(4):1402–11.
73. Wang-Sattler R, Yu Z, Herder C, Messias AC, Floegel A, He Y, et al. Novel biomarkers for pre-diabetes identified by metabolomics. Mol Syst Biol. 2012;8(1):615.
74. Ferrannini E, Natali A, Camastra S, Nannipieri M, Mari A, Adam K-P, et al. Early metabolic markers of the development of dysglycemia and type 2 diabetes and their physiological significance. Diabetes. 2013;62(5):1730–7.
75. Guasch-Ferré M, Hruby A, Toledo E, Clish CB, Martínez-González MA, Salas-Salvadó J, et al. Metabolomics in prediabetes and diabetes: a systematic review and meta-analysis. Diabetes Care. 2016;39(5):833–46.
76. Mahendran Y, Cederberg H, Vangipurapu J, Kangas AJ, Soininen P, Kuusisto J, et al. Glycerol and fatty acids in serum predict the development of hyperglycemia and type 2 diabetes in Finnish men. Diabetes Care. 2013;36(11):3732–8.
77. Ahola-Olli AV, Mustelin L, Kalimeri M, Kettunen J, Jokelainen J, Auvinen J, et al. Circulating metabolites and the risk of type 2 diabetes: a prospective study of 11,896 young adults from four Finnish cohorts. Diabetologia. 2019;62:2298–309.
78. Yuan S, Larsson SC. Association of genetic variants related to plasma fatty acids with type 2 diabetes mellitus and glycaemic traits: a Mendelian randomisation study. Diabetologia. 2020;63:116–23.
79. Organization WH. Obesity and overweight. key facts. Available from: https://www.who.int/news-room/fact-sheets/detail/obesity-and-overweight.
80. Sohn YB. The genetics of obesity a narrative review. Prec Fut Med. 2022;6(4):226–32.
81. Mahmoud R, Kimonis V, Butler MG. Genetics of obesity in humans: a clinical review. Int J Mol Sci. 2022;23:11005.
82. Fall T, Ingelsson E. Genome-wide association studies of obesity and metabolic syndrome. Mol Cel Endocrinol. 2014;382(1):740–57.
83. Pigeyre M, Yazdi FT, Kaur Y, Meyre D. Recent progress in genetics, epigenetics and metagenomics unveils the pathophysiology of human obesity. Clin Sci (Lond). 2016;130(12):943–86.
84. Trang K, Grant SFA. Genetics and epigenetics in the obesity phenotyping scenario. Rev Endocr Metab Disord. 2023;24(5):775–93.
85. Loos RJF, Yeo GSH. The genetics of obesity: from discovery to biology. Nat Rev Genet. 2022;23:120–33.
86. Woldemariam S, Dorner TE, Wiesinger T, Stein KV. Multi-omics approaches for precision obesity management: potentials and limitations of omics in precision prevention, treatment and risk reduction of obesity. Wien Klin Wochenschr. 2023;135(5–6):113–24.
87. Butte NF, Liu Y, Zakeri IF, Mohney RP, Mehta N, Voruganti VS, et al. Global metabolomic profiling targeting childhood obesity in the Hispanic population. Am J Clin Nutr. 2015;102(2):256–67.
88. Wiklund PK, Pekkala S, Autio R, Munukka E, Xu L, Saltevo J, et al. Serum metabolic profiles in overweight and obese women with and without metabolic syndrome. Diabetol Metab Syndr. 2014;6(1):1–9.
89. Primeau V, Coderre L, Karelis A, Brochu M, Lavoie M, Messier V, et al. Characterizing the profile of obese patients who are metabolically healthy. Int J Obes. 2011;35(7):971–81.
90. Rangel-Huerta OD, Pastor-Villaescusa B, Gil A. Are we close to defining a metabolomic signature of human obesity? A systematic review of metabolomics studies. Metabolomics. 2019;15:1–31.
91. Sorrow P, Maguire R, Murphy SK, Belcher SM, Hoyo C. Elevated metabolites of acetaminophen in cord blood of children with obesity. Pediatr Obes. 2019;14(1):e12465.
92. Cirulli ET, Guo L, Swisher CL, Shah N, Huang L, Napier LA, et al. Profound perturbation of the metabolome in obesity is associated with health risk. Cell Metab. 2019;29(2):488–500. e2
93. Newgard CB, An J, Bain JR, Muehlbauer MJ, Stevens RD, Lien LF, et al. A branched-chain amino acid-related metabolic signature that differentiates obese and lean humans and contributes to insulin resistance. Cell Metab. 2009;9(4):311–26.
94. Kang M, Yoo HJ, Kim M, Kim M, Lee JH. Metabolomics identifies increases in the acylcarnitine profiles in the plasma of overweight subjects in response to mild weight loss: a randomized, controlled design study. Lipids Health Dis. 2018;17:1–13.

95. Dapas M, Dunaif A. Deconstructing a syndrome: genomic insights into PCOS causal mechanisms and classification. Endocr Rev. 2022;43(6):927–65.
96. Khan MJ, Ullah A, Basit S. Genetic basis of polycystic ovary syndrome (PCOS): current perspectives. Appl Clin Genet. 2019;12:249–60.
97. Rajska A, Buszewska-Forajta M, Rachoń D, Markuszewski MJ. Metabolomic insight into polycystic ovary syndrome – an overview. Int J Mol Sci. 2020;21(14):4853.
98. Zhao Y, Fu L, Li R, Wang L-N, Yang Y, Liu N-N, et al. Metabolic profiles characterizing different phenotypes of polycystic ovary syndrome: plasma metabolomics analysis. BMC Med. 2012;10(1):1–12.
99. Murri M, Insenser M, Escobar-Morreale HF. Metabolomics in polycystic ovary syndrome. Clin Chim Acta. 2014;429:181–8.
100. Escobar-Morreale HF, Samino S, Insenser M, Vinaixa M, Luque-Ramirez M, Lasuncion MA, et al. Metabolic heterogeneity in polycystic ovary syndrome is determined by obesity: plasma metabolomic approach using GC-MS. Clin Chem. 2012;58(6):999–1009.
101. Chiovato L, Magri F, Carlé A. Hypothyroidism in context: where we've been and where we're going. Adv Ther. 2019;36:47–58.
102. Medici M, Visser TJ, Peeters RP. Genetics of thyroid function. Best Pract Res Clin Endocrinol Metab. 2017;31(2):129–42.
103. Williams AT, et al. Genome-wide association study of thyroid-stimulating hormone highlights new genes, pathways and associations with thyroid disease. Nat Commun. 2023;14:6713.
104. Shao F, Li R, Guo Q, Qin R, Su W, Yin H, et al. Plasma metabolomics reveals systemic metabolic alterations of subclinical and clinical hypothyroidism. J Clin Endocrinol Metabol. 2023;108(1):13–25.
105. Jiang X, Zhao X, Gu X, Luo T, Li P, Wan C, et al. Serum metabolomic analysis in patients with Hashimoto's thyroiditis. Front Endocrinol. 2022;13:1046159.
106. Xia Q, Qian W, Chen L, Chen X, Xie R, Zhang D, et al. Comprehensive metabolomics study in children with graves' disease. Front Endocrinol. 2021;12:752496.
107. Lee HY, Sim BC, Nga HT, Moon JS, Tian J, Linh NT, et al. Metabolite changes during the transition from hyperthyroidism to Euthyroidism in patients with graves' disease. Endocrinol Metab. 2022;37(6):891–900.
108. Jaber MA, Benabdelkamel H, Dahabiyeh LA, Masood A, AlMalki RH, Musambil M, et al. The metabolomics approach revealed a distinctive metabolomics pattern associated with hyperthyroidism treatment. Front Endocrinol. 2022;13:1050201.
109. Coelho M, Raposo L, Goodfellow BJ, Atzori L, Jones J, Manadas B. The potential of metabolomics in the diagnosis of thyroid cancer. Int J Mol Sci. 2020;21(15):5272.
110. Wang Z, Yang Y, Xing Y, Si D, Wang S, Lin J, et al. Combined metabolomic and lipidomic analysis uncovers metabolic profile and biomarkers for papillary thyroid carcinoma. Sci Rep. 2023;13(1):17666.
111. Gauss C, Rowland D, Ergun-Longmire B. An update on genetics of adrenal gland and associated disorders. Endocrine. 2022;3(2):187–97.
112. Storbeck K-H, Schiffer L, Baranowski ES, Chortis V, Prete A, Barnard L, et al. Steroid metabolome analysis in disorders of adrenal steroid biosynthesis and metabolism. Endocr Rev. 2019;40(6):1605–25.
113. Bancos I, Taylor AE, Chortis V, Sitch AJ, Jenkinson C, Davidge-Pitts CJ, et al. Urine steroid metabolomics for the differential diagnosis of adrenal incidentalomas in the EURINE-ACT study: a prospective test validation study. Lancet Diabetes Endocrinol. 2020;8(9):773–81.
114. Eisenhofer G, Durán C, Chavakis T, Cannistraci CV. Steroid metabolomics: machine learning and multidimensional diagnostics for adrenal cortical tumors, hyperplasias, and related disorders. Curr Opin Endocr Metab Res. 2019;8:40–9.
115. Schweitzer S, Kunz M, Kurlbaum M, Vey J, Kendl S, Deutschbein T, et al. Plasma steroid metabolome profiling for the diagnosis of adrenocortical carcinoma. Eur J Endocrinol. 2019;180(2):117–25.
116. Imperiale A, Elbayed K, Moussallieh F-M, Reix N, Piotto M, Bellocq J-P, et al. Metabolomic profile of the adrenal gland: from physiology to pathological conditions. Endocr Relat Cancer. 2013;20(5):705–16.

Chapter 8
Host–Microbiota Interactions in Endocrine Diseases

Azin Pakmehr, Seyed Davar Siadat, and Hanieh-Sadat Ejtahed

8.1 Definition of Human Microbiome and Its Dysbiosis

The human body hosts different microorganisms, mostly bacteria, of various species called microbiota which takes part in a wide range of biological processes. At birth, microorganisms begin to colonize in oral and nasopharyngeal membranes of the newly born baby and manage to increase in number and diversity until they exist in multiple areas of the human body like skin, upper airway, and genital and gastrointestinal tract. The composition of this community is unique in each individual based on factors like diet, lifestyle, hygiene, and genetic background. Since the gastrointestinal tract provides the largest interface with the environment outside the human body, it is the most important site to house a large number of microorganisms [1].

Gut microbiota is highly diverse and plays fundamental roles in the intestine along with the human system as a whole. The majority of microorganisms colonize distal part of the gastrointestinal tract where their abundance surpasses 10^{11} cells per gram content. The bacterial groups in the intestine mostly include Gram-positive Firmicutes and Gram-negative Bacteroidetes. The composition of gut microbiota and the proportion of these two groups can change dynamically following multiple factors such as geographical region, diet, drugs, and health status. This can destroy the balance present in this symbiotic relationship and lead to a condition known as

A. Pakmehr
Endocrinology and Metabolism Research Center, Endocrinology and Metabolism Clinical Sciences Institute, Tehran University of Medical Sciences, Tehran, Iran

S. D. Siadat
Mycobacteriology & Pulmonary Research Department, Pasteur Institute of Iran, Tehran, Iran

H.-S. Ejtahed (✉)
Obesity and Eating Habits Research Center, Endocrinology and Metabolism Clinical Sciences Institute, Tehran University of Medical Sciences, Tehran, Iran

H. Gharib et al. (eds.), *Interdisciplinary Advances in Endocrinology*, https://doi.org/10.1007/978-981-95-2286-6_8

gut dysbiosis which has been found to have significant associations with several pathologies such as metabolic disorders like diabetes mellitus and hypertension, cardiovascular diseases, inflammatory bowel syndromes, and cancers as gut microbiota is involved in maintaining intestinal integrity and regulation of inflammatory responses [2].

On the other hand, physiological changes during life can have impacts on the composition of gut microbiota. Hormonal changes following pregnancy can affect bacterial metabolism, growth, and virulence leading to alterations in gut microbial diversity according to gestational age, nutritional status, and other factors. In addition, gut microbiota seems to decline in diversity and stability as one gets older resulting in inflammatory disturbances and disruption of intestinal integrity. Although gut dysbiosis, an imbalance of microorganisms in the intestines, can play a causative role in developing some diseases, many treatments help to alleviate disorders through modifications in gut microbiota and restore healthy composition. Also, microorganisms contribute to the metabolization and absorption of drugs, so there seems to be a drug–microbiota axis that affects the potential ability of each prescribed drug [3]. Given the fact that gut microbiota is highly involved in human health and therapeutical strategies, it is important to delve into its role and possible effects.

8.2 Host–Microbiome Interaction

This disciplined system has many beneficial effects including maintaining gut integrity, defending against pathogens, regulating inflammatory responses, and harvesting energy. Gut dysbiosis results in alterations in the intra-intestinal environment consisting of immune system cells and enteric neurons which may disturb the homeostasis that stands in the gastrointestinal tract locally and other organs systemically. Consequently, there seems to be an integrated relationship between gut microbiota and extraintestinal parts of the human body shaping interorgan connections like gut–lung axis, gut–skin axis, gut–brain axis, and gut–liver axis (Fig. 8.1). This two-way relationship between microbiota and the host is called host–microbiota interaction [3].

8.2.1 Lung

Respiratory tract contains a normal composition of microbiota which is related to other organs' microbiota. In fact, any changes in gut microbiota composition can lead to a change in the composition of the microbiota existing in the respiratory tract and lead to respiratory diseases. A decline in bacteria producing short-chain fatty acids (SCFAs) may cause disturbances in gut barrier and inflammatory control. This can be seen in patients with tuberculosis and coronavirus disease 2019. The same

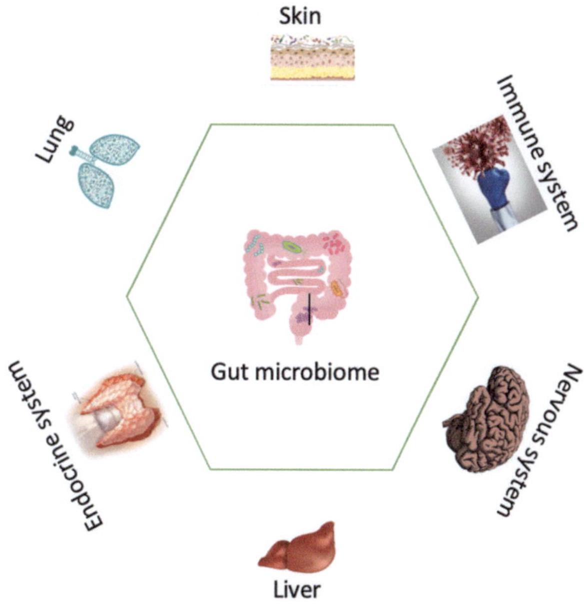

Fig. 8.1 The interaction between gut microbiota and extraintestinal organs

happens for patients with chronic obstructive pulmonary disease, and it seems that they have a depletion in some SCFA-producing genera. Also, those with an abundance of SCFA producers have lower viral load during viral respiratory infections [4].

8.2.2 *Skin*

Skin is the very first defense barrier of the human body with a wide variety of microorganisms which play an important role in educating the immune system to distinguish the pathogenic microbes and properly eliminate them. Also, some commensals are able to produce bactericidal factors and antimicrobial peptides to help inhibit pathogen colonization and growth. The composition of skin microbiota can change during dermatological disorders like psoriasis, acne vulgaris, and atopic dermatitis. Psoriasis is strongly associated with gut dysbiosis in addition to skin dysbiosis since the composition of gut microbiota changes toward a more inflammatory status in patients with psoriasis, and evidence has shown the modulating effects of dietary treatments to modify gut microbiota on this disease [5]. The same pattern exists when it comes to other inflammatory skin disorders like acne vulgaris and atopic dermatitis. Gut microbiota tends to increase in a way that triggers inflammatory responses and fuels the cascade that started in individuals with genetic susceptibility. To confirm this, inflammatory bowel diseases (IBD) are more common in those with inflammatory skin disorders, and administration of prebiotics or probiotics to change the resident gut microbiota seems to alleviate both diseases [5, 6].

8.2.3 Nervous System

Gut microbiota seems to affect nervous system through brain–gut axis in which microorganisms secrete neuroactive compounds like dopamine and serotonin that affect neuron activity. Furthermore, metabolites produced by gut microbiota such as glutamate have been demonstrated to have impacts on behavior and nervous system development [7]. Evidence has supported the role of gut dysbiosis in developing neurodegenerative and neuroinflammatory disorders through different pathways. SCFA-producing bacteria decrease in number in Parkinson's disease which causes higher intestine permeability and creates a larger interface for neural plexus and toxins leading to an inflammatory status, while inflammatory suppression is not as practical as before since SCFA depletion downregulates regulatory T-cells. The same pattern seems to exist for multiple sclerosis [8]. Additionally, glutamate is an excitatory neurotransmitter in the central nervous system of mammalians and plays a substantial role in the nervous system. Gut microbiota seems to interfere with glutamate metabolisms leading to Alzheimer's disease pathogenesis [9]. Regarding psychiatric disorders like depression and bipolarity, an increase in proinflammatory species and subsequent cytokines and a decline in anti-inflammatory butyrate-producing species seem to accompany other factors involved in developing these diseases [10]. Due to the bidirectional communication between the gut and brain, neuropeptide-like proteins produced by bacteria during dysbiosis can cross-react with immunoglobulins secreted under stress. This interaction affects the hunger and satiety centers in the hypothalamus, impairing the patient's ability to regulate food intake and potentially leading to eating disorders [11].

8.2.4 Liver

Since the liver and gastrointestinal tract are linked anatomically and functionally through the portal network, changes in gut microbiota will affect this organ inevitably. Any disruption of the intestinal wall integrity allows pathogens to cross this barrier, triggering an inflammatory response and the production of cytokines. These cytokines, along with antigens, can then enter the portal circulation and reach the liver. This is the possible mechanism involved in the role of gut microbiota in alcoholic liver damage. The stage of injury has shown a correlation with the severity of gut dysbiosis which is determined by the decline in SCFA-producing bacteria. Also, dysbiosis in obesity leads to the abundance of ethanol-producing bacteria which can lead to increased inflammatory status and promote insulin resistance that triggers lipogenesis in the liver regardless of oral alcohol intake, which happens in nonalcoholic fatty liver disease. As gut microbiota plays a pivotal role in transforming bile acids to metabolites, any changes in this pathway result in disturbances in fat metabolization, gut permeability and motility, bacterial overgrowth, and further liver diseases including nonalcoholic steatohepatitis and cirrhosis [12].

8.2.5 Immune System

The dysbiosis of gut microbiota has been detected in many diseases related to a disturbance in the immune system which draws scientists' attention to the role of microbiota in regulating immune responses. Bacterial species that produce SCFA seem to prevent B-cell activation, plasma cell differentiation, and antibody class switching, so their shortage may play a prominent role in developing immune-related disorders that can be seen in systemic lupus erythematosus [13]. It has been found that some lipopolysaccharide (LPS)-producing bacteria can induce the innate immune system and produce inflammatory cytokines which is what happens in inflammatory diseases like gout [14]. Also, as some disorders in the intestine are strongly associated with inflammation in other parts of the body, scientists have been looking for mechanisms which may contribute to this phenomenon. A decrease in microbial diversity and similar changes in the composition of gut dysbiosis in patients suffering from different inflammatory diseases lead us to the undeniable association between microbiota and the immune system [15].

8.2.6 Endocrine System

The world inside human intestine is not only limited to microorganisms existing there but also materials secreted by them. As a result of degrading nutrients, including polyunsaturated fats (PUFA), dietary fibers, carnitine, and bile acids by microbial enzymes during digestion, a myriad of metabolites like short-chain fatty acids (SCFAs), conjugated linoleic acid (CLA), trimethylamine nitrogen oxide (TMAO), secondary bile acids (BAs), tryptophan, choline metabolites, gases, vitamins, and neurotransmitters are yield that can pass through the intestinal barrier and are intimately linked with the human health and diseases. That is why gut microbiota can be addressed as an endocrine organ. In addition, it has been shown that microbiota is able to affect and also be affected by hormone secretion in the body and a pivotal impact on regulating metabolism, appetite, and immune system through different mechanisms. These bidirectional relationships give birth to the term "microbial endocrinology" [16] which is the main focus of this chapter.

8.3 Microbiota Dysbiosis and Metabolic Diseases

8.3.1 Obesity

Gut microbiota has a significant role in extracting energy from food intake and subsequent lipid accumulation. Studies on animal models of mice have shown that germ-free mice increased in body fat and weight when colonized with normal microbiota although mice without microbiota did not change in adiposity even when they were fed with a high-fat diet. Also, the gut microbiota of obese mice codes genes related to harvesting energy from polysaccharides which are not normally digested in thin models leading to more absorption of products. Obesity appears to disrupt the balance of gut microbiota, leading to a higher abundance of the Firmicutes phylum and a reduced presence of the Bacteroidetes phylum compared to normal-weight individuals. This altered microbial composition is thought to be more efficient at extracting energy from the consumed food [17]. Furthermore, gut microbiota is related to subtle chronic inflammation which exists in obesity. Due to gut dysbiosis in obesity, bacterial lipopolysaccharide (LPS) increases in the intestinal lumen and is transported to the bloodstream following disturbances in intestinal permeability through a pathway involving Toll-like receptor (TLR)-4 which fuels the cascade of inflammation. Lipoprotein lipase (LPL), which is synthetized following a high-fat diet and transported via chylomicrons, induces the production of inflammatory cytokines like interleukin-6 (IL-6) and tumor necrosis factor-α (TNF-α), a process called "metabolic endotoxemia." Intestinal microbiota related to obesity suppresses fasting-induced adipose factor (FIAF) which is meant to inhibit LPL activity and prevent triglyceride accumulation. In addition, in germ-free mice, adenosine monophosphate (AMP)-activated protein kinase (AMPK) stimulates fat consumption in other organs like liver and muscles which in turn protects from getting obese [18].

On the other hand, weight loss can reverse the changes in gut microbiota composition. Also, replacement of the high-fat diet could change the ratio toward the high abundance in Firmicutes phylum which suggests the potential role of diet apart from obesity in gut dysbiosis.

As we previously mentioned, gut microbiota acts like an endocrine organ, and the metabolite profile of the human body correlates strongly with microbiota composition. Following the dysbiosis happening in obesity, it has been found that specific metabolites show a significant alteration. As a result of alteration in gut microbiota, branched-chain amino acids and aromatic amino acids seem to increase in obese individuals. This rise in the amount of these amino acids correlated with the decrease in *Bacteroides* which happens in obesity. Different studies have shown that these amino acids are known risk factors for further obesity-related complications like insulin resistance, hyperglycemia, hyperlipidemia, elevated circulating inflammatory factors, diabetes, and cardiovascular diseases. Glutamate is another amino acid which increases significantly in obese individuals compared to lean ones and has a positive relationship with obesity indices like body mass index. Moreover,

SCFAs (acetate, propionate, and butyrate) are microbial metabolites produced through fermenting indigestible starch in the colon and have a prominent role in providing energy, de novo hepatic triglyceride and glucose synthesis, gut motility, and releasing satiety hormones. Butyrate can increase the plasma levels of gastric inhibitory peptide (GIP), glucagon-like peptide 1 (GLP-1), and amylin, which consequently slows down digestion and nutrient intestinal transit and promotes satiety. Acetate seems to increase leptin released by fat cells, and propionate increases GLP-1 in the gut and controls the rates of lipolysis and lipogenesis in fat cells. Studies investigating the role of gut microbiota in obesity indicated a close relationship between dysbiosis in species producing these metabolites with unhealthy fat accumulation and obesity complications. Also, species which happen to increase in obesity are highly related to serum saturated fatty acids, monounsaturated fatty acids, and triglyceride (TG), but the ratio of acetate and polyunsaturated fatty acids to total fatty acids and the postprandial metabolism of TG in diet decline following these changes [19].

Since gut microbiota has a bidirectional relationship with the brain, the perturbation in its composition can affect the appetite-regulating pathways in the brain which results in unhealthy changes in eating behaviors. For example, LPS can cause blood–brain barrier disruption and let inflammatory cytokines enter the brain that ruins the regulatory pattern existing in satiety and hunger centers in the central nervous system. Also, gut bacteria are able to produce peptides that are similar to appetite-regulatory hormones. Then, when the body releases autoantibodies against them, they counteract the host's own hormones and disturb the functional appetite-regulatory pathways [20].

8.3.2 Nonalcoholic Fatty Liver Disease

The accumulation of triglyceride in hepatocytes causes a condition known as nonalcoholic fatty liver disease (NAFLD) which is supposed to be associated with obesity. Gut microbiota composition differs widely in patients with NAFLD and healthy controls. This gut microbiota is carried to the liver through the anatomical pathway of the portal vein and initiates the activation of immune cells in the liver—Kupffer cells—leading to the production of TNF-α and insulin resistance. This increases the accumulation of hepatic triglycerides by promoting triglyceride synthesis, hepatic uptake of free fatty acids, and peripheral lipolysis which happens in NAFLD. Gut dysbiosis and the increase in the ratio of Firmicutes/Bacteroidetes lead to a rise in endogenous ethanol production along with other metabolites like LPS which is not related to oral ethanol consumption. Ethanol concentration helps activate TLRs and ignites a cascade of inflammation and cytokine production including IL-6, IL-12, IL-1β, and TNF-α. On the other hand, gut dysbiosis itself affects intestinal integrity and increases the exposure of endotoxins which promotes the inflammation and oxidative stress caused by ethanol. Exposure of the liver to endotoxin and lipopolysaccharide causes an acute inflammatory response and leads to an early accumulation of inflammatory cells, such as monocytes, neutrophils, and lymphocytes which release proteases, other enzymes, and reactive oxygen metabolites, and the progression of liver injury. Consequently, these mechanisms may help develop steatohepatitis and activate stellate cells leading to hepatic fibrosis and cirrhosis [21].

Gut microbiota plays an important role in modulating primary bile acids to secondary bile acids through various pathways. These secondary bile acids contribute to emulsification and fat solubilization which may be disturbed following any changes in gut microbiota structure. Also, they induce the expression of FXR (farnesoid X receptor) in the ileum which regulates the enterohepatic bile acid circulation. FXR induces the expression of the small heterodimer partner (SHP) in the liver to inhibit the expression of CYP7A1 (cholesterol 7 alpha-hydroxylase) but increases the levels of circulating fibroblast growth factor 19 (FGF19) in the intestine, which decreases the expression of CYP7A1 and cytochrome P450 12a-hydroxylase B1 (CYP8B1). Altogether, this inhibits the production of bile acids which in turn leads to retained bile salts, perpetuation of gut permeability, small bowel translocation, bacterial overgrowth, and liver disease at the time of gut dysbiosis. Additionally, FXR activation reduces triglyceride levels which suppresses the synthesis and uptake of the fatty acids in the liver [12]. Secondary bile acids can help alleviate inflammatory responses as well. Peptidoglycan from Gram-positive bacteria and bacterial DNA promotes inflammatory response primarily through the activation of mitogen-activated protein kinase (MAPK)/nuclear factor kappa-B (NF-κB), and secondary bile acids inhibit NF-κB signaling and cytokine production in macrophages, mainly by activating Takeda-G-protein-receptor-5 [21].

8.3.3 *Diabetes Mellitus*

Type 1 diabetes mellitus (T1DM) is a multifactorial chronic autoimmune disease that occurs mostly in children and younger adults and is characterized by the destruction of pancreatic beta cells that are responsible for producing insulin. A significantly lower diversity of gut microbiota is detected in patients with T1DM as well as significant alteration in some bacterial species. As this diversity is negatively associated with immune-related diseases, it has been suggested to have a role in developing T1DM. Also, because of microbial dysbiosis, oxidative stress and low-grade inflammation occur which leads to pancreatic beta-cell death and a state of insulin resistance. A decrease in Firmicutes/Bacteroidetes (F/B) ratio has been reported in patients with T1DM especially children with autoantibodies. Butyrate, as a SCFA, is produced by some bacterial species in the intestine that can induce T regulatory cells to inhibit inflammatory responses by secreting anti-inflammatory cytokines like IL-10. Also, butyrate can help tighten intestinal junctions and keep the gut integrity. However, a reduction in bacterial species producing butyrate like *Clostridium* has been detected in some studies evaluating T1DM. The same inverse relationship exists between *Bifidobacterium* and T1DM. On the other hand,

Bacteroides produce acetate and propionate which, unlike butyrate, cannot increase mucin production and does not strengthen intestinal integrity. An increase in the abundance of this bacteria may result in thinning the mucus layer, increasing the gut permeability, enhancing translocation of intestinal luminal antigens leading to chronic inflammation, and consequently promoting islet-directed autoimmune responses. Also, LPS from *Bacteroides* may suppress the innate immune signaling and endotoxin tolerance and prevent the normal maturation of the immune system in early life [22].

Type 2 diabetes mellitus (T2DM) is a noncommunicable chronic disease characterized by high blood glucose level which makes the patient susceptible to further complications like kidney failure, retinopathy, neuropathy, cardiovascular diseases, and limb amputations. Studies have shown the potential association between gut microbiota and T2DM stating that a lower gut microbiota diversity and alteration in the structure of gut microbiota may be a contributing factor in developing this disease. As obesity is considered a key factor in developing this disease, an increase in F/B ratio is also expected as the possible mediating factor since Firmicutes seems to be more efficient in harvesting energy from food which has been taken. Moreover, a low-grade inflammatory state that is caused by specific LPS contributes to the insulin resistance and pathogenesis of T2DM. Gut microbiota dysbiosis is undoubtedly followed by alteration of secreted metabolites such as SCFAs which is found to affect the regulation of genes involved in insulin signaling and inflammation. *Faecalibacterium prausnitzii*, *Roseburia*, *Dialister*, and *Flavonifractor* are some of the bacterial species which produce butyrate and have been shown to decrease in T2DM leading to disturbance of intestinal barrier, energy homeostasis, glycemic responses, and inflammation [23, 24].

Hormonal changes during pregnancy can cause physiological alterations in gut microbiota including increased abundance of Actinobacteria and Proteobacteria and reduction of butyrate-producing bacteria and alpha diversity. Proteobacteria induce inflammation by exposing proinflammatory LPS, while butyrate as mentioned before has an anti-obesogenic effect, induces an anti-inflammatory response, and increases insulin sensitivity. This insulin resistance along with an increase in glucogenesis helps meet the energy necessary for the fetus which is replaced by normal status as the pregnancy comes to an end. In case of a higher increase in insulin resistance or a problem with insulin secretion, gestational diabetes mellitus (GDM) occurs which is characterized by a hyperglycemic state [25]. When assessing GDM, the trimesters in which we evaluate it, the treatments the pregnant woman takes and the diagnosis criteria used can affect the results. Nevertheless, since a significant difference in microbiota composition of GDM and non-GDM women has been detected, it raises the question of whether gut dysbiosis is associated with GDM [26]. *Collinsella* which is positively associated with insulin level and homeostatic model assessment for insulin resistance (HOMA-IR) and negatively associated with insulin sensitivity showed an increase in abundance in GDM women which seems to play a role in developing this disease. Also, some species of bacteria have shown a great relationship with glucose metabolism, and studies regarding this issue indicated significant differences in the abundance of these bacteria between GDM and non-GDM women [27]. Given the fact that Verrucomicrobia is associated with the production of short-chain fatty acids (SCFAs) involved in glucose tolerance and insulin sensitivity and reinforces the intestinal barrier by reducing its permeability, the reduction in its abundance seems to affect the metabolic homeostasis and helps develop GDM. Additionally, *Bifidobacterium* which is a beneficial acetate- and lactate-producing bacteria has been shown to diminish in abundance in the GDM group [28].

8.3.4 Hypertension

Hypertension is a prevalent cardiovascular disease that is affected by both endogenous and environmental factors and is a causative factor for many later complications. Investigations into the underlying mechanisms and predisposing factors have led to the idea that gut microbiota composition and diversity play an important role in developing the disease. Studies have found a significant difference in the gut microbiota diversity and composition of patients with and without HTN [29]. A negative association between alpha-diversity and systolic blood pressure was identified after adjusting for other variables. In other words, HTN is associated with a lower richness of the genes. Also, most of the taxonomic changes in gut microbiota belonged to Firmicutes phylum. An increased F/B ratio was seen in hypertensive patients which could be due to an increase in Firmicutes or a decrease in Bacteroidetes. HTN seems to correlate positively with *Rothia*, *Serratia*, Enterobacteriaceae, Leuconostocaceae, and *Fusobacterium*, while a negative correlation exists with *Coprococcus*, *Adlercreutzia*, *Eggerthella*, and *Ralstonia*. SCFAs regulate gut inflammation and metabolism. Thus, a shortage in the production of SCFAs by gut microbiota may act as a risk factor for developing metabolic disorders. SCFAs induce arterial vasodilation when they are attached to G-protein-coupled free fatty acid receptors that exist in renal arteries. However, a negative association has been found between BP and SCFA-producing bacteria. In addition, serum butyrate has shown an inverse relationship with HTN, and butyrate-producing bacteria—*Eubacterium rectale*—was reported to be lower compared with healthy controls [30].

Furthermore, inflammation triggered by proinflammatory LPS has a pivotal role in developing HTN as *Prevotella* and *Klebsiella* which are Gram-negative bacteria that seem to increase in abundance in patients with HTN. There are multiple studies stating that intestinal integrity is also disturbed in HTN and contributes to the inflammatory status which exists in this disease. Zonulin is a protein present in the intestinal tight junctions which can be used as a biomarker to indicate intestinal health. Changes in the soluble form of zonulin seem to correlate with developing this disease. Additionally, genes that degrade choline into trimethylamine and some bacterial genera containing these genes have shown an increase in abundance in HTN leading to the fact that trimethylamine *N*-oxide (TMAO) may affect the pathogenesis of this disease [31].

8.3.5 Dyslipidemia

Dyslipidemia is a metabolic disorder involved in multiple cardio-cerebrovascular diseases. As gut microbiota helps regulate nutritional metabolism, intestinal barrier, and immune system, its role in the pathogenesis of various diseases has been investigated. When the environment inside the intestine changes, mostly because of diet, gut microbiota faces dysbiosis, and the metabolites produced by them change as well which subsequently affects the composition of gut microbiota and aggravates the dysbiosis. Normal bacterial composition in the intestine produces cholesterol oxidase through which it helps degrade cholesterol and prevent cholesterol synthesis. High-fat diet can disturb the balance of gut microbiota leading to further disturbances in lipid metabolism, inflammatory status, intestinal integrity, and metabolite production [32]. Studies have detected a relationship of gut microbiota diversity with triglyceride (TG) and low-density lipoprotein (LDL) and high-density lipoprotein (HDL). On the other hand, modulation of gut microbiota composition is recommended for the treatment of dyslipidemia.

SCFAs play an important role in modulating lipid metabolism. Elevated acetate production by gut microbiota can increase appetite, promote glucose-mediated insulin secretion, and lead to imbalanced lipid metabolism. Propionate induces intestinal gluconeogenesis and the release of satiety hormone peptide YY (PYY) and glucagon-like peptide 1 (GLP-1) which reduces energy intake but triggers insulin secretion that stimulates fat accumulation. These SCFAs are also used as substrates for gluconeogenesis and lipogenesis in the liver. On the other hand, butyrate suppresses the activity of lipase which in turn inhibits fat accumulation and synthesis. Using fermentable fibers helps increase SCFA-producing bacteria which in turn have fat-lowering effects.

Studies demonstrate that gut microbiota plays an important role in cholesterol metabolism, hepatic cholesterol synthesis, and enterohepatic circulation mostly through bile acids. Bile acids act like mediators for metabolic homeostasis, and if primary bile acids are not converted to secondary bile acids, which normally happens using bile-salt hydrolase (BHS) enzyme from the gut microbiome, it can disturb lipid metabolism and promote intestinal inflammation by the growth of *Clostridium difficile.* Some bacterial taxa such as *Bifidobacterium, Lactobacillus acidophilus*, and *Bacteroides* produce bile hydrolytic enzyme (BSH) and regulate the FXR metabolic pathway which affects cholesterol metabolism. On the other hand, Firmicutes, *Streptococcus*, and *Bacillus aerogenes* produce steroid dehydrogenases and catalyze the production of secondary bile acids that regulate lipid metabolism in the liver and whole body. In addition, dietary phosphatidylcholine which contains a part of trimethylammonium is directly converted into trimethylamine (TMA) by gut bacteria which is metabolized in the blood to pro-atherosclerotic molecule of TMAO that interferes with reverse cholesterol transcription (RCT), regulates cholesterol balance, and affects blood lipids. Overall, SCFAs seem to play a protective role in developing dyslipidemia, while bile acids and TMAO may act as contributing factors [33].

8.3.6 Thyroid Disorders

As iodine is the fundamental material used by the thyroid gland to synthesize hormones, and it is prominently absorbed through the intestine, gut microbiota seems to play an important role in iodine metabolism. There is increasing evidence supporting the bidirectional relationship between thyroid function and gut microbiota [34]. A potential site to affect thyroid function is sodium/iodine symporter (NIS) which mediates iodine uptake. LPS increases the expression of NIS by directly stimulating thyroid cells. Also, LPS activates nuclear factor kappa-B (NF-κB) through Toll-like receptor-4 (TLR-4) which acts along with paired box 8 (Pax8) to increase NIS gene expression. On the other hand, LPS inhibits the activity of hepatic type 1 iodothyronine deiodinase and triggers type 2 of this enzyme which facilitates the conversion of thyroxine (T4) to triiodothyronine (T3). Similarly, it has been shown that butyrate may have the same impact on NIS activity. Selenium is another important micronutrient in regulating thyroid function and prevents the secretion of inflammatory cytokines at the time of thyroiditis. Several studies have reported a bidirectional relationship between selenium and gut microbiota, in which gut microbiota induces the upregulation of NIS via increased expression of Pax8, while there is a rise in selenium uptake. Also, gut microbiota can have an impact on the absorption of other micronutrients which may have a regulatory effect on the production of thyroid hormones. Gut microbiota adheres to iodothyronine, acts like a reservoir, and reduces the dose required for levothyroxine treatment. Also, these microorganisms increase the reuptake of thyroid hormones on the one hand and inhibit 5-deiodinase on the other hand leading to the regulation of iodothyronine metabolism [35].

Thyroid gland is considered an organ with a high rate of autoimmune diseases like Hashimoto's thyroiditis (HT) and Graves' disease (GD), which are characterized by the presence of thyrotropin receptor antibody (TRAb), thyroid peroxidase antibody (TPOAb), and thyroglobulin antibody (TGAb). Multiple endogenous and exogenous factors seem to affect the development of these diseases including gut microbiota. One mechanism through which gut microbiota may contribute to thyroid autoimmune diseases is the antigenic cross-reaction between substances secreted or existed in some microbial species, like thyrotropin receptor (TSHR)-like substances from *Yersinia enterocolitica* and TPO Tg-like substances by the *Bifidobacterium* and *Lactobacillus*, with thyroid normal products which can initiate inflammatory responses. Multiple studies revealed an association between gut microbiota composition and Hashimoto's disease. *Prevotella* is associated with anti-inflammatory metabolites, anti-inflammatory T regulatory cells, and reduced proinflammatory Th17 polarization but seems to decrease in abundance in these patients. *Bifidobacterium* and *Lactobacillus*, which are considered beneficial to human health, tend to decrease in number in those with hyperthyroidism although some special strains of these two bacteria have similar amino acid structures to human thyroid peroxidase (TPO) and thyroglobulin, and studies revealed a higher abundance of these strains in anti-TPO antibody-positive patients.

Due to the fact that hypothyroidism reduces gut motility, it provides suitable condition for gut microbiota to colonize and increase in abundance which in turn worsens the impairment of gut motility and promotes gastrointestinal symptoms of hypothyroidism. A distinct composition of gut microbiota is detected in patients with primary hypothyroidism. Consequently, a shortage of SCFA-producing bacteria results in intestinal barrier impairment and higher LPS exposure inducing inflammatory status [36].

8.3.7 Osteoporosis and Sarcopenia

Osteoporosis is a worldwide health challenge that affects middle-aged and older adults leading to structural fractures and lifelong morbidities. Given the fact that gut microbiota has a symbiotic relationship with the human host, disturbances in its composition and diversity can affect the balance between osteoblast and osteoclast via gut–bone axis through multiple hypothesized mechanisms including intestinal permeability, calcium transport, T-cell response, and systemic inflammation via cytokine activation [37]. A relatively lower abundance of *Blautia* has been detected in patients with osteoporosis. These bacteria have an impact on regulatory T-cells promoting the generation of T $CD8^+$ in bone marrow which increases bone mass via upregulating the expression of protein Wnt family member 10b (Wnt10b) [38]. Gram-negative genus *Bacteroides* which seems to increase in patients with osteoporosis correlates negatively with bone marrow densitometry, and it is positively associated with osteoclastogenesis activity. The rise in this genus disrupts the intestinal barrier and promotes the secretion of proinflammatory cytokines like IL-1 and TNF-α leading to immune-mediated bone loss. In addition, SCFA-producing bacteria can interfere with bone reabsorption via inducing G-protein-coupled receptors on the walls of the intestine to suppress the expression of lipopolysaccharide (LPS)-induced cytokines like TNF-α and gamma interferon (IFN-γ), increase the expression of IL-4 and IL-10, induce regulatory T-cell activation in the colon, reduce the production of inflammatory cytokines like NF-κB, and alleviate intestinal inflammation, consequently. Also, butyrate increases the expression of intracellular calcium transporters which drives an increase in intracellular calcium absorption and limits the production of parathyroid hormone reducing bone resorption. *Alistipes*, which is a SCFA-producing bacteria and helps keep the intestinal barrier, tends to decrease in these patients. These changes facilitate the growth of some opportunistic species which pave the way for further bone loss [39].

Sarcopenia is defined as a progressive loss of muscle mass which affects the physical performance of the elderly and makes them susceptible to falls, fractures, and other physical complications. As aging is associated with gut dysbiosis and sarcopenia affects mostly older adults, the question about the causal effect of gut microbiota in sarcopenia has risen. Studies have demonstrated the role of inflammation in the pathogenesis of sarcopenia [40]. On the other hand, aging is accompanied by changes in gut microbiota toward such composition which disturbs intestinal integrity, promotes inflammatory status, and increases circulating proinflammatory cytokines. Additionally, products secreted by microorganisms exert potential positive or negative effects on the host. For example, serum microbiota-derived indoxyl sulfate is positively associated with the expression of myostatin and atrogin-1 which are negative regulators of skeletal muscle mass. Also, the role of gut microbiota in the absorption of macronutrients like amino acids is another mechanism by which gut microbiota can affect muscle metabolism. Microorganisms can increase amino acid bioavailability, modify insulin secretion, and promote the responsiveness of muscles leading to facilitating protein and muscle mass production [41].

8.3.8 Cancers

As cancers have remained a serious health challenge around the world, investigation regarding the factors that may aggravate or alleviate the process of carcinogenesis is still a hot topic of research. An increasing number of studies have revealed the inevitable association between microbiota and diseases including cancers. Inflammation seems to promote DNA damage of the epithelial cells leading to inflammatory-associated cancers and facilitate their invasion and metastasis. Inflammatory cytokines like IL1, IL6, IL10, and TNF-α activate NF-κB, inhibit apoptosis, and induce an oxidative stress state. Also, these inflammatory factors suppress tumor suppressor genes like P53 and activate oncogenes like Kirsten RAS. Gut dysbiosis can affect innate and adaptive immune responses and cause an inflammatory condition which plays a role in carcinogenesis. Metabolites produced by microorganisms can either promote or inhibit inflammation. For example, lipoteichoic acid binds to Toll-like receptor 2 (TLR2) and stimulates the secretion of proinflammatory cytokines, whereas short-chain fatty acids (SCFAs) help regulate the immune response by activating regulatory T cells [42].

8.3.8.1 Gastrointestinal Cancers

Gastric cancer is a typical example of an inflammation-associated cancer in which *Helicobacter pylori* is considered a risk factor, and elevated levels of inflammatory cytokines have been found in infected individuals compared to healthy controls. Furthermore, several studies have reported significant differences in some species related to esophageal cancers. Gram-negative bacteria such as Bacteroidetes, Proteobacteria, Fusobacteria, and Spirochaetes were associated with esophagitis and Barrett's esophagus. LPS from these bacteria can promote inflammation through multiple pathways increasing the risk of carcinogenesis. Regarding colorectal cancers, higher proportions of *Faecalibacterium prausnitzii*, *Eubacterium rectale*, and

Eubacterium eligens were observed in the control group, while higher proportions of *Prevotella copri*, *Ruminococcus torques*, and *Bacteroides vulgatus* were observed in the case group. Also, studies revealed a pathologic role of *Parabacteroides* although they are rare and research on the potential mechanisms is not sufficient. A higher abundance of genus *Anaerotruncus* results in increased tumor-associated metabolites such as *S*-adenosylmethionine (SAM) and *S*-adenosyl-homocysteine (SAH) by influencing steroid, terpene, and bile acid biosynthesis along with increased level of LPS. It has been reported that significantly higher levels of SAM exist in the tumor tissues of these patients compared to normal tissues. Enterotoxigenic *Bacteroides fragilis* (ETBF) which is a Gram-negative anaerobic bacterium has been found to have a close association with colorectal cancer. It can produce a specific toxin, which can promote the activation of Wnt and NF-KB signaling pathways, facilitating cell proliferation and DNA damage, when bound to intestinal mucosal epithelial receptors leading to abnormal cell transformation. It also promotes the release of reactive oxygen species from inflammatory cells and increases the expression of cytokines and chemokines, leading to DNA damage which in turn promotes the development of colorectal cancers [43]. On the other hand, butyrate as a SCFA is utilized by the mitochondria in colonocytes and helps to maintain a healthy energy balance and benefit colonic epithelial cell proliferation. GPR109a, as a receptor of SCFAs, is expressed on immune cells and activates the ligands of BA, and then it inhibits inflammatory cytokines and suppresses the process of inflammation. The host immune response fights back DNA methylation-mediated GPR109a silencing through IFN-γ and encourages anticarcinogenic effects accordingly.

8.3.8.2 Liver Cancers

As liver is highly related to microorganisms and metabolites in the gastrointestinal tract via gut–liver axis and portal vein, gut dysbiosis undoubtedly contributes to the pathogenesis of liver cancers. Gut dysbiosis and intestinal barrier disturbances can be seen from the early stages of chronic liver disease. Leaky gut makes contribution to hepatocellular carcinogenesis through elevated LPS exposure and inflammatory responses. Higher abundance of *E. coli* in the feces of patients with hepatocellular carcinoma compared to healthy controls and a higher population of Dietziaceae, Pseudomonadaceae, and Oxalobacteraceae in the bile duct samples of patients with cholangiocarcinoma than samples from healthy individuals have been detected in several studies. Also, LPS from *H. pylori* increases the levels of IL-8 and TGF-β and can directly promote the growth and migration of liver cancer. Moreover, considering the enterohepatic circulation of bile acids, decreased quantities of bile acids cause uncontrolled growth of gut microbiota which accelerates inflammation, and the enterohepatic circulation of deoxycholic acid produced by *Clostridium* causes DNA damage that promotes cancer [44].

8.3.8.3 Pancreas Cancers

Pancreas can be affected by gut microbiota through portal vein or mesenteric lymph nodes, so their contribution to the pathogenesis of pancreas cancers is undeniable. *H. pylori* has been shown to be an important risk factor in pancreatitis as well as pancreas cancers. These bacteria produce ammonia and LPS and activate inflammatory pathways leading to higher level of inflammatory cytokines. LPS from *H. pylori* stimulates mutations of KRAS genes, which perform an essential role in normal tissue signaling and initiate the process of pancreatic carcinogenesis. In addition, persistent activation of signal transducer and activator of transcription 3 (STAT3), which exerts a significant impact on transforming epithelial cells by *H. pylori* infections, can promote pancreatic cancer progression by upregulating the expression of antiapoptotic and pro-proliferative proteins. Additionally, pancreas cancers have shown a great association with oral microbiome such as *Fusobacterium* spp. and *Porphyromonas gingivalis*. As chronic pancreatitis is an important risk factor for pancreas cancer, it is worth mentioning that infection with *Enterococcus faecalis* is involved in chronic pancreatitis and may result in the development of cancer since lipoteichoic acid is a surface component of Gram-positive bacteria and triggers the oversecretion of proinflammatory factors by binding to CD14 or TLR2. Also, deoxycholic acid, which is produced by 7α-dehydroxylating bacteria and secondary bile acids, promotes the induction of pancreas cancers through increasing DNA damage [45].

8.3.8.4 Thyroid Cancers

Myriads of studies revealed the role of gut microbiota and dysbiosis in thyroid diseases. They affect the secretion of thyroid-stimulating hormone and create chronic inflammation in the thyroid gland through their metabolites leading to thyroid disorders. Changes in gut microbiota can cause chronic inflammation and inflammatory cytokines in other organs as well as local symptoms and induce DNA damage through secreted toxins. Also, they can induce CD8(+) T-cells and promote chronic inflammation and early T-cell failure, consequently reducing antitumor immunity. The fact that gut microbiota composition differs significantly between patients with thyroid cancers and healthy controls raised the question of whether microbiota plays a role in developing this disease other than gastrointestinal cancers. An increase in the abundance of Firmicutes and Proteobacteria and a decrease in Bacteroidetes can be detected in these patients, which also differs along with the stage of disease. Considering that some types of thyroid cancers are more common in areas of high iodine uptake, gut microbiota, which regulates the absorption of micronutrients, can influence in developing this disease as there seems to be an association between selenium and thyroid cancer prevalence, as well. In addition, metabolites secreted by these microorganisms showed to have an important role through butyrate and pyruvate metabolism and disturbances in amino acid degradation. Gut microbiota of patients with thyroid cancer showed a reduced abundance of

SCFA-producing bacteria like Lachnospiraceae and *Butyricimonas*, which is thought to have a regulatory effect on the immune microenvironment and lead to increased cell death and cell renewal, causing a higher risk of malignancies [36]. On the other hand, it has been found that the microorganisms that exist in the thyroid tissue are different from normal non-tumoral tissue. A significant increase in the abundances of Sphingomonas and Aeromonas in tumor tissues, along with a marked rise in Comamonas, Acinetobacter, and Peptostreptococcus in peritumoral tissues, correlates with the expression of inflammatory genes and is associated with higher mutation rates [46]. Relative abundance of Clostridiaceae, *Neisseria*, and *Streptococcus* is significantly higher in thyroid disease, while, in thyroid nodules, *Streptococcus* and *Neisseria* relatively increased in comparison to healthy control groups in one study. Clostridiaceae apparently have carcinogenic effects, *Streptococcus* leads to a higher risk of adenomas and carcinomas, and *Neisseria* has been linked to inflammatory disorders and pancreatic disease [47].

8.4 Microbiota as Biomarkers in Diagnosis and Prediction

Microbiota develops a symbiotic relationship with the host. Evidence has shown their significant changes in composition at the time of a disease, or even changes that happen during one's normal life such as aging and pregnancy. Metabolites produced by these microorganisms are considered a functional arm to perform their role, and alteration in the amount of these chemicals seems to be involved in health disturbances through multiple mechanisms, as well. Given the fact that microbiota is undoubtedly associated with our health, recent studies have focused on whether we can utilize their changes as a tool for early diagnosis of diseases or consider them a biomarker in different health conditions. Myriads of studies have evaluated the Firmicutes/Bacteroidetes ratio in patients with metabolic disorders such as obesity, type 2 diabetes, and cardiovascular diseases. An increase in this ratio typically reflects a higher abundance of Firmicutes relative to Bacteroidetes, while normalization of this ratio often occurs during calorierestricting diets through an increase in Bacteroidetes abundance. Controversies in the results of different studies are mainly due to interpretation biases, and if these were eliminated, the Firmicutes/Bacteroidetes ratio could serve as a reliable hallmark for these diseases [48].

Higher abundances of *Proteus* and *Enterobacter* bacteria and lower abundance of *Ruminococcus* and *Lactobacillus* were remarkably associated with NAFLD along with fecal bile acid composition. As simple steatosis progresses to advanced liver fibrosis, the number of Gram-negative bacteria, especially *Proteus* bacteria, increases. Machine learning models relating microbiota structure to this disease resulted in highly accurate perspectives in using these microorganisms as screening markers [49]. *Prevotella* and *Helicobacter* species have been shown to be significantly different between mouse models of Alzheimer's disease and healthy controls, but Actinobacteria and TM7 phylum seem to be more accurate in diagnosing this disease. Also, significant shifts in the abundance of the families Proteobacteriaceae,

Verrucomicrobiaceae, Bifidobacteriaceae, Erysipelotrichaceae, Prevotellaceae, Bacteroidaceae, and Rikenellaceae could be detected far before any plaque deposition in the brain which suggests a great potentiality for early diagnosis. Changes in microbiota-derived metabolites like TMAO and SCFAs have been evaluated in this disease but are still limited and require later investigations [50]. In addition, studies have discovered a new lipodipeptide derived from gut microbiota called Lipid 654, which acts as a TLR-2 ligand regulating immune responses. Accompanied by changes in the composition of gut microbiota, Lipid 654 is detected significantly less in the serum of patients with multiple sclerosis and can be used as a biomarker for this disease [51].

Some metabolites secreted from *Enterococcus faecalis*, enterotoxin *Bacteroides fragilis*, or *F. nucleatum* bacteria are capable of damaging DNA, and it has been reported that they can induce the proliferation of colon cells in studies of gut microbiota in cancer patients. Also, antibiotic therapy or the absence of the gut microbiota reduces the incidence of tumors in several animal models. Fusobacteria exists in cancerous tissue much more than normal colon tissue, and most of the time it does not exist in a normal colon environment as a normal flora. This bacterium enhances the expression of inflammatory markers and modulates immune responses through several virulence factors leading to increasing expression of oncogenes. *Fusobacterium* species is considered a risk factor in the onset and progression of colorectal cancers, and it is used as a biomarker for this disease [52].

8.5 Role of Microbiota in Disease Treatment (Microbiota Medicine)

According to what has been mentioned since now, changes in the composition of gut microbiota can cause disturbances in the metabolism and immune system of an individual leading to developing or aggravating a disease as numerous studies revealed the association between gut microbiota and different diseases. So, modification of gut microbiota seems to be a potential strategy to reverse the balance and regulate its composition since normal composition keeps the intestinal integrity and protects against opportunistic pathogens (Fig. 8.2).

8.5.1 Prebiotics

Prebiotics are nondigestible dietary substances which are selectively used within the small intestine by host microbiota. They can be derived from natural sources like peas, beans, cow's milk, human breast milk, soybean, rye, tomato, barley, wheat, honey, banana, onion, chicory, garlic, sugar beet, asparagus, and artichoke and are mostly subsets of carbohydrate groups especially oligosaccharide carbohydrates

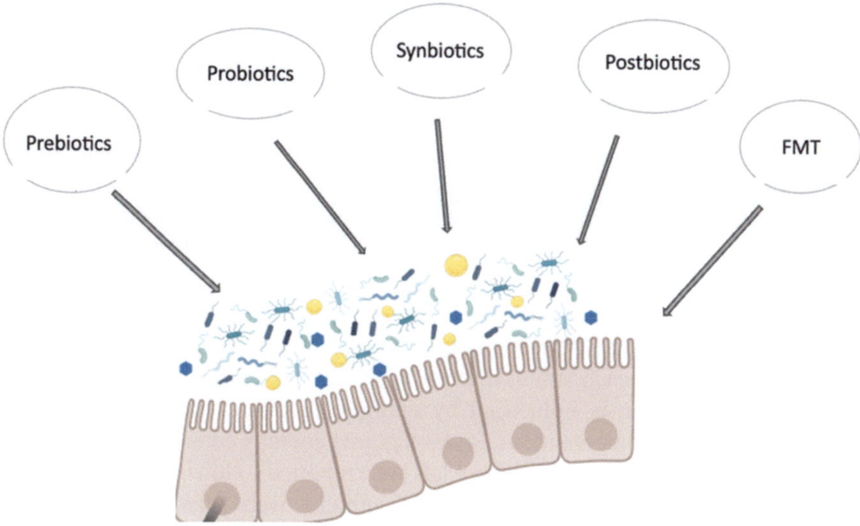

Fig. 8.2 Modulatory approaches to alter gut microbiota composition and improve dysbiosis. *FMT* fecal microbiota transplantation

including fructans like inulin and fructo-oligosaccharides, galacto-oligosaccharides, starch, and glucose-derived oligosaccharides like resistant starch and polydextrose, other oligosaccharides like pectic-oligosaccharide, and noncarbohydrate oligosaccharides like cocoa-derived flavanols. Gut microbiota ferments prebiotics and secrets useful metabolites which facilitate their functions. Also, they provide a lower pH in the gastrointestinal environment leading to an increase in the amount of butyrate and a decrease in the number of acid-sensitive species [53]. Polyphenols as prebiotics are derived from plants, fruits, and nuts and are able to increase microbiota diversity and improve the relevant abundance of some genera including *Akkermansia*, *Bacteroides*, *Blautia*, and *Roseburia. Blautia* as a butyric-producing genus which inversely associated with visceral adiposity can be improved with grape seed proanthocyanidin extract, resveratrol, Rutgers scarlet lettuce, green tea, oolong tea and black tea, rapeseed oil with sinapine, and tea polyphenols. *Roseburia*, another butyrate-producing genus which is decreased in T2DM, is improved with grape seed proanthocyanidin extract, a combination of resveratrol and sinapic acid, Rutgers scarlet lettuce, grape seed extract, tea polyphenols, and grape pomace extract [54]. Polyphenols also seem to increase brain-derived neurotrophic factors and improve cognitive function including memory and planning and reduce mental fatigue [55]. In addition, curcumin, a polyphenol derived from the ginger family, has been shown to have significant effects on inflammatory cytokines and oxidative stress markers as it improves TNF-α, C-reactive protein, and malondialdehyde and significantly affects body composition indices, serum lipid, and glucose factors in patients with metabolic syndrome [56].

8.5.2 Probiotics

Probiotics are live microorganisms that seem to have health benefits when they are used in sufficient doses. *Lactobacillus*, *Bifidobacterium*, *Saccharomyces*, *Streptococcus*, *Enterococcus*, *Escherichia*, and *Bacillus* are the organisms found commonly in these products, which affect the gut microbiota composition modifying inflammatory state and food absorption. They affect the host via TLRs and nucleotide-binding oligomerization domain-containing protein-like receptors and modulate important key signaling pathways, such as nuclear factor-κB and mitogen-activated protein kinase, to enhance or suppress immunity pathways. This effect is dependent on the dosage, frequency of consumption, sole or multi-strain product and the proportion of each strain, severity of the disease, and so on. Although the dose of administration is influenced by multiple factors, it ranges from 10^8 to 10^{11} CFU/day in most interventions. Probiotics are generally considered as harmless interventions, and no serious side effect has been reported following these products; however, mild to moderate gastrointestinal symptoms were seen. *Bifidobacterium* and *Lactobacillus* strains have been commonly evaluated for their effects on cognitive function and indicated a significant influence on cognition possibly through improvement in inflammatory and oxidative stress status [57]. The majority of probiotic strains used in obesity are from the genera *Lactobacillus* and *Bifidobacterium*, and high doses of common single- and multispecies of these bacteria can at least affect one or several key clinical and anthropometric variables [58]. Utilizing probiotics in patients with T2DM showed a significant effect as they can reduce fasting blood glucose, HbA1C, and insulin resistance following the intervention. This effect is associated with changes in gut microbiota leading to secretion of useful SCFA and lower LPS in blood. *L. plantarum* A7, *L. acidophilus* La-5, and *B. animalis* subsp. *lactis* BB-12 administration in patients with T2DM showed a significant effect on antioxidant status, inflammatory responses, and glucose markers. In addition, supplementation with *L. gasseri* SBT2055 in obese adults resulted in a reduction in BMI, waist circumference, abdominal visceral fat area, and hip circumference. It has been indicated that probiotic-enriched cheese containing *Lactobacillus plantarum* reduced the BMI in Russian adults with obesity and hypertension. Furthermore, treatment with *L. bulgaricus* and *S. thermophilus* revealed a decrease in alanine aminotransferase (ALT), aspartate aminotransferase (ASP), and γ-GTP levels as indicators of improving liver function, so supplementation with probiotic yogurt containing *L. acidophilus* La5 and *B. lactis* Bb12 in patients with nonalcoholic fatty liver disease resulted in a reduction in the serum levels of ALT, ASP, total cholesterol, and low-density lipoprotein compared with the control group [59]. Also, studies revealed the beneficial role of probiotics in alleviating predisposing factors and management of colorectal cancers. Using probiotic bacteria from *Lactobacillus* and *Bifidobacterium* species increases the abundance of beneficial bacteria such as *Lactobacillus, Eubacterium, Peptostreptococcus, Bacillus*, and *Bifidobacterium* and decreases the abundance of potentially harmful bacteria such as *Fusobacterium, Porphyromonas, Pseudomonas*, and *Enterococcus* leading to promoting intestinal permeability, tight junction function, and suppressing inflammatory disturbances in these patients which could influence the postoperative outcomes as well as the treatment of this disease [60].

Thanks to gene sequencing methods, beneficial bacterial strains can be identified, extracted, and used in sufficient dosage without being concerned about their culture difficulties and safety. Some species including *Akkermansia muciniphila, Faecalibacterium prausnitzii, Bacteroides fragilis, Eubacterium hallii*, and *Roseburia* spp. have shown great potential in this regard for disease intervention and treatment. The probiotics manufactured in this way are called next-generation probiotics (NGPs). As microbiota composition is different from one person to the other, and it is difficult to understand the unique interaction between microbiota and the host individually, it seems rational that the same probiotic does not have the same effects in different patients. Thus, personalized treatment based on identifying involved strains, developing pure cultures in vitro, and administering NGPs after successful clinical trials is an attractive issue that has been taken into account in recent research studies [61].

8.5.3 Synbiotics

Synbiotics are a combination of live microorganisms and prebiotics with the aim of achieving more benefits than each of them alone. It is intended that the prebiotic part enhance the probiotic growth and colonization. Live microorganisms use oligosaccharides, the prebiotic part, as a major nutrient source and also ferment them to produce short-chain fatty acids that prevent opportunistic bacteria growth, modulate intestinal epithelial integrity, and improve barrier function. Synbiotics composed of common probiotic strains (*Lactobacillus* and *Bifidobacterium*) seem to alleviate abdominal pain, urgency, and flatulence in patients with irritable bowel syndrome [62]. Also, synbiotics containing *Lactobacilli* or *Bifidobacteria* (or both) combined with fructo-oligosaccharides (FOS) and galacto-oligosaccharides (GOS) or inulin seem to reduce the occurrence of necrotizing enterocolitis in preterm infants as the prebiotic part induces the growth of non-pathogen probiotic part leading to restored balance in gut microbiota and improved intestinal integrity [63]. Moreover, synbiotics reduce C-reactive protein, TNF-α, and IL-6; increase GSH, NO, and total antioxidant capacity; and decrease MDA in patients with prediabetes and T2DM which suggest its beneficial role in modulating cardiometabolic risk factors in these patients [64].

8.5.4 Postbiotics

Rare reports of probiotics-related infections, inflammatory responses, bacterial translocation to unwanted tissues, the possibility of developing antibiotic resistance and transferring its genes to gut microorganisms, and limitations to the use of probiotics in immunosuppressed patients have encouraged scientists to utilize postbiotics instead of live microorganisms. Postbiotics, also called paraprobiotics or ghost probiotics, are killed or inactivated microorganisms, cell-free supernatants, and bioactive compounds produced during a fermentation process including microbial cell constituents like capsule, bacterial carbohydrates (lipopolysaccharides), bacterial nucleic acids (DNA or RNA), bacterial peptides (flagellin), lipoproteins, lipoteichoic acids, peptidoglycans, S-layer proteins, and metabolites like vitamins, organic acids, short-chain fatty acids, secreted proteins/peptides, bacteriocins, neurotransmitters, secreted biosurfactants, amino acids, flavonoid-derived postbiotics, and so on that seem to maintain the beneficial characteristics of a live microorganism and confer health benefits when administered in sufficient dose. They stimulate the host immune system through the interaction between TLRs and nucleotide-binding oligomerization domain-like receptors (NLR) with bacterial components and contribute to the activation of immunity cells leading to regulating inflammatory responses. Heat-killed *L. paracasei* seems to reduce the episodes of diarrhea and prevent respiratory tract infections in children younger than 5 years old [65].

Although recent studies address the effects of postbiotics more than before, the number of published articles particularly systematic reviews and meta-analyses is not enough; however, there are several original papers in this regard. Heat-killed probiotics are able to fight against diarrheal and food-borne pathogens because of their ability to compete for adhesion sites on gut enterocytes. Several heat-killed strains of *Lactobacillus* have demonstrated the ability to suppress the inflammatory markers like IL-6 and TNF-α, enhance anti-inflammatory cytokines like IL-10, and scavenge the free radicals at in vitro and in vivo experimental models. Exopolysaccharides (EPS) are extracellular biopolymers synthesized or secreted by microorganisms during their growth. The EPS of lactic acid bacteria has been shown to contribute to some anti-oxidative (ability to scavenge a wide range of free radicals), cholesterol-lowering (ability to bind free cholesterol), immunomodulatory, and antiaging functions, gut microbiota modulation, antitoxic effect, anti-biofilm effect, and antitumor effects [66]. The cell surface proteins of bacteria including S-layer protein contribute to adhesion and further interaction with the host as the surface proteins of *L. rhamnosus* GG have been reported to alleviate the inflammatory cytokines and TLR activation at mRNA level and attenuate lipopolysaccharide (LPS)-induced signaling pathways. Teichoic acids are glycopolymers that exist in the cell walls of Gram-positive bacteria including lipoteichoic acid (LTA) and wall teichoic acid (WTA). LTA is a microbe-associated molecular pattern (MAMP) recognized by pattern recognition receptor (TLR-2) on the surface of gut enterocytes and induces inflammatory cytokine response. On the contrary, the administration of LTA extracted from *L. paracasei* D3-5 strain ameliorates the high-fat diet-induced metabolic dysfunctions, maintains intestinal integrity, decreases inflammation, and improves physical and cognitive functions in mice models. The LTA from *L. delbrueckii*, *L. sakei*, and *L. rhamnosus* GG suppressed the viral double-stranded RNA-induced proinflammatory cytokine (IL-8) in the intestinal epithelial cell line [67]. The peptidoglycan extracted from probiotic bacteria demonstrated in vitro and in vivo anticancer effects and anti-inflammatory effects as peptidoglycan from *L. rhamnosus* CRL1505 significantly improved lung $CD3^{+}CD4^{+}IFN\text{-}\gamma^{+}$ and $CD3^{+}CD4^{+}IL\text{-}10^{+}$ T-cells as well as $CD11c^{+}SiglecF^{+}IFN\text{-}\beta^{+}$ alveolar macrophages with the consequent increases of IFN-γ, IL-10, and IFN-β in the respiratory tract [68]. Cell-free supernatant of *L. rhamnosus* GG modulated anti-inflammatory cytokines such as interleukin (IL)-4, IL-5, and IL-10, and the cell-free supernatant of *L. acidophilus*, *L. casei*, *L. lactis*, *L. reuteri*, and *Saccharomyces boulardii* appeared to demonstrate anti-oxidative effects. Also, the cell-free soluble factors of some bacteria show antipathogenic effects and protective effects such as *E. coli* Nissle 1917 against enteropathogenic *E. coli* preventing intestinal epithelial barrier disturbance by triggering the expression of tight junction (ZO-1, claudin-14, and claudin-2) gene expression [69]. Bacteriocins are antimicrobial peptides produced by both Gram-positive bacteria and Gram-negative bacteria that inhibit closely related species such as *L. lactis* subsp. *lactis* bacteriocin that has been found to have inhibitory actions against food-borne enteropathogens including *Clostridium difficile.* In addition, bacteriocins can be used in the clinical sector to prevent opportunistic bacterial infections [68].

Prebiotics are selectively fermented by probiotic bacteria in the gut to produce various products including short-chain fatty acids (SCFAs), primarily acetate, propionate, and butyrate through which they can perform some of their functions. Supplementation with a mix of acetate, propionate, and butyrate was found effective against the growth of gastrointestinal pathogens like *Clostridium difficile* (involved in antibiotic-associated diarrhea) and *E. coli.* On the other hand, humans are incapable of biosynthesizing most of the vitamins, and therefore they subsequently have to be supplemented exogenously. The use of microorganisms is an economically viable alternative to reach an adequate amount of vitamins, particularly vitamin B12 utilized through a whey-based liquid medium from *Propionibacterium freudenreichii* 2067, than fortification with chemically synthesized pseudo-vitamins. Also, supplementation with *B. animalis* subsp. *lactis* HNO19 (DR10™) in pregnant women resulted in a significant increase in vitamin B6 and vitamin B12 in the second and third trimesters [68].

Extracellular vesicles (EVs) are defined as nano-vesicles which may contain signaling molecules such as DNA, RNA, microRNA, proteins, peptidoglycan, and lipids secreted by live cellular organisms such as gut bacteria which help them modulate their function in the intestinal environment. EVs like those of *Bifidobacterium longum* can carry adhesion factors that promote intestinal bacterial colonization, and polysaccharide-degrading enzymes like EVs of *Bacteroides thetaiotaomicron* and *Bacteroides fragilis* break down complex polysaccharides and provide a source of nutrition for the intestinal bacteria. EVs secreted by mesenchymal stromal cells of patients with myelodysplastic syndrome contain microRNAs in different proportions compared to normal human which can alter the hematopoietic stem cells' fate leading to the development of the disease [70]. Also, these EVs may reduce the host's innate immune response, as *V. cholerae* does, and reduce the expression of inflammatory cytokines in order to colonize the intestine. Studies have shown the role of EVs in intestinal barrier disruption, immune disturbance, and developing the disease consequently. Since these structures contain information from the releasing bacteria, detecting them can help investigate changes in microbiota composition and metabolites of the patient. For example, a significant increase in the abundance of EVs secreted by Firmicutes phyla, such as *Eubacterium, Faecalibacterium*, those of the Ruminococcaceae family, and *Catenibacterium*, was found in the fecal samples of patients with colon cancer. On the other hand, EVs can be utilized for therapeutic purposes to promote probiotic growth or prevent pathogen colonization. Their influence on the immune system makes them a perfect target for vaccine production, and they can stimulate the immune system to defend against tumor cells as *S. typhimurium* EVs can induce the maturation of human monocyte-derived dendritic cells (DCs) and $CD11c^+$ splenic DCs, which in turn activate $CD8^+$T-cell responses that is a key factor in treating viruses and tumors. In addition, these vesicles can be modified in order to perform the desired role for therapeutical purposes as EVs containing LPS are co-incubated with a lysosome in order to reduce its toxicity, or they can be combined with drugs and enhance their therapeutic effect considering EV characteristics [71].

8.5.5 *Fecal Microbiota Transplantation (FMT)*

FMT refers to the transfer of intestinal microbiota from a healthy donor after screening for pathogens to a recipient through oral capsule, endoscopic approaches like oral or nasal tubes, colonoscopy, or enema. Thus, beneficial microorganisms colonize the intestine and produce useful metabolites in order to restore immunity balance and intestinal integrity and help overcome dysbiosis-related diseases. Potential factors that may affect the efficacy of FMT include modality of FMT delivery, fresh or frozen stool FMT, single or mixed donor sample, and FMT dosage. Despite multiple challenges in finding and screening suitable donors and recipients, FMT is now being utilized in the treatment process of a variety of diseases affecting infections, gut diseases, gut–liver axis, gut–brain axis, metabolic diseases, oncology, hematological diseases, and other diseases [72]. The *Clostridioides difficile* infection, urinary tract infections, and antibody-associated diarrhea indicated a significant decrease following FMT. Patients with inflammatory bowel disease, irritable bowel syndrome, and constipation also have been shown to benefit from this procedure. FMT in patients with NAFLD seems to improve inflammatory genes and lipid metabolism similar to what could be detected in patients with cirrhosis. In addition, this treatment has been reported to improve autism symptoms as well as psychiatric and other neurological disorders. The BMI of obese patients reduced, and the necessary dose of insulin in patients with T2DM decreased following FMT. Severe adverse events including infection are not seen commonly, but frequent adverse events include mild gastrointestinal symptoms which occur in a very few percent of patients [73]. Studies also revealed the role of FMT in Alzheimer's disease as it restores beneficial microorganisms and enhances the level of useful SCFAs which in turn influence brain function, strengthen blood–brain barrier, and inhibit the secretion of proinflammatory cytokines [74].

8.6 Precision Medicine and Omics Studies

Considering the fact that each patient is different from others in terms of demographic characteristics, family history, genomic background, and so on, individualized medicine has developed in order to enhance the efficacy of the medical processes taking patient profile into account. As microbiota play numerous metabolic functions and have an inevitable association with health, data regarding microorganisms colonizing our body should be introduced into precision medicine other than the host's characteristics. The next-generation sequencing and other high-throughput methods which are ways to analyze the microbial composition and function in a specific site of the body should be considered in this regard. Thus, the association between microbiota and diseases can be tracked from functions encoded by microorganisms, and the information can be used to supplement the individual with the proper probiotic, gene product, or metabolites to restore health [75]. Despite the profound influence these methods have in medical sciences, there are still challenges to overcome. One is the understanding of the association between microbiota dysbiosis and disease across the population as most of the times not only one bacterial strain but multiple strains are involved in developing a disease. The same treatment of the same disease in different patients may result in different outcomes as it is affected by different bacterial taxa and related to host–microbiota interaction. In addition, as microbiota is involved in the metabolism of drugs, their profile may help in making decisions about prescribing a drug, or continuing its prescription. Of course omics studies including genomics, epigenomics, transcriptomics, proteomics, microbiomics, and metabolomics should be considered as well as host phenotypic characteristics and other information so that scientists are able to identify biomarkers, stratify patients, and assign the best treatment to each group in order to achieve the highest efficiency [76].

Genomic studies the organisms' whole genome which could be the host or the microorganisms living in the body. Thus, it is possible to determine the genetic biomarkers of different diseases and the association between microbiota dysbiosis and these diseases using data from microbiota profiling as *Bacteroides* are found to be associated with nonalcoholic steatohepatitis and *Ruminococcus* with fibrosis in NAFLD. In addition, genetic characteristics of a host along with microbiota composition are engaged in treatment outcomes and help draw a map for individualized medicine which gives rise to the concept of pharmacogenomics. Genetic variants lead to coding different proteins that are involved in absorption and metabolism of drugs and result in different treatment responses. Since the presence of a gene does not necessarily mean that it is being expressed, transcriptomic, epigenomic, and proteomic studies developed to focus on factors influencing the expression of genes which can affect the host's susceptibility to a disease even more than the genetic background. Genomic studies may identify potential species involved in a specific disease, while proteomics and transcriptomics do not match the results which emphasizes the importance of measuring the functional capacity [77].

Proteomics relates to studying the whole proteins of an organism, so it would be possible to establish an association between the protein profile secreted by the host or microorganisms and diseases. Studies revealed significant differences in 12 protein peaks produced by gut microbiota in patients with NAFLD compared with obese patients without NAFLD. Also, protein profile has entered the pharmacology area, pharmacoproteomics that may affect every stage of treatment effectiveness. Metabolomics evaluates the metabolites of humans, animals, and microorganisms to search for changes and biomarkers related to a disease. Changes in metabolite profiles like bile acids can predict the risk of T2DM years before the onset of the disease. Also, branch-chained amino acids seem to upregulate in these patients more than normal controls and can be considered a biomarker for this disease. As gut microbiota is associated with NAFLD, metabolomic studies revealed the association between metabolites and this disease as well. Primary/secondary bile acid ratio is higher in NAFLD patients, and bile acid metabolism faces disturbances since deoxycholic acid which is an antagonist of FXR, a key factor in bile acid metabolism, increases in these patients. Given the fact that multiple pathways are disturbed in metabolic syndrome, metabolite changes are undoubtable. Utilizing data from metabolomics, TMAO from gut microbiota seems to be associated with BMI, visceral adiposity, insulin resistance, and developing metabolic syndrome, and branch-chained amino acids are also involved in this disease.

Another important side of introducing microbiota in precision medicine is to develop methods to alter microbiota with the aim of benefiting the host without destroying beneficial species. Considering the role of microbiota and their metabolites in metabolic diseases and treatment outcomes, editing microbiota composition or administration of drugs restoring the metabolic pathways influenced by these microorganisms and their metabolites is beneficial. Patients who are undergoing treatment for disorders like cancers may have their microbiota profiled to assess their inflammatory status, so that they can receive microbiota-editing treatment prior to radiotherapy. On the other hand, drugs can modulate gut microbiome and affect further mechanisms performed by them, as antibiotics change the composition and proportion of gut microorganisms. New potential targets in the microbiome are being identified, and new methods to selectively manipulate them such as NGPs are now being evaluated to be able to be administered in ex vivo and in vivo models [1].

Omics studies are important in understanding the role of microorganisms in the prediction, pathogenesis, diagnosis, and treatment of diseases. For example, treatment outcome is highly influenced by the host's initial microbiota composition, and omics studies help predict and enhance the efficacy of the prescribed drugs. Patients with T2DM can be stratified into two groups based on microbiota profile, one dominated by *Prevotella* and the other by *Bacteroides*, and each group is more responsive to a particular treatment strategy. Also, specific antitumor treatments are effective in patients whose intestine is colonized with certain immune-regulating bacterial species like *Akkermansia muciniphila*. Consequently, multi-omics studies combining different omics studies provide the opportunity to optimize various aspects of medical care as utilizing genomic and metabolomic information along with clinical characteristics [78].

In summary, microorganisms in different organs create a complex network through which they communicate with each other and influence the function of human body. Also, changes in their composition and metabolites produced by them are associated with disturbances in endocrine system. Therefore, identifying their characteristics can help prevent, diagnose, and treat disorders being affected by them. As this system is unique to every individual, this approach could be a great step toward personalized medicine.

References

1. Zhang X, Li L, Butcher J, Stintzi A, Figeys D. Advancing functional and translational microbiome research using meta-omics approaches. Microbiome. 2019;7(1):154.
2. Singh RK, Chang HW, Yan D, Lee KM, Ucmak D, Wong K, et al. Influence of diet on the gut microbiome and implications for human health. J Transl Med. 2017;15:73.
3. Microbiota medicine: towards clinical revolution. [cited 2023 Sep 4]. Available from: https://pubmed.ncbi.nlm.nih.gov/35255932/
4. Woodall CA, McGeoch LJ, Hay AD, Hammond A. Respiratory tract infections and gut microbiome modifications: a systematic review. PLoS One. 2022;17(1):e0262057.
5. Benhadou F, Mintoff D, Schnebert B, Thio HB. Psoriasis and microbiota: a systematic review. Diseases. 2018;6(2):47.
6. Daou H, Paradiso M, Hennessy K, Seminario-Vidal L. Rosacea and the microbiome: a systematic review. Dermatol Ther. 2020;11(1):1–12.
7. Is There Any Link between Cognitive Impairment and Gut Microbiota? A Systematic Review | Gerontology | Karger Publishers [Internet]. [cited 2024 Jan 7]. Available from: https://karger.com/ger/article/68/11/1201/823877/Is-There-Any-Link-between-Cognitive-Impairment-and
8. Parkinson's Disease and Gut Microbiota [Internet]. [cited 2023 Sep 5]. Available from: https://pubmed.ncbi.nlm.nih.gov/34500451/
9. Chang CH, Lin CH, Lane HY. D-glutamate and gut microbiota in Alzheimer's disease. Int J Mol Sci. 2020;21(8):2676.
10. Nikolova VL, Hall MRB, Hall LJ, Cleare AJ, Stone JM, Young AH. Perturbations in gut microbiota composition in psychiatric disorders. JAMA Psychiatry. 2021;78(12):1–12.
11. Carbone EA, D'Amato P, Vicchio G, De Fazio P, Segura-Garcia C. A systematic review on the role of microbiota in the pathogenesis and treatment of eating disorders. Eur Psychiatry. 2020;64(1):e2.
12. Milosevic I, Vujovic A, Barac A, Djelic M, Korac M, Radovanovic Spurnic A, et al. Gut-liver Axis, gut microbiota, and its modulation in the Management of Liver Diseases: a review of the literature. Int J Mol Sci. 2019;20(2):395.
13. Xiang S, Qu Y, Qian S, Wang R, Wang Y, Jin Y, et al. Association between systemic lupus erythematosus and disruption of gut microbiota: a meta-analysis. Lupus Sci Med. 2022;9(1):e000599.

14. Shirvani-Rad S, Khatibzade-Nasari N, Ejtahed HS, Larijani B. Exploring the role of gut microbiota dysbiosis in gout pathogenesis: a systematic review. Front Med. 2023;10:1163778.
15. Salem F, Kindt N, Marchesi JR, Netter P, Lopez A, Kokten T, et al. Gut microbiome in chronic rheumatic and inflammatory bowel diseases: similarities and differences. United Eur Gastroenterol J. 2019;7(8):1008–32.
16. Neuman H, Debelius JW, Knight R, Koren O. Microbial endocrinology: the interplay between the microbiota and the endocrine system. FEMS Microbiol Rev. 2015;39(4):509–21.
17. Angoorani P, Ejtahed HS, Ettehad Marvasti F, Taghavi M, Mohammadpour Ahranjani B, Hasani-Ranjbar S, et al. The effects of probiotics, prebiotics, and synbiotics on polycystic ovarian syndrome: an overview of systematic reviews. Front Med. 2023;10:1141355.
18. da Silva ST, dos Santos CA, Bressan J. Intestinal microbiota; relevance to obesity and modulation by prebiotics and probiotics. Nutr Hosp. 2013;28(4):1039–48.
19. Ejtahed HS, Angoorani P, Soroush AR, Hasani-Ranjbar S, Siadat SD, Larijani B. Gut microbiota-derived metabolites in obesity: a systematic review. Biosci Microbiota Food Health. 2020;39(3):65–76.
20. Lam YY, Maguire S, Palacios T, Caterson ID. Are the gut bacteria telling us to eat or not to eat? Reviewing the role of gut microbiota in the etiology, disease progression and treatment of eating disorders. Nutrients. 2017;9(6):602.
21. Pan X, Wen SW, Kaminga AC, Liu A. Gut metabolites and inflammation factors in non-alcoholic fatty liver disease: a systematic review and meta-analysis. Sci Rep. 2020;10:8848.
22. Zhou H, Zhao X, Sun L, Liu Y, Lv Y, Gang X, et al. Gut microbiota profile in patients with type 1 diabetes based on 16S rRNA gene sequencing: a systematic review. Dis Markers. 2020;2020:3936247.
23. Sadagopan A, Mahmoud A, Begg M, Tarhuni M, Fotso M, Gonzalez NA, et al. Understanding the role of the gut microbiome in diabetes and therapeutics targeting leaky gut: a systematic review. Cureus. 15(7):e41559.
24. Letchumanan G, Abdullah N, Marlini M, Baharom N, Lawley B, Omar MR, et al. Gut microbiota composition in prediabetes and newly diagnosed type 2 diabetes: a systematic review of observational studies. Front Cell Infect Microbiol. 2022;12:943427.
25. Farhat S, Hemmatabadi M, Ejtahed HS, Shirzad N, Larijani B. Microbiome alterations in women with gestational diabetes mellitus and their offspring: a systematic review. Front Endocrinol. 2022;13:1060488.
26. Pakmehr A, Ejtahed HS, Shirzad N, Hemmatabadi M, Farhat S, Larijani B. Preventive effect of probiotics supplementation on occurrence of gestational diabetes mellitus: a systematic review and meta-analysis of randomized controlled trials. Front Med. 2022;9:1031915.
27. Rold LS, Bundgaard-Nielsen C, Niemann Holm-Jacobsen J, Glud Ovesen P, Leutscher P, Hagstrøm S, et al. Characteristics of the gut microbiome in women with gestational diabetes mellitus: a systematic review. PLoS One. 2022;17(1):e0262618.
28. Teixeira RA, Silva C, Ferreira AC, Martins D, Leite-Moreira A, Miranda IM, et al. The association between gestational diabetes and the microbiome: a systematic review and meta-analysis. Microorganisms. 2023;11(7):1749.
29. Ejtahed HS, Ardeshirlarijani E, Tabatabaei-Malazy O, Hoseini-Tavassol Z, Hasani-Ranjbar S, Soroush AR, et al. Effect of probiotic foods and supplements on blood pressure: a systematic review of meta-analyses studies of controlled trials. J Diabetes Metab Disord. 2020;19(1):617–23.
30. Qin Y, Zhao J, Wang Y, Bai M, Sun S. Specific alterations of gut microbiota in Chinese patients with hypertension: a systematic review and meta-analysis. Kidney Blood Press Res. 2022;47(7):433–47.
31. Naik SS, Ramphall S, Rijal S, Prakash V, Ekladios H, Mulayamkuzhiyil Saju J, et al. Association of gut microbial dysbiosis and hypertension: a systematic review. Cureus. 2022;14(10):e29927.

32. Hoseini-Tavassol Z, Ejtahed HS, Larijani B, Hasani-Ranjbar S. Trimethylamine N-oxide as a potential risk factor for non-communicable diseases: a systematic review. Endocr Metab Immune Disord Drug Targets. 2023;23(5):617–32.
33. Lei L, Zhao N, Zhang L, Chen J, Liu X, Piao S. Gut microbiota is a potential goalkeeper of dyslipidemia. Front Endocrinol. 2022;13:950826.
34. Ejtahed HS, Angoorani P, Soroush AR, Siadat SD, Shirzad N, Hasani-Ranjbar S, et al. Our little friends with big roles: alterations of the gut microbiota in thyroid disorders. Endocr Metab Immune Disord Drug Targets. 2020;20(3):344–50.
35. Gong B, Wang C, Meng F, Wang H, Song B, Yang Y, et al. Association between gut microbiota and autoimmune thyroid disease: a systematic review and meta-analysis. Front Endocrinol. 2021;12:774362.
36. Jiang W, Lu G, Gao D, Lv Z, Li D. The relationships between the gut microbiota and its metabolites with thyroid diseases. Front Endocrinol. 2022;13:943408.
37. Malmir H, Ejtahed HS, Soroush AR, Mortazavian AM, Fahimfar N, Ostovar A, et al. Probiotics as a new regulator for bone health: a systematic review and meta-analysis. Evid-Based Complement Altern Med. 2021;2021:3582989.
38. Huang R, Liu P, Bai Y, Huang J, Pan R, Li H, Su Y, Zhou Q, Ma R, Zong S, Zeng G. Changes in the gut microbiota of osteoporosis patients based on 16S rRNA gene sequencing: a systematic review and meta-analysis. J Zhejiang Univ Sci B. 2022;23(12):1002–13.
39. Akinsuyi OS, Roesch LFW. Meta-analysis reveals compositional and functional microbial changes associated with osteoporosis. Microbiol Spectr. 2023;11(3):e0032223.
40. Nikkhah A, Ejtahed HS, Ettehad Marvasti F, Taghavi M, Pakmehr A, Hajipour F, et al. The critical role of gut microbiota dysbiosis in skeletal muscle wasting: a systematic review. J Appl Microbiol. 2023;134(1):lxac014.
41. Ticinesi A, Nouvenne A, Cerundolo N, Catania P, Prati B, Tana C, et al. Gut microbiota, muscle mass and function in aging: a focus on physical frailty and sarcopenia. Nutrients. 2019;11(7):1633.
42. Meng C, Bai C, Brown TD, Hood LE, Tian Q. Human gut microbiota and gastrointestinal cancer. Genomics Proteomics Bioinformatics. 2018;16(1):33–49.
43. Xiang Y, Zhang C, Wang J, Cheng Y, Wang L, Tong Y, et al. Identification of host gene-microbiome associations in colorectal cancer patients using mendelian randomization. J Transl Med. 2023;21:535.
44. Yu LX, Schwabe RF. The gut microbiome and liver cancer: mechanisms and clinical translation. Nat Rev Gastroenterol Hepatol. 2017;14(9):527–39.
45. Li Q, Jin M, Liu Y, Jin L. Gut microbiota: its potential roles in pancreatic cancer. Front Cell Infect Microbiol. 2020;10:572492.
46. Liu Q, Sun W, Zhang H. Interaction of gut microbiota with endocrine homeostasis and thyroid cancer. Cancer. 2022;14(11):2656.
47. Knezevic J, Starchl C, Berisha AT, Amrein K. Thyroid-gut-Axis: how does the microbiota influence thyroid function? Nutrients. 2020;12(6)
48. Magne F, Gotteland M, Gauthier L, Zazueta A, Pesoa S, Navarrete P, et al. The Firmicutes/Bacteroidetes ratio: a relevant marker of gut Dysbiosis in obese patients? Nutrients. 2020;12(5):1474.
49. Fang J, Yu CH, Li XJ, Yao JM, Fang ZY, Yoon SH, et al. Gut dysbiosis in nonalcoholic fatty liver disease: pathogenesis, diagnosis, and therapeutic implications. Front Cell Infect Microbiol. 2022;12:997018.
50. Varesi A, Pierella E, Romeo M, Piccini GB, Alfano C, Bjørklund G, et al. The potential role of gut microbiota in Alzheimer's disease: from diagnosis to treatment. Nutrients. 2022;14(3):668.
51. Farrokhi V, Nemati R, Nichols FC, Yao X, Anstadt E, Fujiwara M, et al. Bacterial lipodipeptide, lipid 654, is a microbiome-associated biomarker for multiple sclerosis. Clin Transl Immunol. 2013;2(11):e8.

52. Ranjbar M, Salehi R, Haghjooy Javanmard S, Rafiee L, Faraji H, et al. The dysbiosis signature of Fusobacterium nucleatum in colorectal cancer-cause or consequences? A systematic review. Cancer Cell Int. 2021;21:194.
53. Cooper TE, Scholes-Robertson N, Craig JC, Hawley CM, Howell M, Johnson DW, et al. Synbiotics, prebiotics and probiotics for solid organ transplant recipients. Cochrane Database Syst Rev. 2022;2022(9):CD014804.
54. Moorthy M, Sundralingam U, Palanisamy UD. Polyphenols as prebiotics in the management of high-fat diet-induced obesity: a systematic review of animal studies. Foods. 2021;10(2):299.
55. Ammar A, Trabelsi K, Boukhris O, Bouaziz B, Müller P, Glenn JM, et al. Effects of polyphenol-rich interventions on cognition and brain health in healthy young and middle-aged adults: systematic review and meta-analysis. J Clin Med. 2020;9(5)
56. Qiu L, Gao C, Wang H, Ren Y, Li J, Li M, et al. Effects of dietary polyphenol curcumin supplementation on metabolic, inflammatory, and oxidative stress indices in patients with metabolic syndrome: a systematic review and meta-analysis of randomized controlled trials. Front Endocrinol. 2023;14:1216708.
57. Den H, Dong X, Chen M, Zou Z. Efficacy of probiotics on cognition, and biomarkers of inflammation and oxidative stress in adults with Alzheimer's disease or mild cognitive impairment – a meta-analysis of randomized controlled trials. Aging. 2020;12(4):4010–39.
58. López-Moreno A, Suárez A, Avanzi C, Monteoliva-Sánchez M, Aguilera M. Probiotic strains and intervention total doses for modulating obesity-related microbiota dysbiosis: a systematic review and meta-analysis. Nutrients. 2020;12(7):1921.
59. Sáez-Lara MJ, Robles-Sanchez C, Ruiz-Ojeda FJ, Plaza-Diaz J, Gil A. Effects of probiotics and synbiotics on obesity, insulin resistance syndrome, type 2 diabetes and non-alcoholic fatty liver disease: a review of human clinical trials. Int J Mol Sci. 2016;17(6):928.
60. Wierzbicka A, Mańkowska-Wierzbicka D, Mardas M, Stelmach-Mardas M. Role of probiotics in modulating human gut microbiota populations and activities in patients with colorectal cancer – a systematic review of clinical trials. Nutrients. 2021;13(4):1160.
61. Zhang H, Duan Y, Cai F, Cao D, Wang L, Qiao Z, et al. Next-generation probiotics: microflora intervention to human diseases. Biomed Res Int. 2022;2022:e5633403.
62. Asha MZ, Khalil SFH. Efficacy and safety of probiotics, prebiotics and synbiotics in the treatment of irritable bowel syndrome. Sultan Qaboos Univ Med J. 2020;20(1):e13–24.
63. Sharif S, Heath PT, Oddie SJ, McGuire W. Synbiotics to prevent necrotising enterocolitis in very preterm or very low birth weight infants. Cochrane Database Syst Rev. 2022;2022(3):CD014067.
64. Naseri K, Saadati S, Ghaemi F, Ashtary-Larky D, Asbaghi O, Sadeghi A, et al. The effects of probiotic and synbiotic supplementation on inflammation, oxidative stress, and circulating adiponectin and leptin concentration in subjects with prediabetes and type 2 diabetes mellitus: a GRADE-assessed systematic review, meta-analysis, and meta-regression of randomized clinical trials. Eur J Nutr. 2023;62(2):543–61.
65. Malagón-Rojas JN, Mantziari A, Salminen S, Szajewska H. Postbiotics for preventing and treating common infectious diseases in children: a systematic review. Nutrients. 2020;12(2):389.
66. Lindström C, Holst O, Nilsson L, Öste R, Andersson KE. Effects of Pediococcus parvulus 2.6 and its exopolysaccharide on plasma cholesterol levels and inflammatory markers in mice. AMB Express. 2012;2:66.
67. Jeon B, Kim HR, Kim H, Chung DK. In vitro and in vivo downregulation of C3 by lipoteichoic acid isolated from lactobacillus plantarum K8 suppressed cytokine-mediated complement system activation. FEMS Microbiol Lett. 2016;363(14):fnw140.
68. Nataraj BH, Ali SA, Behare PV, Yadav H. Postbiotics-parabiotics: the new horizons in microbial biotherapy and functional foods. Microb Cell Factories. 2020:19.
69. Escamilla J, Lane MA, Maitin V. Cell-free supernatants from probiotic lactobacillus casei and lactobacillus rhamnosus GG decrease colon cancer cell invasion in vitro. Nutr Cancer. 2012;64(6):871–8.

70. Meunier M, Laurin D, Park S. Extracellular vesicles and MicroRNA in myelodysplastic syndromes. Cells. 2023;12(4):658.
71. Liang X, Dai N, Sheng K, Lu H, Wang J, Chen L, et al. Gut bacterial extracellular vesicles: important players in regulating intestinal microenvironment. Gut Microbes. 2022;14(1):2134689.
72. Pakmehr A, Mousavi SM, Ejtahed HS, Hoseini-Tavassol Z, Siadat SD, Hasani-Ranjbar S, et al. The effect of fecal microbiota transplantation on Cardiometabolic risk factors: a systematic review and meta-analysis. Clin Ther. 2023;(23):S0149–2918.
73. Wang Y, Zhang S, Borody TJ, Zhang F. Encyclopedia of fecal microbiota transplantation: a review of effectiveness in the treatment of 85 diseases. Chin Med J. 2022;135(16):1927–39.
74. Nassar ST, Tasha T, Desai A, Bajgain A, Ali A, Dutta C, et al. Fecal microbiota transplantation role in the treatment of Alzheimer's disease: a systematic review. Cureus. 2022;14(10):e29968.
75. Shirvani Rad S, Nikkhah A, Orvatinia M, Ejtahed HS, Sarhangi N, Jamaldini SH, Khodayari N, Aghaei Meybodi HR, Hasanzad M. Gut microbiota: a perspective of precision medicine in endocrine disorders. J Diabetes Metab Disord. 2020;19(2):1827–34.
76. Petrosino JF. The microbiome in precision medicine: the way forward. Genome Med. 2018;10(1):12.
77. Ejtahed HS, Hasani-Ranjbar S, Larijani B. Human microbiome as an approach to personalized medicine. Altern Ther Health Med. 2017;23(6):8–9.
78. Hu C, Jia W. Multi-omics profiling: the way toward precision medicine in metabolic diseases. J Mol Cell Biol. 2021;13(8):576–93.

Chapter 9
Precision Medicine in Endocrinology

Marzieh Nosrati, Homa Hemati, George P. Patrinos, Negar Sarhangi, Mandana Hasanzad, and Shekoufeh Nikfar

9.1 Introduction

Endocrine disorders have a noticeable impact on individuals' quality of life, as they can affect patients' cellular metabolism and the functioning of different organs in the body. These disorders are risk factors for developing other diseases. Furthermore, these disorders also account for the fifth cause of mortality worldwide (5% in women and 4% in men) [1]. Endocrine disorders impose a significant social and economic burden on the healthcare system. Therefore, effective prevention, early diagnosis, and treatment of these diseases play an essential role in improving public health [2].

M. Nosrati
Personalized Medicine Research Center, Endocrinology and Metabolism Clinical Sciences Institute, Tehran University of Medical Sciences, Tehran, Iran

Faculty of Pharmacy, Department of Pharmacoeconomics and Pharmaceutical Administration, Tehran University of Medical Sciences, Tehran, Iran

H. Hemati
Faculty of Pharmacy, Department of Pharmacoeconomics and Pharmaceutical Administration, Tehran University of Medical Sciences, Tehran, Iran

G. P. Patrinos
School of Health Sciences, Department of Pharmacy, University of Patras, Patras, Greece

College of Medicine and Health Sciences, Department of Genetics and Genomics, United Arab Emirates University, Abu Dhabi, UAE

Zayed Center for Health Sciences, United Arab Emirates University, Abu Dhabi, UAE

Faculty of Medicine and Health Sciences, Department of Pathology, Clinical Bioinformatics Unit, Erasmus University Medical Center, Rotterdam, the Netherlands

N. Sarhangi
Personalized Medicine Research Center, Endocrinology and Metabolism Clinical Sciences Institute, Tehran University of Medical Sciences, Tehran, Iran

H. Gharib et al. (eds.), *Interdisciplinary Advances in Endocrinology*,
https://doi.org/10.1007/978-981-95-2286-6_9

Precision medicine also named as personalized medicine is revolutionizing the field of endocrinology by employing treatment strategies tailored to individual patients based on their unique genetic makeup, lifestyle factors, and specific disease characteristics. This approach allows for a more precise and targeted management of endocrine disorders, such as diabetes, thyroid, and adrenal disorders. By leveraging advancements in genomics, molecular diagnostics, and other technologies, personalized medicine offers the potential for improved treatment outcomes, reduced side effects, and enhanced patient adherence and satisfaction. It represents a paradigm shift from a one-size-fits-all approach to a more individualized and effective strategy in endocrinology, ultimately improving patient care and long-term health outcomes [3]. While personalized medicine has made significant strides in certain diseases, its application in endocrine disorders is still evolving and requires further research and development. Nonetheless, personalized medicine offers a promising approach to address the complex and diverse nature of endocrine disorders.

Diabetes, obesity, and endocrine cancers are some important endocrine diseases affected by personalized medicine interventions.

In this chapter, we focus on the advancements of personalized medicine in prevention, diagnosis, and treatment of these mentioned diseases. Moreover, we discuss new interventions that may be utilized in the near future for the management of them.

9.2 Diabetes

Diabetes is one of the most critical concerns of health systems due to its significant prevalence and the subsequent remarkably high costs. In recent decades, its prevalence has been increasing considerably, and it has been predicted that 783 million people worldwide will be affected by diabetes by 2045 [4]. Diabetes healthcare expenditures were estimated to be $966 billion globally in 2021, and these costs are projected to increase to $1028 billion by 2030 [5]. Despite the availability of recent diabetes treatments and technologies in healthcare markets, achieving the target blood glucose level is still very challenging due to individual disparities in responding to treatments. This challenge underscores the importance of applying the

M. Hasanzad
Personalized Medicine Research Center, Endocrinology and Metabolism Clinical Sciences Institute, Tehran University of Medical Sciences, Tehran, Iran

Medical Genomic Research Center, TeMS.C., Islamic Azad University, Tehran, Iran

S. Nikfar (✉)
Faculty of Pharmacy, Department of Pharmacoeconomics and Pharmaceutical Administration, Tehran University of Medical Sciences, Tehran, Iran

Endocrinology and Metabolism Research Center, Endocrinology and Metabolism Clinical Sciences Institute, Tehran University of Medical Sciences, Tehran, Iran strategy of personalized medicine in the prevention, diagnosis, and treatment of diabetes [6].

According to the summary report by ADA and EASD, there are five fundamental pillars in personalized diabetes care: personalized diabetes, personalized prevention, personalized treatment, personalized prognostic, and personalized monitoring [7]. Based on these five pillars, it is understood that in the personalized medicine approach by identifying the circulating biomarkers, genomic sequencing, and other types of biomarker metrics as well as considering the manifestations of the disease, diabetic patients can be divided into various types of subgroups. In each subgroup specially, the risk of diabetic complication is predicted, treatment goals are defined, and tailored treatment is prescribed [8, 9]. Moreover, by considering this approach, a more favorable outcome is obtained, and it will lead to more efficient healthcare resource utilization. Diabetes is classified into four main types: type 1, type 2 (polygenic diabetes), gestational, and monogenic diabetes. So far, about 80 genetic loci have been identified on chromosomes that are effective in the occurrence of type 1 and 2 diabetes [10].

9.2.1 Personalized Medicine in Type 1 Diabetes

With the development of pharmaceutical formulation of insulin, type 1 diabetes changed from an unmanageable disease to a chronic and controllable condition. In-depth knowledge about the pathogenesis of type 1 diabetes will help to reveal the importance of the role of personalized medicine interventions in the better management of this type of diabetes.

One of the essential functions of personalized medicine in diabetes type 1 is the prediction of its occurrence in newborns (or in other words, finding at-risk patients) via the examination of HLA variants. It means that by obtaining different types of genetic risk combination and measuring polygenic (or genetic) risk score (PRS) of HLA and non-HLA with genome-wide association studies (GWAS), the occurrence of type 1 diabetes in newborn would be predictable or the disease could be classified into different types [11]. In general, PRS is defined as: "a single value estimate of an individual's common genetic liability to a phenotype, calculated as a sum of their genome-wide genotypes, weighted by corresponding genotype effect size estimates (or Z-scores) derived from summary statistics GWAS data" [12]. It should be noted that many high-risk individuals will probably not develop type 1 diabetes. Presently, the primary biomarkers associated with an increased susceptibility to this disease include genetics, age, number, types and titres of autoantibodies, and the age at which these autoantibodies appear, dysglycemia and C-peptide level.

Type 1 diabetes is an autoimmune disease. Presently, the FDA is focusing on teplizumab as a disease-modifying therapy in diabetes type 1. Studies have shown that consumption of this medicine at the second stage of type 1 diabetes can delay the onset of clinical presentation. However, the response rate to this treatment is associated with heterogeneity. More studies are needed to clarify how age and type of autoantibodies influence the response to such therapies. A new analysis in young type 1 diabetes patients has shown that this disease can be categorized in ten subgroups (seven subgroups based on the presence of different autoantibodies and three subgroups based on the absence of various ones). Identifying the pathogenesis of type 1 diabetes and its correct grouping would be helpful in selecting more accurate treatment strategies. Therefore, ADA and EASD guidelines have recommended islet autoantibody tests when diagnosing type 1 diabetes. Moreover, determining the genetic risk score in type 1 diabetes can be effective in differentiating among type 1 and 2 and other types of diabetes.

Another crucial role of the personalized type 1 diabetes care is its considerable role in the treatment. One of the important issues in the treatment of type 1 diabetes patients is administration of insulin and management of blood glucose levels (with the aim of preventing the occurrence of hypo- and hyperglycemia). Presently, various forms of insulin, resulted from the variation in formulation and delivery (such as continuous subcutaneous insulin infusion systems), have made it possible to achieve individualized insulin therapy. Management of blood glucose level is very substantial in diabetic patients because the incidence of many micro- and macrovascular complications would be resulted from dysglycemia. Controlling blood glucose level with laboratory methods such as HbA1c is not possible at any moment. The use of continuous glucose monitoring (CGM), which can measure the level of blood glucose every 5 to 15 minutes using sensors, will make individualized blood glucose monitoring achievable. Individualized monitoring of blood glucose has proven effective in minimizing the time spent in hypo- and hyperglycemia and improving the quality of life. The result of using GCM along with advanced insulin delivery methods has led to more precise control of blood glucose at any moment in type 1 diabetes patients. Besides, in the personalized type 1 diabetes care, the concept of individualized glycemic target should be considered, which means that the optimal blood glucose level is different in various patients and depends on factors such as the duration of diabetes, patient's age and life expectancy, other comorbidities, and complications.

Considering educational strategies for type 1 diabetes with the aim of matching the diet and insulin required dose in different conditions for each patient is another instance of the application of a personalized diabetes care in the management of type 1 diabetes. For example, using programs such as Dose Adjustment for Normal Eating (DAFNE) will help patients to be aware of the amount of carbohydrates in their meal and adjust the amounts more accurately. In-depth educational strategies help to improve the behaviors of type 1 diabetes patients, especially regarding exercise, and have a possible crucial role in better control and management of the disease [11].

9.2.2 Personalized Medicine in Type 2 Diabetes

Today, type 2 diabetes can be identified in any patient who does not have monogenic or type 1 diabetes. A genetic syndrome linked to abnormalities in blood glucose metabolism is type 2 diabetes. Its incidence is attributed to several environmental factors, including stress, diet, and lifestyle. It is estimated that genetics accounts for 30–70% of diabetes cases.

There is significant heterogeneity in the phenotype of individuals with type 2 diabetes, and these variations are frequently ignored in the management of these patients [13, 14]. Until now, the number of variants associated with type 2 diabetes has exceeded four hundreds [14]. It will be possible to divide type 2 diabetes patients (as well as those with type 1 diabetes) into several subgroups and develop strategies for treatment and prevention in each group by considering genetic variations. Research indicates that even with inadequate glycemic control, many individuals are less vulnerable to the consequences of diabetes. This example indicates that patients should be categorized into several categories, with consideration for treatment objectives in each grouping.

Studies revealed that several gene variations can play a role in developing type 2 diabetes, its prevention, and how the human body responds to certain hypoglycemic medications [15]. The *TCF7L2* variant known as rs7903146 will raise the risk of type 2 diabetes by 41%, according to the findings of a meta-analysis that aggregated data from 28 studies. This particular variant is among the most significant ones linked to the risk of type 2 diabetes when compared to others. *PPARG* is another gene associated with type 2 diabetes. Studies' findings have indicated that this gene's Pro alleles are linked to an increased risk of type 2 diabetes. The genetic knowledge of type 2 diabetes will become clearer to us as a result of GWAS research. These studies provide more precise results with stronger statistical power about common variants that enhance risk of diabetes mellitus by incorporating data relating to many ethnic groups and races and by adding a sizable sample size. An increase in blood glucose after fasting and 2 hours after eating and a raised HbA1c level in comparison to normal are indicators of diabetes. Numerous variations have been found in GWAS studies that are linked to fasting insulin, fasting glucose, fasting proinsulin, and fasting insulin resistance. With this knowledge, diabetes's heterogeneity and pathogenesis in various individuals can be better understood, allowing for the planning of more precise treatment strategies and objectives for each subgroup. Typically, certain conditions like type 2 diabetes, fasting glucose levels, fasting insulin levels, and BMI are associated with specific genetic regions. These identified regions primarily influence the development of type 2 diabetes. However, some genetic variations can play multiple roles [16]. In Table 9.1, the genes that are effective in type 2 diabetes and have at least one additional association are mentioned.

Table 9.1 Effective genes in type 2 diabetes and other associated glycemic traits [17]

	Associated glycemic trait		
Genes	Fasting glucose	Fasting insulin	BMI
ADCY5	+		
C2CD4A	+		
CDKAL1	+		
CDKN2A	+		
DGKB	+		
GCK	+		
GLIS3	+		
IGFBP2A	+		
IGF2BP2	+		
MTNR1B	+		
PROX1	+		
RREB1	+		
SLC30A8	+		
TCF7L2	+		
ZBED3	+		
GCKR	+	+	
IRS1		+	
PPARG		+	
ANKRD55		+	
ARL15		+	
GRB14		+	
COBLL1		+	
FTO		+	+
MC4R			+
QPCTL			+
GIPR			+

9.2.3 *Personalized Medicine in Monogenic Diabetes*

Monogenic diabetes, which resembles type 2 diabetes in its symptoms, results from the deficiency of a single gene and is observed in younger individuals. Because the characteristics of monogenic diabetes and type 1 and 2 diabetes overlap, misdiagnosis is frequent. Treatment is based on the underlying cause and necessitates genetic analysis. Monogenic diabetes is categorized in three types: maturity-onset diabetes of the young (MODY), neonatal diabetes mellitus (NDM), and syndromic diabetes [9].

MODY, the prevalent form of monogenic diabetes, encompasses a range of endocrine disorders that impact 1–5% of individuals diagnosed with diabetes mellitus. This form of monogenic diabetes usually demonstrates inheritance through autosomal dominant patterns, although occasional spontaneous mutations can arise. Key clinical traits of MODY comprise early-onset high blood glucose, signs of ongoing pancreatic function, and absence of beta cell autoimmunity or insulin resistance [18].

Some of the key concepts and characteristics of this kind of diabetes were elucidated by research on rarer MODY subtypes, as follows:

- So far, 14 types of MODY have been recognized.
  - Various researches utilize different MODY criteria for genetic testing.
- The two most often reported variants are found in the *ABCC8*-(MODY12) and *INS*-(MODY10) genes.
- Less common MODY subtypes have characteristics including diabetic ketoacidosis and obesity that are assumed to be absent from MODY.
- Oral hypoglycemic agents, or more recent medications, are also used in the treatment of uncommon MODY subtypes, while insulin is the mainstay. Insulin is largely needed by rarer MODY subtypes such as IPF1/PDX1-(MODY4), CEL-(MODY8), INS-(MODY10), and APPL1-(MODY14). Individuals with variants in ABCC8-(MODY12) frequently transition from insulin therapy to sulfonylurea therapy. In certain instances, newer medications like sitagliptin and dapagliflozin have been employed. Sitagliptin and rosiglitazone were administered to an HNF1A-(MODY3) patient who had received insulin treatment in the past. Future research ought to look into these patients' use of more recent antidiabetic medications. Sulfonylureas are recommended as treatment for HNF1A-(MODY3) and HNF4A-(MODY3) patients.
- Insufficient information about macrovascular and microvascular problems in less common MODY subtypes [19].

9.2.4 Pharmacogenomics of Diabetes

Individuals respond differently to medicines for different reasons, both hereditary and nongenetic. The fields of pharmacogenetics and pharmacogenomics study the relationship between an individual's genetic makeup and their particular pharmacological responses. Drug pharmacokinetics and pharmacodynamics may vary depending on the expression levels of drug receptors, transporters, metabolic enzymes, and other proteins that are determined by gene polymorphisms. Single-nucleotide polymorphisms (SNPs) and other biological biomarkers are taken into account when making therapeutic and diagnostic decisions [20]. As diabetic patients respond variably to pharmacotherapy, it is possible to avoid the waste of resources and related costs by applying the pharmacogenetic approach in the field of diabetes. The role of pharmacogenomics on the pharmacodynamic and pharmacokinetic characteristics in each class of hypoglycemic medications is discussed in the following section.

9.2.4.1 Metformin

The first-line therapy for people with type 2 diabetes that is frequently administered and offers additional benefits such as improved insulin sensitivity [21], reduced hepatic gluconeogenesis [21, 22], weight loss, and cardioprotective properties is metformin [23]. Although its mode of action and potential adverse effects are still being investigated, this medicine may offer further benefits in terms of reducing the risk of cancer and aging. The pharmacogenomics of metformin can be examined through two aspects: intolerance and drug's effectiveness.

Some of the important identified genes that influence the response to metformin include *SLC22A1*, *SCL22A2*, and *SLC22A3* [20, 24]:

- Research findings indicated a correlation between the efficacy of metformin in individuals with type 2 diabetes and certain *SLC22A1* variants in several racial groups [20, 24]. For example, the rs622342 variant in South India was linked to metformin efficacy. Moreover, rs122083571 and rs72552763 variants are associated with metformin intolerance [24].
- Changes in *SLC22A2* can influence the elimination of metformin from the blood. The organic cation transporter 2 (OCT2), a protein responsible for transporting metformin from the blood to the kidneys, is encoded by this gene [20]. For example, the *SLC22A2* c.808G > T variant has been shown to increase the glucose-lowering effectiveness of metformin in Chinese patients with type 2 diabetes by delaying the entry of metformin into the kidney [25]. Also, according to the study in Pakistani patients, the *SLC22A2* rs201919874 variant is associated with how effectively metformin works in managing HbA1c levels, as well as random blood glucose and fasting plasma glucose (FPG) concentrations [26].
- Organic cation transporter 3 (OCT3), the protein encoded by the s*SLC22A3* gene, has the main role in metformin absorption in the liver and gut [20]. Therefore, different variants of this gene have various effects on metformin response treatment. For instance, rs3088442G in Pakistani type 2 diabetes patients has demonstrated a significant correlation with metformin response [27]. Another example is rs12194182 in Jordanian type 2 diabetic patients, which was associated with a lower mean HbA1c but not in male Caucasians [28, 29].

The primary reason for metformin intolerance is its transportation into enterocytes from the intestinal lumen. In the human intestines, three main transporters facilitate this process: the serotonin transporter (from the *SLC6A4* gene), the plasma membrane monoamine transporter (PMAT, from the *SLC29A4* gene), and the organic cation transporter 1 (OCT1, from the *SLC22A1* gene). As a result, variations in these genes have been linked to metformin intolerance. In the IMI-DIRECT[1] consortium, metformin intolerance was self-reported by patients, leading to the cessation of metformin or an inability to increase the dose beyond 1 gram. Considering

[1] DIRECT is a European collaborative group focused on diabetes research, initially supported by the European Union's Innovative Medicines Initiative (IMI).

that decreasing the dosage can affect the drug's effectiveness in controlling diabetes, employing a pharmacogenetic strategy in prescribing metformin can be of significant importance [23].

9.2.4.2 Sulfonylurea

Sulfonylureas influence glucose regulation by stimulating pancreatic β-cells to secrete more insulin [20]. Responses may be impacted by mutations in target receptors or metabolic enzymes since one of the enzymes in cytochrome P450 (CYP2C9) metabolizes these compounds in the liver. CYP2C9*2 (p.I359L) and CYP2C9*3 (p.R114C) are two variants that have been linked to higher serum-sulfonylurea levels. Carriers of loss-of-function CYP2C9*2 or CYP2C9*3 alleles had 3.4 times the probability of achieving glycemic control compared to carriers of wild-type alleles based on the GoDARTS64 retrospective study involving 1073 participants [23, 24].

Moreover, variants in some genes like *ABCC8* (encodes SUR1 protein which is a subunit constituting the ATP-sensitive potassium channel [KATP channel] and has a main role in insulin secretion) or *KCJN11* (encodes Kir6.2 protein which is another subunit of the KATP channel) are associated with the response of sulfonylurea. Variants of these genes can cause reduction on the level of HbA1c or increase the risk of hypoglycemia [20, 24]. The response to sulfonylureas has also been connected to other genes. Variants in the *TCF7L2* gene are connected to decreased β-cell function and consequently decreased the effectiveness of sulfonylurea [20, 23, 24].

9.2.4.3 Dipeptidyl Peptidase 4 (DPP4) Inhibitors and Glucagon-Like Peptide-1 (GLP-1) Analogues

GLP1-receptor agonists and DPP4 inhibitors regulate blood glucose levels by affecting the body's incretin system. This regulation is impacted by DPP4's inactivation of GLP1 and gastric inhibitory polypeptide (GIP). These groups are recommended as a second-line treatment for management of type 2 diabetes [24]. The efficacy of this class was linked with the *CTRB1* and *CTRB2* genes, which both encode the digestive enzyme chymotrypsin, a crucial modulator of the incretin pathway [30].

9.2.4.4 Sodium–Glucose Cotransporter 2 Inhibitors

During renal filtration, 99% of the filtered glucose was reabsorbed by sodium–glucose transporters, which are found in the renal tubules. Because sodium–glucose transporter type 2 is the predominant class of these transporters in the renal tubules, SGLT-2 inhibitors lower hyperglycemia by facilitating the excretion of glucose in the urine [30]. The *SLC5A2* gene, which is found on human chromosome 16p11.2, encodes SGLT2 [24]. The rs9934336 G allele of the *SLC5A2* gene is associated with increased 30-min plasma glucose, 120-min insulin concentrations, and AUC120 glucose on oral glucose tolerance test in 907 nondiabetic Sorbs [31].

9.2.4.5 Thiazolidinediones

Peripheral tissue contains proliferator-activated receptor c (PPARc), which is regulated by thiazolidinediones, a peripheral insulin sensitizer that increases peripheral tissue sensitivity to insulin and controls glucose metabolism. Pancreatic islet β-cells are not the target of this class of medications [20]. Studies investigated some of the genetic variants that have effects on pharmacokinetic and pharmacodynamic features of this group such as SLCO1B1, AQP2, SLC12A1, and PPARG. The hepatic drug transporter OATP1B1, which is encoded by the *SLCO1B1*, is involved in thiazolidinedione metabolism. The *SLCO1B1* c.521 T > C variant is significantly associated with improved glycemic response in type 2 diabetic patients receiving rosiglitazone but not in normal population [20]. In rosiglitazone users, edema has been related to the rs296766 T allele of *AQP2* and the rs12904216 G allele of *SLC12A1*. The effect of rosiglitazone is linked to variants in PPARG C1A and PPARG P12A. Carriers of the minor allele of rs1801282 in *PPARG* had a greater probability of responding to pioglitazone than carriers of wild-type alleles, according to an Asian study that included 250 patients. Furthermore, individuals who bear the A allele of rs6467136 in *PAX4* responded to rosiglitazone more favorably. CYP2C8 is a key thiazolidinedione metabolizer, and the *CYP2C8*3* variant responds to insulin less favorable because of the reduced rosiglitazone plasma concentration [24].

9.2.4.6 Glinides

Glinides or meglitinides are a class of insulin secretagogues that affect the KATP channel to increase insulin secretion and lower blood glucose levels similar to sulfonylurea [20]. The study in the Chinese population has shown that the response to meglitinide is linked to *SLCO1B1, CYP2C8, CYP3A4, TCF7L2, SLC30A8, IGF2BP2, KCNJ11, KCNQ1, UCP2, NAMPT, MDR1, PAX4*, and *NEUROD1*. For example, *CYP2C8*1/*3* genotypes reduce repaglinide plasma concentrations [24].

In reality, routinely applying pre-prescription PGx tests needs adequate infrastructure. Collaboration among researchers from various health sectors, ongoing updates, and engagement with manufacturing firms are essential. Additionally, consolidating all clinically relevant variants onto a single platform facilitates processing in an efficient way in Clinical Laboratory Improvement Amendments (CLIA)-certified laboratories [21].

9.3 Obesity

Obesity is a major risk factor for the development of various endocrine disorders, including type 2 diabetes, cardiovascular disease, and certain cancers. The prevalence of obesity has reached alarming levels globally, necessitating effective management strategies [32, 33]. Personalized medicine can aid in the identification of personalized treatment approaches for obesity by considering factors such as body fat distribution and individual health risks [34].

9.3.1 Obesity Diagnosis and Classification

Traditionally, obesity classification is based on body mass index (BMI). All obese people have excess body fat, but there is significant heterogeneity within this population. Therefore, anthropometric obesity classification has limitations in guiding clinical decisions for patients. Research over the past decades has generated new insights that have led to the identification of different subtypes of obese patients.

These classifications provided important information about the underlying pathophysiological mechanisms that cause obesity and its complications and helped pave the way to accurate obesity medicine.

9.3.1.1 BMI and Waist Circumference

Individuals with obesity are traditionally identified by measuring BMI and waist circumference. Using BMI, people are classified from overweight to morbid obesity. Waist circumference is recommended to be considered because central obesity increases the risk of complications like cardiovascular diseases. Although the present classification is widely used, it does not consider several factors that contribute to obesity [34, 35].

9.3.1.2 The Edmonton Obesity Staging System (EOSS)

The EOSS system takes into account metabolic, physical, and psychological factors and how these affect patients' health and treatment options. This system helps have a more individualized approach to obesity and is a better mortality predictor than BMI [36].

9.3.1.3 Genetics

Genetic variants cause only 5% of obesity cases, and these cases can either be monogenic or polygenic. While only a single mutation causes monogenic obesity, polygenic obesity is a result of the interplay between multiple loci. Monogenic obesity is the rare type with a severe early onset and is caused by mutations in genes of the leptin/melanocortin axis involved in food intake regulation (genes encoding for leptin [LEP] and leptin receptor [LEPR], proopiomelanocortin [POMC], proconvertase 1 [PC1]) or in specific genes linked to these pathways. Although targeted therapy plays an important role in the treatment of monogenic obesity, this type is usually not considered in diagnosis and therefore underdiagnosed [37].

9.3.1.4 Obesity Personalized Medicine Initiatives

Genetic and environmental factors influence the two main processes that lead to obesity: calorie intake and physical activity levels. Genetic variants cannot alone explain the obesity epidemic; these days, high-resolution biotechnologies have aided in the characterization of additional biologic variants that may offer a detailed fingerprint of an individual's phenotype and how they might react to various anti-obesity treatments. These variants include transcripts, proteins, metabolites, microbiota, and epigenetic markers. This information can significantly enhance obesity prediction, prevention, and therapy. We have outlined below the potential targets for these biologic variations in order to treat obesity on an individual basis [34].

9.3.1.5 Phenotypes

One approach of personalized medicine has been focusing on pathophysiologic processes that cause energy balance dysregulation and result in excessive storage of calories. Energy balance relies on energy expenditure and energy intake that each have determinants that determines regulation or dysregulation of these two processes. Determinants of the energy expenditure are resting energy expenditure (REE), non-exercise physical activity, the thermogenic effect of food, and exercise. As for the energy intake, its determinants are the homeostatic and hedonic drives to eat. These aspects are quantitative and could be measured. Quantifying these has enabled researchers to identify different gastrointestinal and behavioral traits in obese individuals compared to people with normal weight which include a higher fasting gastric volume for both solids and liquids, accelerated gastric emptying for solids and liquids, a higher volume and/or calories to reach fullness, higher anxiety and depression scores, and lower body image satisfaction. These traits have been utilized to identify four different phenotypes: abnormal satiation associated with abnormal hypothalamic brain perfusion, abnormal satiety associated with intestinal enteroendocrine cell dysfunction, abnormal emotional eating characterized by uncontrolled hedonic eating and associated with abnormal nucleus accumbens perfusion, and abnormal resting energy expenditure associated with decreased REE by indirect calorimetry.

9.3.1.6 Epigenetics

Epigenetics refers to gene activity alteration with modification of nucleotide sequence. Epigenetic changes can be reversed as environmental interventions result in switching on or off the genes. Studies have shown that epigenetic modifications, e.g., mainly DNA methylation, histone modifications, and noncoding RNAs, can provide explanation for the alterations in physiological and pathological processes and contribute to obesity. Discoveries of potential epigenetic biomarkers associated with obesity have proved the potentials effect of epigenetics on obesity. Furthermore, epigenetic profiling is available, thanks to inexpensive microarrays. However, further studies need to be conducted to fully understand the role of epigenetic in obesity [38].

9.3.1.7 Metabolomics

Metabolomics aims to analyze metabolites in biological samples, in qualitative and quantitative ways [39]. By the help of this tool, we can identify changes in the profiles and levels of low molecular weight metabolites (<1500 Da) in cells, tissues, organs, systems, or whole organisms in response to a genetic variation or physiological or pathological condition [40]. So, considering obesity, this tool can be used to detect changes in metabolites at cellular and body fluid levels. There has been a growing attention to metabolomics, and several studies have been conducted to evaluate the association of changes in metabolite profile and obesity. For example, the levels of leucine, isoleucine, valine (branched-chain amino acids), tyrosine, tryptophan, methionine, phenylalanine (aromatic amino acids), and their metabolites have been detected to rise in obese patients. In comparison, the levels of glutamine and glycine are decreased. The metabolites that increase or decrease in obesity could serve as biomarkers of pathophysiological processes of obesity. Therefore, they could be used to screen individuals or to inform about the prognosis of obesity. Moreover, previous studies suggest some metabolomic patterns of obesity are associated with increased risk of comorbid diseases like cardiovascular diseases and type 2 diabetes. However, there are still deficiencies in metabolomic studies, and there need to be further studies to better understand the association of metabolomic signatures and obesity [41].

9.3.1.8 Microbiome

Human gut microbiota is the community of microorganisms in human digestive tracts that consists of trillion microorganisms, and its function in the digestive tracts is microbiome. Gut microbiota and microbiome are under the influence of internal (e.g., genetics) and external (e.g., diet, exercise) factors. As for obesity, researchers have investigated the association between microbiota and this disease and have identified some difference of microbiota composition in obese patients compared to normal-weight people. For example, in obese subjects' gut, there is an increase in short-chain fatty acid-producing bacteria, such as *Roseburia intestinalis* and *Eubacterium ventriosum*, and a decrease in glutamate-fermenting bacteria, such as *Bacteroides thetaiotaomicron* [42].

The mentioned difference affects the metabolic profile of individuals. For instance, the intestinal microbiota contributes to metabolism of bile acids and transforming them to secondary ones. Secondary bile acids increase the production of GLP-1, a hormone that modulates glucose homeostasis and energy metabolism. As the enzymatic action of microbiota is changed in obesity, the composition of bile acids changes (the proportion of secondary bile acids decreases). This results in lower GLP-1 and insulin resistance in obese patients. Considering the role of microbiome in metabolic processes, some studies suggest microbiome manipulation by consuming probiotics and fecal microbiota transplantation could result in the treatment of obesity [34]. Nevertheless, the efficacy of the mentioned interventions has not been fully investigated.

9.3.2 *Treatment*

Weight loss is a key component of obesity management, and it has been shown to reduce the risk of obesity-related diseases in a dose-related manner. Various weight loss interventions, including lifestyle modification programs, diets, exercise programs, medications, and surgery, have been found to be effective [35]. However, weight regain is expected in all patients, highlighting the need for long-term management strategies [43]. Personalized medicine can help tailor these interventions to individual patients, taking into account their unique characteristics and needs.

9.3.2.1 Individualized Obesity Treatments

There is a hypothesis that anti-obesity medications could be used in a targeted way to treat obese people with different phenotypes. For example, patients with abnormal satiation phenotype could benefit from phentermine–topiramate that modulates the adrenergic and GABAergic pathways resulting in satiation. Furthermore, those patients that have abnormal emotional hunger phenotype could benefit from naltrexone/bupropion sustained release, a medication that modulates the dopamine and opioid pathways. A large real-world study reported that after 12 months of phenotype-guided treatment, 79% of patients lost >10% compared to 34% of patients who were in the non-phenotype-guided treatment. Therefore, more studies should be conducted to fully understand the benefits of phenotype-based treatment in obese patients, and physicians should be informed to utilize this approach [44].

9.3.2.2 Individualized Treatment of Monogenic Obesity

The most successful role of targeted therapy is in the treatment of monogenic diabetes. For example, for the obese cases with variants of *LEPR* gene or its receptor, recombinant leptin has been a successful treatment. Similarly, setmelanotide (a melanocortin 4 receptor agonist) is approved for the treatment of obesity due to mutations in proopiomelanocortin (POMC), proprotein convertase subtilisin/kexin type 1 (PCSK1), or LEPR confirmed by genetic testing [44–46].

9.4 Endocrine Cancers

In the field of endocrine cancers, personalized medicine has made progress in the evaluation and treatment of these cancers in recent years. This approach has been particularly successful in the field of oncology, where it has improved cancer screening and treatment by identifying genetic mutations and choosing a treatment considering them. Targeted therapies that target specific molecular pathways have been introduced that are helpful in patients that become refractory to certain treatments or have deficiencies in metabolic pathways due to genetic alterations [47]. Therefore, it has remarkably contributed in improving patient outcomes and reducing the burden of endocrine cancers [48].

Endocrine cancers pose significant challenges in terms of diagnosis and treatment with thyroid cancer being the most common endocrine cancer [49]. Since the impact of personalized medicine in the management of thyroid cancer has been widely studied, we will explore its role in thyroid cancer, focusing on the use of molecular epidemiology, theranostic radioiodine, and predictive markers of endocrine therapy response. By understanding the molecular characteristics of these cancers and utilizing advanced diagnostic and therapeutic techniques, personalized medicine opens new avenues for more effective and targeted management of thyroid cancer [48]. This section provides a summary of the role played by personalized medicine in three types of thyroid cancer: differentiated, medullary, and anaplastic.

9.4.1 Differentiated Thyroid Cancer

Differentiated thyroid cancer (DTC), which includes papillary thyroid cancer (PTC) and follicular thyroid cancer, is the most common type of thyroid cancer, and accurate evaluation is crucial for appropriate management and treatment decisions. Molecular testing, such as cytomolecular testing, has been developed to improve the accuracy of fine-needle aspiration (FNA) biopsies in distinguishing between benign and malignant thyroid nodules. By molecular testing, specific gene mutations associated with thyroid cancer can be identified. This could help confirm malignancy when mutation is present and provide reassurance when malignancy is absent [50]. One of the most well-known variants in DTC is the c.T1799A *BRAF* variant, which occurs exclusively in PTC. This variant serves as a specific diagnostic marker for PTC when identified in cytological and histological specimens [51]. However, there is presently no molecular test that can definitively rule in or rule out malignancy because there is a lack of outcome data on using molecular testing [52].

Molecular testing has not only improved the accuracy of thyroid nodule evaluation but also enhanced our understanding of thyroid nodule formation and progression. By identifying specific gene variants, cytomolecular testing can guide the need for and extent of thyroid surgery in the setting of indeterminate thyroid nodules [50]. This can lead to improved patient care and more personalized treatment plans. The c.T1799A *BRAF* variant, in particular, has been shown to have prognostic value in the risk evaluation of thyroid cancer. It is associated with a poorer clinicopathological outcome and serves as an independent molecular prognostic marker [51]. Presently, mortality risk assessment systems do not consider molecular testing. As several studies have evaluated the impact of different markers in disease progression and recurrence, molecular markers might be used in risk stratification of thyroid cancer in the future.

Furthermore, additional diagnostic molecular marker strategies are also under development. Specifically, mRNA markers, as well as miRNA markers, have shown initial diagnostic utility in FNA samples with indeterminate cytological diagnoses, but they have not been thoroughly validated [52].

Personalized medicine in the management of DTC also involves the use of theranostic approaches. Theranostic combines diagnostic and therapeutic modalities to provide personalized treatment options based on individual patient characteristics. In the context of DTC, theranostic radioiodine molecular imaging has shown promise in guiding treatment decisions and predicting response to therapy [53]. This approach involves the use of molecular imaging techniques, such as positron emission tomography (PET), to assess the expression of specific molecular targets in DTC cells and determine the suitability of radioiodine therapy [54].

One of the key aspects of personalized medicine in the management and treatment of DTC is the use of radioiodine (I-131) therapy. Radioiodine therapy is a well-established and effective treatment option for DTC, particularly for patients with high-risk features or residual disease after initial surgery [55]. RAI takes advantage of the expression of the sodium-iodide symporter (NIS) in thyroid cells, which allows the uptake of radioactive iodine. This therapy has been used for more than eight decades and is still being used to eliminate remnants after thyroid surgery and treat tumor metastases [56].

Moreover, previous studies have suggested that intratumoral heterogeneity contributes to resistance to therapies and poor prognosis. Therefore, considering intratumoral phenotypic and molecular heterogeneity can help characterize thyroid cancer pathogenesis, guide effective treatment, and improve survival [57].

In addition to molecular imaging, artificial intelligence (AI) has emerged as a promising tool in personalized medicine for thyroid cancer. AI algorithms can analyze large amounts of patient data and assist in risk stratification and treatment decision-making. By integrating AI with molecular imaging techniques, clinicians can obtain a more comprehensive and accurate assessment of the disease, leading to improved personalized treatment strategies [58].

Only less than 5% of all cases, but 60–70% of metastatic DTC, lose the ability to uptake and concentrate RAI and to produce thyroglobulin (Tg), becoming RAI refractory (RR)-DTC [59]. The understanding of the molecular pathogenesis of thyroid cancer has improved with the discovery of new biomarkers, allowing for more personalized treatments. Targeted therapies have been developed to inhibit the known oncogenic mechanisms involved in thyroid cancer initiation and progression, such as the MAPK pathway, PI3K/Akt-mTOR pathways, and vascular endothelial growth factor (VEGF) [60]. These targeted therapies aim to specifically target the dysregulated pathways in thyroid cancer cells, providing a more tailored approach to treatment.

In addition to targeted therapies and immunotherapy, other treatment modalities are being explored for RAI-refractory thyroid cancer. These include kinase inhibitors, angiogenesis inhibitors, and combination therapies [61]. The goal is to develop personalized treatment strategies that take into account the specific genetic alterations and dysregulated pathways in each patient's tumor. Nowadays, sorafenib and lenvatinib are the only multi-kinase inhibitors (MKIs) which have received approval for the treatment of patients with progressive RR-DTC. Unfortunately, MKI treatment is burdened with important adverse effects, potentially affecting patients' quality of life. Thus, evaluating the risk–benefit ratio is mandatory before starting treatment [59].

9.4.2 Medullary Thyroid Cancer

Medullary thyroid cancer (MTC) is a type of thyroid cancer that arises from the neural crest-derived C-cells. It can occur sporadically or as part of a genetic or familial condition, such as multiple endocrine neoplasia (MEN) 2A and 2B. The RET proto-oncogene is important for the diagnosis of MTC, including screening for hereditary MTC [62, 63]. Activating germline variants in the RET proto-oncogene are responsible for hereditary MTC syndromes. Evaluating the specific RET variants associated with hereditary MTC enables clinicians to treat patients based on their level of risk [64]. Genetic screening can identify individuals at risk for hereditary MTC, allowing for early detection and prophylactic thyroidectomy to prevent the development of MTC [65]. Therefore, the American Thyroid Association (ATA) has recommended screening for hereditary MTC in individuals that have RET germline mutation in their family [63].

Total thyroidectomy is the standard treatment for patients with sporadic or hereditary MTC. However, patients are occasionally diagnosed with MTC following a unilateral hemithyroidectomy. In these patients, total thyroidectomy following hemithyroidectomy is not indicated unless the patient has a RET germline variant.

Furthermore, targeted therapies have shown efficacy in the treatment of MTC. Selective RET inhibitors have demonstrated effectiveness in the treatment of MTC with limited systemic toxicity compared to non-specific tyrosine kinase inhibitors. These targeted therapies specifically inhibit the abnormal signaling pathways associated with MTC, leading to improved outcomes for patients [66].

9.4.3 Anaplastic Thyroid Cancer

Anaplastic thyroid cancer (ATC), also known as undifferentiated thyroid cancer, is a subtype of thyroid cancer that is characterized by the loss of differentiation and aggressive behavior. Genetic analysis helps in understanding the underlying molecular mechanisms and identifying potential therapeutic targets. However, none of the genetic alterations found in ATC are specific for ATC and therfore are not sufficient to diagnose ATC [63].

One of the key molecular alterations associated with the development of poorly differentiated thyroid tumors, including ATC, is the loss of the p53 tumor suppressor gene. The loss of p53 function can lead to uncontrolled cell growth and division, contributing to the aggressive nature of ATC. Genetic analysis can detect variants in the p53 gene, providing valuable information for the management of ATC [67].

In addition to p53, other genetic alterations have been associated with the progression from well-differentiated to undifferentiated thyroid carcinomas. Distinct molecular alterations have been identified at specific stages of follicular cell carcinogenesis, driving the transformation from well-differentiated to undifferentiated thyroid cancer. These molecular alterations can be detected through genetic analysis, such as the analysis of proto-oncogene proteins C-RET and B-RAF [68]. Understanding these genetic alterations can help in the classification and prognosis of ATC, as well as guide targeted therapies.

Furthermore, the concept of cancer stem-like cells has been proposed in the development of ATC. According to this theory, a small subpopulation of stem cells undergoes genetic and epigenetic transformations, giving rise to phenotypically different cancer cells [68]. Genetic analysis can help in identifying these stem cells and understanding the mechanisms by which they contribute to the development and progression of ATC.

Undifferentiated thyroid cancer is resistant to conventional treatments such as surgery, radioiodine therapy, and chemotherapy. However, targeted therapy has emerged as a promising approach for the treatment of ATC [67]. Among ATCs, *BRAF* p.V600E is the most commonly encountered productively actionable variant, seen in 50–70% of cases. When PTC coexists in the pathology specimen with ATC, over 90% may harbor a *BRAF* p.V600E variant. In 2018, the BRAF/MEK inhibitor combination,[2] dabrafenib plus trametinib, was approved by the U.S. FDA for ATC patients harboring a *BRAF* p.V600E (but not other) variant. BRAF-directed therapy can induce prompt and impressive tumor regression in these patients, and therefore the use of these drugs in stage IVC patients is recommended in *BRAF* p.V600E patients. In p.BRAF *V600E*-variant ATC patients with unresectable stage IVB disease, however, consideration of upfront chemoradiation is the present standard. Alternatively, when upfront chemoradiation may be contraindicated or not desired by the patient, systemic therapy with BRAF-directed therapy can be considered. Neoadjuvant use of dabrafenib plus trametinib is also being explored as a way to convert an unresectable primary tumor to a resectable one [69].

Another potential target for targeted therapy in undifferentiated thyroid cancer is the p53 family proteins, including p63 and p73. These proteins play a crucial role in regulating cell growth, differentiation, and apoptosis, and their dysregulation has been implicated in thyroid cancer progression. In recent years, there has been a growing understanding of the complex network of interactions among p53 family members and other factors involved in thyroid cancer progression. This knowledge has paved the way for the development of therapeutic strategies that target these proteins and their associated signaling pathways [67].

Multiple clinical trials have been conducted to evaluate the efficacy of multikinase inhibitors (MKIs) in the treatment of undifferentiated thyroid cancer. Sorafenib and lenvatinib are two MKIs that have been approved by the FDA and EMA for the treatment of undifferentiated thyroid cancer. These drugs target multiple kinases involved in tumor growth and angiogenesis, thereby inhibiting cancer cell proliferation and promoting tumor regression. In addition to MKIs, other targeted therapies such as SP600125, a reversible ATP-competitive MKI, have also shown promise in preclinical studies. Another targeted therapy that has been used for the treatment of undifferentiated thyroid cancer is radioiodine therapy (RAI) [56, 67].

[2] A MEK inhibitor is a chemical or drug that inhibits the mitogen-activated protein kinase kinase enzymes MEK1 and MEK2.

9.5 Conclusions

Personalized medicine is a strategy that optimizes the diagnosis, prevention, and treatment of endocrine disorders by considering factors like hormone profiles, genetic makeup, lifestyle, and environmental impacts. It is instrumental in diabetes, obesity, and endocrine malignancies. In diabetes, a personalized medicine approach involves identifying the risk of diabetes and its complications for tailoring preventive strategies and early interventions. Moreover, other personalized medicine approach in diabetes such as personalized blood glucose targets based on factors like age, comorbidities, and lifestyle, personalized lifestyle modification, and pharmacogenomic tests has a significant role in the precise prevention, diagnosis, and treatment strategies for better management of diabetes.

Personalized medicine in obesity considers genetic, environmental, and lifestyle factors to create more effective and sustainable interventions. These factors include genetic predisposition, metabolic profiling, lifestyle interventions, selecting the strategy for treatment, gut microbiome analysis, and psychosocial factors. By considering the multifaceted nature of obesity and tailoring interventions to individual characteristics, personalized medicine aims to improve the effectiveness of weight management strategies and promote long-term success in achieving and maintaining a healthy weight.

In endocrine cancer, personalized medicine has a major role in the diagnosis and treatment of thyroid cancer. Personalized medicine in thyroid cancer involves tailoring diagnostic and treatment strategies to each individual's specific thyroid cancer characteristics. Thyroid cancer is a diverse group of malignancies, and personalized approaches take into consideration factors such as the type of thyroid cancer, genetic mutations, tumor characteristics, and individual patient factors. It aims to improve treatment outcomes by tailoring interventions to the specific characteristics of the individual's cancer and considering their overall health and preferences. As our understanding of the molecular and genetic basis of thyroid cancer advances, the implementation of personalized approaches is likely to become more refined and effective.

References

1. Crafa A, Calogero AE, Cannarella R, Mongioi LM, Condorelli RA, Greco EA, et al. The burden of hormonal disorders: a worldwide overview with a particular look in Italy. Front Endocrinol (Lausanne). 2021;12:694325.
2. Shriraam V, Mahadevan S, Anitharani M, Sathiyasekaran BWC. National health programs in the field of endocrinology and metabolism – miles to go. Indian J Endocrinol Metab. 2014;18(1):7–12.
3. Bidlingmaier M, Gleeson H, Latronico AC, Savage MO. Applying precision medicine to the diagnosis and management of endocrine disorders. Endocr Connect. 2022;11(10)
4. https://diabetesatlas.org/.
5. Magliano DJ, Boyko EJ. IDF diabetes atlas. 2022.

6. Scheen AJ. Precision medicine: the future in diabetes care? Diabetes Res Clin Pract. 2016;117:12–21.
7. Nolan JJ, Kahkoska AR, Semnani-Azad Z, Hivert M-F, Ji L, Mohan V, et al. ADA/EASD precision medicine in diabetes initiative: an international perspective and future vision for precision medicine in diabetes. Diabetes Care. 2022;45(2):261.
8. Klonoff DC. Precision medicine for managing diabetes. Los Angeles: SAGE Publications; 2015. p. 3–7.
9. Zhang H, Colclough K, Gloyn AL, Pollin TI. Monogenic diabetes: a gateway to precision medicine in diabetes. J Clin Invest. 2021;131(3)
10. Kleinberger JW, Pollin TI. Personalized medicine in diabetes mellitus: current opportunities and future prospects. Ann N Y Acad Sci. 2015;1346(1):45–56.
11. Carr AL, Evans-Molina C, Oram RA. Precision medicine in type 1 diabetes. Diabetologia. 2022;65(11):1854–66.
12. Choi SW, Mak TS-H, O'Reilly PF. Tutorial: a guide to performing polygenic risk score analyses. Nat Protoc. 2020;15(9):2759–72.
13. Laakso M, Fernandes SL. Genetics of type 2 diabetes: past, present, and future. Nutrients. 2022;14(15):3201.
14. Prasad RB, Groop L. Precision medicine in type 2 diabetes. J Intern Med. 2019;285(1):40–8.
15. Prasad RB, Groop L. Genetics of type 2 diabetes – pitfalls and possibilities. Genes. 2015;6(1):87–123.
16. Grarup N, Sandholt CH, Hansen T, Pedersen O. Genetic susceptibility to type 2 diabetes and obesity: from genome-wide association studies to rare variants and beyond. Diabetologia. 2014;57:1528–41.
17. Merino J, Udler MS, Leong A, Meigs JB. A decade of genetic and metabolomic contributions to type 2 diabetes risk prediction. Curr Diab Rep. 2017;17(12):135.
18. Nkonge KM, Nkonge DK, Nkonge TN. The epidemiology, molecular pathogenesis, diagnosis, and treatment of maturity-onset diabetes of the young (MODY). Clin Diabetes Endocrinol. 2020;6(1):1–10.
19. Aarthy R, Aston-Mourney K, Mikocka-Walus A, Radha V, Amutha A, Anjana RM, et al. Clinical features, complications and treatment of rarer forms of maturity-onset diabetes of the young (MODY)-a review. J Diabetes Complicat. 2021;35(1):107640.
20. Zeng Z, Huang S-Y, Sun T. Pharmacogenomic studies of current antidiabetic agents and potential new drug targets for precision medicine of diabetes. Diabetes Therapy. 2020;11:2521–38.
21. Huang C, Florez JC. Pharmacogenetics in type 2 diabetes: potential implications for clinical practice. Genome Med. 2011;3:1–9.
22. Nasykhova YA, Tonyan ZN, Mikhailova AA, Danilova MM, Glotov AS. Pharmacogenetics of type 2 diabetes – progress and prospects. Int J Mol Sci. 2020;21(18):6842.
23. Pearson ER. Diabetes: is there a future for pharmacogenomics guided treatment? Clin Pharmacol Ther. 2019;106(2):329–37.
24. Venkatachalapathy P, Padhilahouse S, Sellappan M, Subramanian T, Kurian SJ, Miraj SS, et al. Pharmacogenomics and personalized medicine in type 2 diabetes mellitus: potential implications for clinical practice. Pharm Personal Med. 2021;Volume 14:1441–55.
25. Hou W, Zhang D, Lu W, Zheng T, Wan L, Li Q, et al. Polymorphism of organic cation transporter 2 improves glucose-lowering effect of metformin via influencing its pharmacokinetics in Chinese type 2 diabetic patients. Mol Diagn Ther. 2015;19:25–33.
26. Moeez S, Khalid Z, Jalil F, Irfan M, Ismail M, Arif MA, et al. Effects of SLC22A2 (rs201919874) and SLC47A2 (rs138244461) genetic variants on metformin pharmacokinetics in Pakistani T2DM patients. JPMA. 2019;69(2):155–63.
27. Moeez S, Riaz S, Masood N, Kanwal N, Arif MA, Niazi R, et al. Evaluation of the rs3088442 G> a SLC22A3 gene polymorphism and the role of microRNA 147 in groups of adult Pakistani populations with type 2 diabetes in response to metformin. Can J Diabetes. 2019;43(2):128–35.
28. Al-Eitan LN, Almomani BA, Nassar AM, Elsaqa BZ, Saadeh NA. Metformin pharmacogenetics: effects of SLC22A1, SLC22A2, and SLC22A3 polymorphisms on glycemic control and HbA1c levels. J Personal Med. 2019;9(1):17.

29. Tzvetkov MV, Vormfelde SV, Balen D, Meineke I, Schmidt T, Sehrt D, et al. The effects of genetic polymorphisms in the organic cation transporters OCT1, OCT2, and OCT3 on the renal clearance of metformin. Clin Pharmacol Ther. 2009;86(3):299–306.
30. Meybodi HRA, Hasanzad M, Larijani B. Path to personalized medicine for type 2 diabetes mellitus: reality and hope. Acta Med Iran. 2017:166–74.
31. Andrulionytè L, Zacharova J, Chiasson J-L, Laakso M. Common polymorphisms of the PPAR-? 2 (Pro12Ala) and PGC-1a (Gly482Ser) genes are associated with the conversion from impaired glucose tolerance to type 2 diabetes in the STOP-NIDDM trial. Diabetologia. 2004;47(12):2176.
32. Sarmiento-Andrade Y, Suárez R, Quintero B, Garrochamba K, Chapela SP. Gut microbiota and obesity: new insights. Front Nutr. 2022;9:1018212.
33. World Health Organization. Obesity and overweight. 2021.
34. Hurtado AMD, Acosta A. Precision medicine and obesity. Gastroenterol Clin N Am. 2021;50(1):127–39.
35. Jensen MD, Ryan DH, Apovian CM, Ard JD, Comuzzie AG, Donato KA, et al. 2013 AHA/ACC/TOS guideline for the management of overweight and obesity in adults: a report of the American College of Cardiology/American Heart Association task force on practice guidelines and the obesity society. Circulation. 2014;129(25 Suppl 2):S102–38.
36. Sharma AM, Kushner RF. A proposed clinical staging system for obesity. Int J Obes. 2009;33(3):289–95.
37. Huvenne H, Dubern B, Clément K, Poitou C. Rare genetic forms of obesity: clinical approach and current treatments in 2016. Obes Facts. 2016;9(3):158–73.
38. Wu F-Y, Yin R-X. Recent progress in epigenetics of obesity. Diabetol Metab Syndr. 2022;14(1):171.
39. Clish CB. Metabolomics: an emerging but powerful tool for precision medicine. Cold Spring Harb Mol Case Stud. 2015;1(1):a000588.
40. Gibney MJ, Walsh M, Brennan L, Roche HM, German B, van Ommen B. Metabolomics in human nutrition: opportunities and challenges. Am J Clin Nutr. 2005;82(3):497–503.
41. Rangel-Huerta OD, Pastor-Villaescusa B, Gil A. Are we close to defining a metabolomic signature of human obesity? A systematic review of metabolomics studies. Metabolomics. 2019;15(6):93.
42. Cifuentes L, Hurtado AM, Eckel-Passow J, Acosta A. Precision medicine for obesity. Dig Dis Interv. 2021;5(3):239–48.
43. Bray GA, Heisel WE, Afshin A, Jensen MD, Dietz WH, Long M, et al. The science of obesity management: an endocrine society scientific statement. Endocr Rev. 2018;39(2):79–132.
44. Sacoto D, Hurtado MD, Acosta A. Precision medicine and obesity. Handb Exp Pharmacol. 2022;274:467–85.
45. Hocking S, Sumithran P. Individualised prescription of medications for treatment of obesity in adults. Rev Endocr Metab Disord. 2023;24(5):951–60.
46. Clément K, van den Akker E, Argente J, Bahm A, Chung WK, Connors H, et al. Efficacy and safety of setmelanotide, an MC4R agonist, in individuals with severe obesity due to LEPR or POMC deficiency: single-arm, open-label, multicentre, phase 3 trials. Lancet Diabetes Endocrinol. 2020;8(12):960–70.
47. Khatami F, Larijani B, Nikfar S, Hasanzad M, Fendereski K, Tavangar SM. Personalized treatment options for thyroid cancer: current perspectives. Pharmgenomics Pers Med. 2019;12:235–45.
48. Ronchi CL, Altieri B. Special issue: present and future of personalised medicine for endocrine cancers. J Pers Med. 2022;12(5)
49. Nguyen QT, Lee EJ, Huang MG, Park YI, Khullar A, Plodkowski RA. Diagnosis and treatment of patients with thyroid cancer. Am Health Drug Benefits. 2015;8(1):30–40.
50. Roth MY, Witt RL, Steward DL. Molecular testing for thyroid nodules: review and current state. Cancer. 2018;124(5):888–98.
51. Xing M. BRAF mutation in thyroid cancer. Endocr Relat Cancer. 2005;12(2):245–62.

52. Haugen BR, Alexander EK, Bible KC, Doherty GM, Mandel SJ, Nikiforov YE, et al. 2015 American Thyroid Association management guidelines for adult patients with thyroid nodules and differentiated thyroid cancer: the American Thyroid Association guidelines task force on thyroid nodules and differentiated thyroid cancer. Thyroid. 2016;26(1):1–133.
53. Ahn B-C. Personalized medicine based on Theranostic radioiodine molecular imaging for differentiated thyroid cancer. Biomed Res Int. 2016;2016:1680464.
54. Giovanella L, Deandreis D, Vrachimis A, Campenni A, Petranovic OP. Molecular imaging and Theragnostics of thyroid cancers. Cancers (Basel). 2022;14(5)
55. Tuttle RM, Ahuja S, Avram AM, Bernet VJ, Bourguet P, Daniels GH, et al. Controversies, consensus, and collaboration in the use of (131)I therapy in differentiated thyroid cancer: a joint statement from the American Thyroid Association, the European Association of Nuclear Medicine, the Society of Nuclear Medicine and Molecular Imaging, and the European thyroid association. Thyroid. 2019;29(4):461–70.
56. De la Vieja A, Riesco-Eizaguirre G. Radio-iodide treatment: from molecular aspects to the clinical view. Cancers (Basel). 2021;13(5)
57. Ieni A, Vita R, Pizzimenti C, Benvenga S, Tuccari G. Intratumoral heterogeneity in differentiated thyroid tumors: an intriguing reappraisal in the era of personalized medicine. J Pers Med. 2021;11(5)
58. Li L-R, Du B, Liu H-Q, Chen C. Artificial intelligence for personalized medicine in thyroid cancer: current status and future perspectives. Front Oncol. 2021:10.
59. Feola T, Cozzolino A, Centello R, Pandozzi C, Tarsitano MG, Giannetta E. Predictors of response and survival to multikinase inhibitors in radioiodine resistant differentiated thyroid cancer. J Pers Med. 2021;11(7)
60. Laha D, Nilubol N, Boufraqech M. New therapies for advanced thyroid cancer. Front Endocrinol. 2020;11
61. Kim TY, Kim WG, Kim WB, Shong YK. Current status and future perspectives in differentiated thyroid cancer. Endocrinol Metab (Seoul). 2014;29(3):217–25.
62. Segura S, Ramos-Rivera G, Suhrland M. Educational case: endocrine neoplasm: medullary thyroid carcinoma. Acad Pathol. 2018;5:2374289518775722.
63. Wells SA Jr, Asa SL, Dralle H, Elisei R, Evans DB, Gagel RF, et al. Revised American Thyroid Association guidelines for the management of medullary thyroid carcinoma. Thyroid. 2015;25(6):567–610.
64. Ogilvie JB, Kebebew E. Indication and timing of thyroid surgery for patients with hereditary medullary thyroid cancer syndromes. J Natl Compr Cancer Netw. 2006;4(2):139–47.
65. Rosenthal MS, Diekema DS. Pediatric ethics guidelines for hereditary medullary thyroid cancer. Int J Pediatr Endocrinol. 2011;2011(1):847603.
66. Araque KA, Gubbi S, Klubo-Gwiezdzinska J. Updates on the management of thyroid cancer. Horm Metab Res. 2020;52(08):562–77.
67. Manzella L, Stella S, Pennisi MS, Tirrò E, Massimino M, Romano C, et al. New insights in thyroid cancer and p53 family proteins. Int J Mol Sci. 2017;18(6)
68. Prete A, Borges de Souza P, Censi S, Muzza M, Nucci N, Sponziello M. Update on fundamental mechanisms of thyroid cancer. Front Endocrinol. 2020:11.
69. Bible KC, Kebebew E, Brierley J, Brito JP, Cabanillas ME, Clark TJ Jr, et al. 2021 American Thyroid Association guidelines for management of patients with anaplastic thyroid cancer. Thyroid. 2021;31(3):337–86.

Chapter 10
Traditional Medicine and Endocrinology

Mohammad Sadegh Adel-Mehraban, Narges Lavari, Zahra Aghabeiglooei, Niusha Esmaealzadeh, and Ozra Tabatabaei-Malazy

10.1 Introduction

Noncommunicable diseases (NCDs) consisting of high blood pressure, central obesity, diabetes, metabolic syndrome (MetS), dyslipidemia, and osteoporosis are the most common endocrinology problems in general population that have high

M. S. Adel-Mehraban
Department of Traditional Medicine, School of Persian medicine, Tehran University of Medical Sciences, Tehran, Iran

Traditional Persian Medicine and Complementary Medicine (PerCoMed) Student Association, Students' Scientific Research Center, Tehran University of Medical Sciences, Tehran, Iran
e-mail: sadeghadel@gmail.com

N. Lavari
The Persian Gulf Tropical Medicine Research Center, The Persian Gulf Biomedical Sciences Research Institute, Bushehr University of Medical Sciences, Bushehr, Iran
e-mail: narges.lavari@yahoo.com

Z. Aghabeiglooei
Department of Traditional Medicine, School of Persian Medicine, Shahed University, Tehran, Iran
e-mail: aghabeiglooei@gmail.com

N. Esmaealzadeh
Department of Traditional Medicine, School of Persian medicine, Tehran University of Medical Sciences, Tehran, Iran
e-mail: niushaesmaealzadeh@yahoo.com

O. Tabatabaei-Malazy (✉)
Non-Communicable Diseases Research Center, Endocrinology and Metabolism Population Sciences Institute, Tehran University of Medical Sciences, Tehran, Iran

Endocrinology and Metabolism Research Center, Endocrinology and Metabolism Clinical Sciences Institute, Tehran University of Medical Sciences, Tehran, Iran
e-mail: tabatabaeiml@sina.tums.ac.ir

H. Gharib et al. (eds.), *Interdisciplinary Advances in Endocrinology*,
https://doi.org/10.1007/978-981-95-2286-6_10

economic cost and burden and also can increase the risk of mortality [1, 2]. On the other hand, polycystic ovary syndrome (PCOS) is defined as clinical manifestations of ovarian dysfunction and elevated level of androgens that in the long term may lead to endometriosis, high blood pressure, hyperlipidemia, MetS, cardiovascular disease (CVD), infertility, and psychological problems [2]. It is known MetS and PCOS are responsible for more than 30% of adult health issues, worldwide [3]. Management of MetS requires tremendous changes in lifestyle and behaviors which is poorly accepted by patients. Moreover, although there are numerous pharmacological treatments for the management of abovementioned disorders, concern about the adverse effects of present medicines still remains [4]. For instance, the basic treatment of dyslipidemia is statins, whereas, besides myopathy, they multiply the risk of diabetes [5]. As well, despite the use of hypoglycemic agents, even exogenous insulin, long-term vascular adverse events of diabetes (nephropathy, retinopathy, and neuropathy) are avoidable [6] that results in a growing tendency to use complementary treatments such as herbal medicines [1]. For example, *Crocus sativus Linn*, known as saffron, with its bioactive components such as crocetin, crocin, and *safranal*, is a famous medicinal plant in both traditional and conventional medicine. A recent study showed that saffron improves diabetes and insulin resistance, hyperlipidemia, hypertension, and overweight as well as modulates inflammatory condition and oxidative stress [7]. Another example is grape, *Vitis vinifera L.*, that contains high amounts of polyphenols such as flavonoids and flavanols and shows remarkable lipid-modifying, anti-inflammatory, anti-oxidant, and insulin-mimetic actions [8]. Furthermore, flaxseed with scientific name of *Linum usitatissimum L.* is rich in lignan, soluble fiber, and mucilage that slow down the gastric passage of foods and glucose absorption leading to protective effects on diabetes and diabetic complications [9]. Besides, herbal remedies used for PCOS or hyperprolactinemia such as flaxseed, soy isoflavones, *Vitex agnus-castus L.*, and other medicinal plants affect the number of germ cells, support folliculogenesis, reduce menstrual cramps, and improve serum level of prolactin, progesterone, and luteinizing hormone (LH). According to the emphasis of World Health Organization (WHO) on the complementary use of herbal treatments [10], in this chapter, we aimed to summarize high level of evidence of the herbal treatments in management of these metabolic disorders.

10.2 Herbal Medicines for Management of Diabetes

Diabetes mellitus (DM) is a metabolic disorder characterized by insulin malfunction, inadequate secretion, or resistance to insulin function which induced hyperglycemia [6]. By the year 2021, over 500 million patients have been diagnosed with diabetes, and it is estimated to reach about 643 million diabetic patients by 2030 [11]. Economic growth and urbanization have altered the lifestyle of individuals and resulted in increasing obesity, dyslipidemia, and diabetes [5]. Chronic hyperglycemia in poorly managed diabetic patients leads to progressive macro- and microvascular diseases such as cardiovascular symptoms, renal failure, atherosclerosis, retinopathy, and neuropathy and increases risk of sexual dysfunction, mental disorders, and gastrointestinal symptoms [6, 12]. Common synthetic drugs such as oral hypoglycemic medications or exogenous insulin and other drugs like statins are often useful in the management of different aspects of diabetes. Despite the beneficial effects, this combination imposes an economic burden on the health system (approximately 1 trillion dollars was spent by 2015 for medical costs of managing diabetes) [13]; side effects such as myopathy, dehydration, and headache and side effects of DM, nephropathy, retinopathy, and neuropathy still remain [5, 6, 12]. WHO informed that compared to synthetic drugs, most of the patients preferred alternative medicine, especially medicinal plants, for glycemic control because of fewer side effects and greater satisfaction [10, 14].

Comprehensive search in international web databases with keywords relevant to "diabetes," "insulin resistance," and "herb" shows that a large number of studies have been done to evaluate the effects of plant-derived products on hyperglycemia. Some of these studies are published as systematic review and meta-analysis studies that are known as the top level of evidence-based medicine. The details of these findings are described as follows:

10.2.1 Cinnamomum Cassia *(L.) J. Presl*

Cinnamon is obtained from the bark of *Cinnamomum verum* J. Presl, from the Lauraceae family, and is a worldwide popular spice [15]. Bark, leaf, and root of the cinnamon have been used in both traditional and Western medicines. Animal and clinical studies have indicated antimicrobial, antioxidant, anti-inflammatory, antihypertensive, antidiabetic, anti-obesity, anticancer, and antihyperlipidemic effects [15–17]. The main active components of cinnamon are volatile oils, coumarin, camphor, eugenol, cinnamate, cinnamaldehyde, cinnamyl acetate, cinnamic acid, and cinnamyl alcohol [15, 17]. Its polyphenolic compounds show anti-inflammatory activities by regulating serum level of interleukin (IL)-1, IL-6, C-reactive protein (CRP), and tumor necrosis factor (TNF)-a [18].

Systematic review and meta-analysis of Davis et al. showed that cinnamon significantly decreased fasting blood glucose (FBG) compared to control group [19]. Previous studies showed that cinnamon can improve insulin sensitivity and decline glycosylated hemoglobin (HbA1C) [20]. Furthermore, cinnamon enhances the process of adipose tissue browning by increasing uncoupling protein (UCP) 1 expression and mitochondrial protein biogenesis [21]. Cinnamon increases the production of glucose transporter 4 (GLUT4) in muscles and adipose tissues resulting in glucose uptake; promotes liver glycogen synthesis; inhibits gluconeogenesis, pancreatic α-amylase, and α-glucosidase; and affects insulin signaling pathways as an insulin mimetic [22].

Systematic review studies indicated that consuming 1–2 g/d of cinnamon for 3 months and up to 6 g/d for 4 months was safe; however, excessive amounts (beyond 6 grams daily) can lead to adverse effects, including potential harm to the liver, decreased blood sugar levels, and oral ulcers [23]. Also, taking high doses of cinnamon, which is more than the recommended dose, must be avoided two weeks before surgery. In topical use, it may cause allergic reaction or irritation. No sufficient data is available on pregnancy and breastfeeding. Cinnamon may interact with some drugs such as blood sugar-lowering medications, Benadryl (diphenhydramine), Crestor (rosuvastatin), Cymbalta (duloxetine), and aspirin. Due to its hypoglycemic effects, blood glucose close monitoring is needed while using other hypoglycemic agents [24]. It also has interaction with antihypertensive drugs. It can inhibit the enzyme CYP2A6 that potentially changes the metabolism of various drugs. Furthermore, high dose of cinnamon shows hepatotoxic effects, particularly in combination with drugs that have hepatic metabolism [25].

10.2.2 Camellia Sinensis (L.) Kuntze

Tea, the most commonly used beverage worldwide next to water, which is collected from leaves of the plant *Camellia sinensis* (L.) Kuntze, has been consumed as green, black, or oolong tea, depending on the fermentation: unfermented, partially fermented, and complete fermented, respectively [26]. The effects of green tea on hypercholesterolemia (HCL), prevention of some cancers, atherosclerosis, hyperglycemia, HbA1C, fasting insulin, obesity, and arthritis have been demonstrated [26–28]. Polyphenolic compounds, constituting approximately 30% of the dry weight of it, have a diverse range of physiological and pharmacological effects. Its main phytochemicals are catechins, i.e., epicatechin, catechin, epigallocatechin, epicatechin gallate, and EGCG, and black tea and oolong tea mainly contain theaflavins and thearubigins [27].

Green tea shows antidiabetic activities by means of its active components such as polyphenols that are attributed to scavenge free radicals and modulate oxidative stress. Recent studies indicated that green tea declines oxidative stress biomarkers, such as lipid peroxidase, and enhances antioxidants, such as superoxide dismutase and glutathione activities. Epigallocatechin gallate inhibits starch hydrolysis, restricts α-amylase and α-glucosidase activity, regulates glucose homeostasis, and restrains liver gluconeogenesis and lipogenesis [29]. Treatment with *C. sinensis* enhances glucose uptake and declines insulin resistance by means of increasing GLUT2, adipose tissue browning, and ameliorating TNF-α-induced insulin resistance [29]. Green tea increases insulin sensitivity, promotes insulin secretion, and improves lipid distribution by altering gene expression and hypermethylation of DNA related to glucose and lipid metabolism [30, 31]. Moreover, *C. sinensis* reduces diabetic complications such as heart disease, dyslipidemia, and neural tube defects [31].

The possible side effects of green tea are insomnia, vomiting, dizziness, hepatotoxicity, heart palpitations, diarrhea, anorexia, and dizziness. The National Center for Complementary and Integrative Health (NCCIH) states that green tea as a beverage or dietary supplement is promoted for improving mental alertness, relieving digestive symptoms and headaches, and promoting weight loss [32]. Overall, moderate intake of green tea (8 cups per day) seems to be safe [32]. Overindulging in green tea can result in various adverse effects, such as sleep disturbances, nausea, vomiting, diarrhea, headaches, dizziness, palpitations, elevated blood pressure, and, in rare instances, liver damage. An important consideration is that green tea supplements might contain elevated levels of catechins, which can heighten the likelihood of encountering these adverse reactions.

Research findings regarding safety of green tea consumption during pregnancy and breastfeeding are inconclusive. Studies suggest potential impacts on maternal inflammatory responses, offspring metabolism, lipid profiles, and kidney-related inflammation, especially with a protein-restricted maternal diet. Furthermore, there are concerns for substantial caffeine intake during these periods. In pregnancy, up to 6 cups per day (300 mg/d caffeine) is considered to be safe, and intake of more caffeine increases the rate of miscarriage and birth complications due to folic acid deficiency. While breastfeeding, intake of green tea must be limited to 2–3 cups per day because caffeine goes through breast milk and may cause irritability, sleep difficulties, and bowel problems in nursing infant. However, due to the limited data on the use of this plant in children, pregnancy, and breastfeeding, they should consume green tea with caution [33]. Green tea consumption should be monitored in anemia, anxiety, bleeding, heart conditions, diarrhea, seizure, glaucoma, hypertension, irritable bowel disease, liver disease, and osteoporosis. It is contraindicated in kidney problems, liver problems, and stomach ulcers. Green tea shows lots of major drug interactions; thus, abovementioned disorders must take care of its use [24]. Some medications including adenosine, beta-lactam, beta-blockers, benzodiazepines, monoamine oxidase inhibitors, quinolone antibiotics, clozapine, digoxin, atorvastatin, simvastatin, and chemotherapy agents have interactions with consumed green tea, potentially leading to reduced drug efficacy or increased drug toxicity. Patients who consume warfarin should not drink green tea or check the level of the international normalized ratio (INR) more frequently. Patients who take calcium channel blockers, sildenafil, or statins should avoid drinking green tea or consume it with caution [34].

10.2.3 Aloe Barbadensis Mill

Aloe vera is a perennial plant mostly famous for its leaves with two major parts: green outer rind and colorless inner gel-like parenchyma that have pharmacological and cosmetic applications. Different studies reported therapeutic effects on cancer, oxidative stress, asthma, glaucoma, skin disease, hyperlipidemia, and diabetes. *Aloe barbadensis* is composed of more than 70 constituents such as vitamins, minerals, fatty acids, hormones, and other components [35]. In meta-analysis study conducted by Dick et al. which pooled data of nine RCTs on diabetic patients, a significant reduction of FBG and HbA1C by *Aloe vera* gel powder, juice, or extract was reported [36] through increasing serum insulin, reducing resistance to insulin, improving pancreatic islets, and increasing liver gluconeogenesis [37]. *Aloe vera* prevents diabetic complications such as nephropathy, neuropathy, and depression by modulating oxidative stress (reducing reactive oxygen species [ROS] production). *Aloe barbadensis* polysaccharides prohibit apoptosis of pancreatic β-cells and endoplasmic reticulum stress [35]. Phytosterols derived from aloe gel reduce serum level of fatty acids and triglycerides, as well as inhibit visceral fat accumulation. Phytosterols cannot go through the intestinal barrier to absorb; hence, they bind to and prevent cholesterol absorption [38]. In short-time usage, aloe gel is safe in dose of 15 cc/d for 6 weeks; however, oral intake of aloe latex can cause stomach pain in high doses. Long-term use of high-dose aloe latex (more than 1 g/d) may cause kidney or heart damage or be fatal. *Aloe vera* is not safe in pregnancy due to its association with miscarriage and risk of birth defects. Patients with intestinal conditions such as ulcerative colitis must avoid aloe latex, but topical use of aloe vera is safe. Major drug interactions of aloe vera include digoxin, antidiabetic agents, laxatives, warfarin, diuretics, anticoagulants, and antiplatelet medicines [24].

10.2.4 Trigonella Foenumgraecum L.

The seed of *Trigonella foenumgraecum* L., known as fenugreek seed (family: Fabaceae), has shown therapeutic properties such as antihyperlipidemic, anti-obesity, antidiabetic, anti-inflammatory, antioxidant, anti-arthritic, antimicrobial, and anticancer activities [39, 40]. Fenugreek in traditional and folklore medicine is used for aiding digestion, lactation, lower limb edema, lung congestion, sinusitis, male baldness, and hair conditioning. On the other hand, recent studies showed effectiveness of fenugreek against oxidative stress, inflammatory conditions, diabetes, obesity, cancer, liver problems, dyslipidemia, climacteric symptoms, and sexual impairments [41]. Therapeutic effects of fenugreek are contributed to various active components, including saponins, terpenes, 4-hydroxyisoleucine, galactomannan, steroidal sapogenins (diosgenin), dietary fibers, alkaloids, amino acids, flavonoids, phenolic acid derivatives, vitamins and minerals, lipids, fatty acids, and esters [42].

Several meta-analysis studies on effects of fenugreek in diabetes have been conducted. Although Suksomboon et al. (2011) reported that fenugreek does not change FBG and Hb A1C [43], further investigations including more studies showed that fenugreek can reduce FBG, 2-h postprandial blood glucose (2hppBG), and HbA1C [39, 44]. Acute hypoglycemic effect of fenugreek seems to be due to its gum fraction. Also, its soluble fiber compound declines digestive enzymes and impairs gastrointestinal glucose absorption. *Trigonelline* increases insulin sensitivity and reduces early glucose response to oral glucose tolerance tests, and amino acids of fenugreek seeds stimulate glucose-dependent insulin secretion from pancreatic islets [44]. Fenugreek delays gastric emptying, reduces glucose and fat absorption selectively, inhibits glucose transportation, and directly constrains lipid accumulation in pancreatic β-cells. As ROS induce impairment of cell membrane fluidity, membrane lipid peroxidation, loss of cellular protein functions, and DNA damage, bioactive components of fenugreek, such as polyphenols, can attenuate oxidative stress by reducing production of thiobarbituric acid reactive substances (TBARS) and lipid peroxidation (LPO), scavenging free radicals, reducing hydrogen peroxide (H_2O_2), and increasing antioxidant enzymes such as superoxide dismutase (SOD), catalase (CAT), glutathione peroxidase (GPx), and glutathione S-transferases (GST). Moreover, fenugreek amino acids, such as hydroxyisoleucine, show anti-inflammatory activities by hindering nuclear factor-kB (NF-kB) activity, inflammation-stimulated insulin receptor (IRS-1), TNF-a-induced insulin resistance, and cyclooxygenase (COX) enzyme [41].

Fenugreek is commonly safe in dose of 5–10 g/d of powdered seed up to 3 years but may cause side effects such as diarrhea, stomach pain, and bloating, and at least 2 weeks before surgery taking fenugreek should be stopped due to its reducing effect on blood clotting time. Higher amounts of fenugreek may lead to malformation or early contractions in pregnant women. It is used to aid breast milk production in a safe dose of 1725 mg/d for 3 weeks, and in children it may just alter the urine and body odor. People who has history of allergic reactions to Fabaceae family such as soybean and peanut, might have allergy to fenugreek, too. Patients that take antidiabetic agents especially metformin, anticoagulants, antiplatelets, warfarin, theophylline, clopidogrel, and metoprolol should consult their physician while consuming fenugreek [24]. Patients with thyroid diseases and diabetes should use fenugreek under physician's supervision.

10.2.5 Catha Edulis (Vahl) Endl

Catha edulis, known as khat, is a flowering plant with a diverse phenotype and genotype species in different parts of the world, probably with different phytochemical contents depending on the region of cultivation. Active components of *C. edulis* can be summarized as alkaloids (phenylalkylamines and cathidulins), flavonoids (flavonols, kaempferol, quercetin, and myricetin), tannins, and sterols [45]. Green leaves of *C. edulis* are a natural source of psychostimulants due to its phenylalkylamine substances, cathinone. Chewing *C. edulis* relieves fatigue, ameliorates depression, and improves the efficacy of special tasks among students while studying such as preparing for exams.

Although Al-Sharafi and Gunaid (2015) reported its anti-obesity and hypoglycemic effects [46], others reported hyperglycemic effects of *C. edulis* [47]. Due to conflicting reports, meta-analysis of Alsahahi et al. summarized 11 clinical trials and 13 animal studies on antihyperglycemic effect of *C. edulis*. They reported antihyperglycemic effect when used for short term in animal studies but hyperglycemic effect in human studies and also when used for long term in animal studies [48]. They suggested that antihyperglycemic effects of *C. edulis* could be contributed to its cathinone component that indirectly stimulates sympathetic system to release noradrenaline and provoke glycogenolysis [48]. According to its euphoric effects, WHO listed *C. edulis* as medicine which makes psychological dependency, so in some countries such as Canada it is banned. It can cause some side effects such as aggression, anxiety, paranoia, hypertension, sleep disturbance, impaired concentration, headache, and hemorrhage. Hence, it is possibly unsafe for diabetic patients and should be avoided in pregnancy and breastfeeding. It has drug interactions with stimulant agents, hypertension medicines, and warfarin [24].

10.2.6 Polyherbal Treatments

Besides studies that evaluated a specific herb in diabetes, a review study of Ghorbani (2014) investigated different herbal mixtures in management of insulin sensitivity and hyperglycemia [49]. This study summarized 16 polyherbal formulas used in animal studies and five polyherbal products used in clinical trials, of which the most commonly used constituents were *Momordica charantia*, *Gymnema sylvestre*, *Trigonella foenum-graecum*, *Curcuma longa*, and *Syzygium cumini* resulting in satisfying management of BG and diabetes' complications [49].

10.2.7 Other Herbal Treatments

Different cultures and traditional medical systems use diverse types of herbal treatments in management of diabetes. In this section, we just discussed about a small number of medicinal plants; however, effects of a large number of herbs have been investigated by meta-analysis studies, including *Nigella sativa L.*, *Stevia rebaudiana (Bertoni) Bertoni*, *Zingiber officinale Roscoe*, *Capsicum annuum L.*, *Anacardium occidentale L.*, *Rhus coriaria L.*, *Phaseolus vulgaris L.*, *Artemisia*, *Sesamum indicum* L., *Juglans regia L.*, *Linum usitatissimum L.*, *Sesamum indicum L.*, *Morus alba L.*, *Curcuma longa L.*, *Crocus sativus L.*, *Coffea arabica L.*, *Malus domestica Borkh.*, and *Vitis vinifera L.* Furthermore, some studies evaluated effects of a polyherbal treatment on diabetes, e.g., combination of (1) *Gymnema sylvestre*, *Syzygium jambolanum*, and *Cephalandra indica*; (2) *Gymnema sylvestre*, *Syzygium cumini, Pterocarpus marsupium*, *Gurcuma longa*, *Emblica officinalis*, *Melia azadirachta*, *Trivang Bhasma*, and *Shilajit*; (3) *Tinospora cordifolia*, *Berberis aristata*, *Pterocarpus marsupium*, *Rubia cordifolia*, *Gymnema sylvestre*, and *Trigonella foenum-graecum*; or (4) *Urtica dioica*, *Silybum marianum Gaertn*, *olibanum gum*, or other formulations.

We summarized these findings in Table 10.1.

Table 10.1 Meta-analyses of RCTs evaluating the effects of some common herbal medicines on diabetes

ID	Author, year	Herbal medicine/ control	Meta-analyzed studies (n)/ disorders	Participants			Intervention		Significant main outcome	Effective dose
				Sample size (n)	Age (yr)	Sex	Dose/frequency	Duration		
1	Davis et al. [19]	*Cinnamomum cassia* (L.) J. Presl/placebo	8/T2DM	186	NR	NR	250–6000 mg/d	14–16 w	↓ FBG	NR
2	Liu et al. [27]	*Camellia sinensis* (L.) Kuntze/ placebo, water	17/DM, obese, healthy	1133	18–73	NR	208–1207 mg/d catechins or 75–236.7 mg/d caffeine or 9 g/d crude green tea	8–24 w	↓ FBG, HbA1C	> 457 mg/d catechins
3	Alsahahi et al. [48]	*Catha edulis* (Vahl) Endl./NR	11/diabetic, healthy	528	NR	NR	100–250 mg/d	60 min to >20 y	↑ FBG in diabetic subjects	NR
4	Dick et al. [36]	*Aloe barbadensis* mill./NR	9/diabetic	283	18–70	NR	100–1400 mg/d powder or 30–600 mL/d juice	4–14 w	↓ FBG, and HbA1C	NR
5	Gong et al. [39]	*Trigonella foenum-graecum* L./diet, exercise, medicine	12/DM	1173	30–72	NR	1–100 g/d	1 w to 3 y	↓ FBG, 2hpp BG, HbA1C	NR
6	Li et al. [27]	*Camellia sinensis* (L.) Kuntze/water, placebo	10/T2DM	608	20–73	NR	Not applicable to summarize	4–16 w	↑ Fins	NR
7	Daryabeygi-Khotbehsara et al. [50]	*Nigella sativa* L./ placebo, metformin	7/T2DM	505	47.5 intervention group, 49 control group	NR	0.5–2 g/d powder or 1–5 mL/d oil	2–12 m	↓ FBG, HbA1C	NR

(continued)

Table 10.1 (continued)

ID	Author, year	Herbal medicine/ control	Meta-analyzed studies (n)/ disorders	Participants			Intervention		Significant main outcome	Effective dose
				Sample size (n)	Age (yr)	Sex	Dose/frequency	Duration		
8	Mohammadi-Sartang et al. [9]	*Linum usitatissimum* L./ placebo, other plant oils (corn, safflower, etc.), wheat	25/T2DM, obese, healthy	2080	Mean range: 29.4–67.6	Both	1–15.9 g/d a-linolenic acid or 21–640 mg/d lignans or 10–60 g/d whole	2–48 w	↓ FBG, insulin, HOMA-IR ↑ QUICKI	NR
9	Bundgaard Anker et al. [51]	*Stevia rebaudiana* (Bertoni) Bertoni/ placebo	7/hypertension, diabetes, hyperlipidemia, healthy	462	NR	NR	200–1500 mg/d	4 h to 2 y	Non-sig. Effect	NR
10	Huang et al. [52]	*Zingiber officinale* roscoe/NR	8/T2DM	454	Mean range: 45.2–55.2	Both	1600–4000 mg/d	8–12 w	↓ HbA1C	NR
11	Huang et al. [53]	*Curcuma longa* L./placebo	14/T2DM, MetS, hyperlipidemia	1277	Mean range: 40.38–64.3	Both	2–3 g/d turmeric or 294–2000 mg/d curcuminoids or 70–1890 mg/d curcumin	4–12 w	↓ FBG, HbA1C, HOMA-IR	>300 mg/d curcuminoids
12	Asbaghi et al. [8]	*Vitis vinifera* L./ placebo	15/T2DM, hyperlipidemia, healthy, hypertension	825	Mean range: 19.8–63.6	Both	100–2000 mg/d	4–25 w	↓ FBG	NR
13	Ding et al. [54]	Algae/placebo	27/DM, obese, hyperlipidemia, healthy	1221	3–79	Both	c	2–28 w	↓ HbA1C ↑ insulin	NR

14	Jang et al. [55]	*Capsicum annuum* L./placebo	11/MetS	609	>18	Both	1–34.5 g/d fresh or 3–9 mg/d dihydrocapsiate or 2–9 mg/d capsinoids	4–12 w	Non-sig. effect	NR
15	Morvaridi et al. [3]	Green coffee/ placebo	27/NR	992	>18	Both	200–2000 mg/d	2–24 w	↓ FBG, insulin	> 400 mg/d
16	Jamshidi et al. [56]	*Anacardium occidentale* L./ placebo	6/MetS, T2DM	521	25–75	NR	28–108 g/d	4–12 w	Non-sig. effect	NR
17	Mohit et al. [57]	*Rhus coriaria* L./ NR	6/T2DM, dyslipidemia, obese	278	Mean range: 41.4–57.2	NR	1–6 g/d	6–12 w	Non-sig. effect	> 2 g/d
18	Nchanji and Ageyo [58]	*Phaseolus vulgaris* L./ NR	7/diabetes	195	18–70	Both	50–275 g/d	0.2–24 w	↓ 2hpp BG	NR
19	Sasani et al. [14]	Artemisia (different families)/placebo	6/NR	419	Mean range: 30–50	NR	0.4–4 g/d	30–90 d	↓ HOMA-IR	NR
20	Yargholi et al. [59]	*Sesamum indicum L./* placebo, glibenclamide	8/MetS, T2DM	517	18–70	Both	200 mg/d sesamin or 30–35 mL/d oil or 28–30 g/d grounded	6–12 w	↓ FBG, HbA1C	NR
21	Kim et al. [60]	*Malus domestica* Borkh./placebo	18/obese, hyperlipidemia, healthy, T2DM	1427	NR	Both	Not applicable to summarize	1–12 w	↓ FBG, insulin	NR
22	Mirzababaei et al. [61]	*Juglans regia* L./ placebo	4/T2DM	195	Mean range: 49.9–58.1	Both	200–750 mg/d	8–12 w	↓ FBG ↑ Fins	NR

(continued)

Table 10.1 (continued)

ID	Author, year	Herbal medicine/ control	Meta-analyzed studies (n)/ disorders	Participants			Intervention		Significant main outcome	Effective dose
				Sample size (n)	Age (yr)	Sex	Dose/frequency	Duration		
23	Musazadeh et al. [62]	*Curcuma longa* L./NR	12/T2DM, fatty liver, MetS	168–2629	Mean range: 29–57.5	NR	80–1500 mg/d	6–19 w	↓ FBG, HOMA-IR, HbA1C, insulin	> 1 g/d
24	Sohouli et al. [12]	*Sesamum indicum* L./placebo, glibenclamide, other oils	8/MetS, T2DM, hypertension	510	18–70	Both	Not applicable to summarize	45 d-9 w	↓ FBG, HbA1C	NR
25	Zamani et al. [7]	*Crocus sativus* L./ placebo	32/T2DM and different types of disease	1674	Mean range: 27–57.95	Both	5–1000 mg/d	1–12 w	↓ FBG, HbA1C, HOMA-IR	NR
26	Cui et al. [4]	*Morus alba* L./ placebo	12/T2DM, obese, healthy	615	18–75	Both	200–5000 mg/d or 0.7% beverage	4–24 w	↓ FBG, HbA1C, Fins	NR
27	Shabil et al. [63]	*Trigonella foenum-graecum* L./placebo or no comparison	14/T2DM, obese	894	25–70	NR	0.5–50 g/d	1 w to 3 y	↓ HbA1C	NR

FBG fasting blood glucose, *HbA1C* glycated hemoglobi, *Fins* fasting insulin, *NR* not reported, *DM* diabetes mellitus, *T1* type 1, *T2* type 2, *BG* blood glucose, *2hpp* 2 hours postprandial, *HOMA-IR* homeostatic model assessment for insulin resistance, *min* minute, *d* day, *m* month, *y* year, *QUICKI* quantitative insulin sensitivity check index, *MetS* metabolic syndrome, ↑ significant increase, ↓ significant decrease, ↔ no significant change

10.3 Role of Herbal Medicines in Improving Dyslipidemia

Dyslipidemia (DLP), as one of the major risk factors of CVD, is characterized by an increase in the serum levels of triglycerides (TG), total cholesterol (TC), or abnormal levels of related lipoprotein species such as low-density lipoprotein cholesterol (LDL-C) and high-density lipoprotein cholesterol (HDL-C). CVD is estimated to cause 25 million deaths annually by 2030 [64]. Besides, the global burden of DLP has increased over the last 30 years [65]. Genetic, some medications, diet, obesity, type 2 diabetes mellitus (T2DM), and MetS can be etiology of DLP. The treatment options for DLP include lifestyle modifications and medications. Lipid-lowering medications can have negative effects on neurocognitive, gastrointestinal, musculoskeletal, liver function, and nervous systems. Therefore, the discovery of new hypolipidemic agents with fewer adverse effects is necessary.

Several studies have shown the beneficial effects of herbal medicines as complementary and alternative medicines (CAM) on DLP. An umbrella review study of 141 meta-analyses of randomized controlled trials (RCTs) showed the efficacy of plant-derived medicines such as polyphenolic compounds, phytosterols, vegetable oils, plant proteins, nuts, and teas in the management of DLP [64].

Some common herbal medicines, including green tea, garlic, ginger, black seed, cinnamon, and saffron, have demonstrated antihyperlipidemic effects in numerous studies. Some of the possible mechanisms of these herbs in improving serum lipids consist of stimulating bile acid production, reducing carbohydrate-responsive element-binding protein (ChREBP) expression, elevating of activity of the lipoprotein lipase (LPL) enzyme and lecithin cholesterol acyltransferase (LCAT), and increasing hepatic LDL-C receptors, as well as reducing the synthesis and absorption of cholesterol by inhibiting squalene monooxygenase and 3-hydroxy-3-methylglutaryl-coenzyme A (HMG-CoA) reductase [64–66]. The effects of these common herbs on lipid parameters are represented in Table 10.2.

In this section, some common medicinal plants with multiple studies on lipid serums, i.e., green tea, garlic, ginger, fenugreek, black seed, cinnamon, and saffron, will be reviewed. Besides, some main phytochemicals of these plants, such as epigallocatechin gallate (EGCG), diosgenin, allicin, thymoquinone, and crocin, will be mentioned in this section (Fig. 10.1).

10.3.1 Camellia sinensis *(L.) Kuntze*

Two meta-analyses of RCTs indicated significant effects of green tea on TC and LDL-C with a dose of 6000 mg/d (Table 10.2) [28, 68]. Furthermore, an umbrella review study that evaluates six meta-analyses of the RCTs has shown the powerful effects of green tea on TC, TG, and LDL-C with the effective doses between 625 and 6000 mg/d [64].

Table 10.2 Meta-analyses of RCTs evaluating the effects of some common herbal medicines on dyslipidemia

Author, year	Plant name	Herbal medicine/ control	Meta-analyzed studies (n)/ disorders	Participants: Sample size (n)	Participants: Age (yr)	Participants: Sex	Intervention: Dose/frequency	Intervention: Duration	Significant main outcome	Effective dose
Hartley et al. [28]	Green tea (leaf of *Camellia sinensis* (L.) Kuntze)	Black tea, green tea/ placebo	11/ high-risk CVD, healthy	821	25–75	Both	One to three capsules daily Two tablets TDS	12–96 w	↓ TC LDL-C	NR
Payab et al. [68]		Green tea/ placebo	16/ obesity, MetS	NR	NR	NR	300–6000 mg/d	8–12 w	↓ TC LDL-C	6000 mg/d
Silagy et al. [72]	Garlic (bulb of *Allium sativum* L.)	Garlic/ placebo	16/HLP, CHD	952	NR	Both	0.6–10 g/d	4–40 w	↓ TG TC	600–900 mg/d
Ried, et al. [71]		Garlic/ placebo	39/HLP, CAD, others	2298	20–60	NR	*Powder*: 600–5600 mg/d *Oil*: 9–18 mg/d *Extract*: 1000–7200 mg/d *Raw*: 4–10 g/d	2–48 w	↓ TC LDL-C ↑ HDL-C	NR
Asghari-Jafarabadi and Khalili [67]	Ginger (rhizome of *Zingiber officinale* roscoe)	Ginger (capsule, ethanolic extract, tablet)/ placebo	21/NR	NR	34.54–59.1	Both	200–3000 mg/d	2–24 w	↓ TG TC LDL-C ↑ HDL-C	Both ≤1500 and > 1500 mg/d for both of ≤8 and > 8 w *In the case of weight control*: >1500 mg/d for >8 w

Askarpour et al. [40]	Fenugreek (seed of *Trigonella foenumgraecum* L.)	Fenugreek/ placebo	12/ T2DM, HLP, healthy	560	22–70	Both	*Powder*: 5–100 g/d *Hydroalcoholic extract*: 0.588–1.176 g/d	2–162 w	↓ TC TG LDL-C ↑ HDL-C	>10 g/d for >8 w
Fakhr et al. [82]		Fenugreek (powder, seed extract, seed)/ placebo	29/ healthy, T2DM, NAFLD, HLP, PCOS	1910	18–70	Both	25–60,000 mg/d	2–144 w	↓ TG ↑ HDL-C	*For HDL-C and TG*: 15 g/d
Sahebkar et al. [86]	Black seed (seed of *Nigella sativa* L.)	Black seed/ placebo	17/HTN, MetS, others	1185	29–59	Both	*Powder*: 1–8 g/d *Oil*: 5 ml/d 1–3 g/d	4–12 w	↓ TG TC LDL-C	NR
Hallajzadeh et al. [83]		Black seed/ placebo	50/ T2DM, HTN, others	3679	26–72	Both	*Extract*: 0.2–3 g/d *Oil*: 1.5–5 ml/d	2–48 w	↓ TG TC LDL-C ↑ HDL-C	NR

(continued)

Table 10.2 (continued)

				Participants			Intervention			
Author, year	Plant name	Herbal medicine/ control	Meta-analyzed studies (n)/ disorders	Sample size (n)	Age (yr)	Sex	Dose/frequency	Duration	Significant main outcome	Effective dose
Zamani et al. [7]	Saffron (flower of *Crocus sativus* L.)	Saffron, crocin/ placebo	32/MetS, T2DM, healthy, OW, NAFLD, others	1674	27–57.95	Both	5–1000 mg/d	1–12 w	↓ TG TC LDL-C	<100 mg/d for ≥12 w
Roshanravan et al. [88]		Saffron/ placebo	8/HTN, CAD, DM, MetS, others	205	41–56	Both	30–1000 mg/d	8–12 w	↓ LDL-C TC TG ↑ HDL-C	30–100 mg/d 12 w and 1000 mg/d 8 w
Wu et al. [89]	Cinnamon (bark of *Cinnamomum verum* J. Presl)	Cinnamon (capsules, extract)/ placebo	12/MetS, PCOS, obese, NAFLD, T2DM, PD, OW	773	Mean age: 27.5–73.0	Both	500–3000 mg/d	2–4 m	↓ TC TG LDL-C ↑ HDL-C (subgroup analysis)	*For HDL-C*: ≥1.5 g/d

CAD coronary artery disease, *CHD* coronary heart disease, *CVD* cardiovascular disease, *DM* diabetes mellitus, *HDL-C* high-density lipoprotein cholesterol, *HLP* hyperlipidemia, *LDL-C* low-density lipoprotein cholesterol, *m* month, *MetS* metabolic syndrome, *NAFLD* nonalcoholic fatty liver disease, *NR* not reported, *OW* overweight, *PCOS* polycystic ovary syndrome, *PD* prediabetes, *T2DM* type 2 diabetes mellitus, *TC* total cholesterol, *TDS* three times a day, *TG* triglyceride, *yr* year, ↓ significant reduction (p value <0.05), ↑ significant elevation (p value <0.05), ↔ no significant change

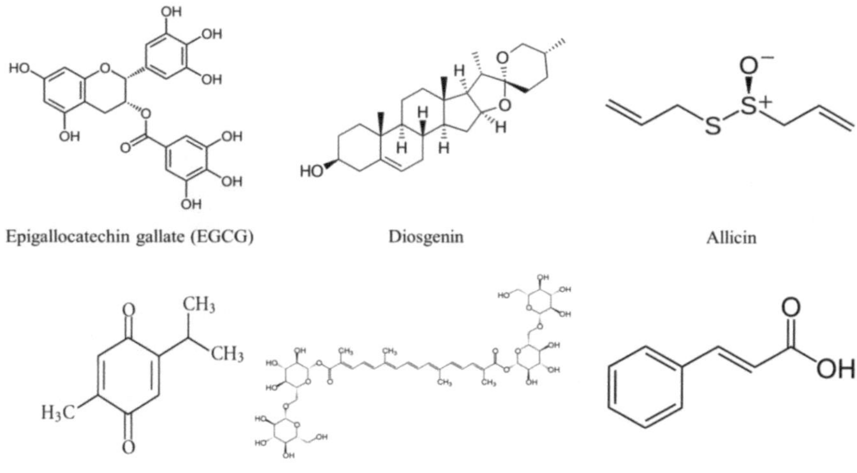

Fig. 10.1 Chemical structure of some main phytochemicals of common plants effective on dyslipidemia

10.3.2 Allium sativum *L.*

Garlic, as the bulb of *Allium sativum* L., belongs to the Amaryllidaceae family and is one of the most commonly used herbal remedies in many countries [69]. It has been shown that it attunes blood lipid and glucose [70]. Some research suggests that the major bioactive components responsible for the management of DLP are organosulfur compounds such as allicin and ajoene [69, 70]. A meta-analysis of 33 RCTs has shown that 500 mg to 20,000 mg doses of garlic decrease TC, LDL-C, and TG as well as increase HDL-C compared to placebo in 1273 patients with hyperlipidemia (HLP) and T2DM [70]. Ried et al., in a meta-analysis of 39 RCTs, concluded that powder, oil, extract, or raw garlic significantly decreased TC and LDL-C, as well as increased HDL-C in 2298 patients with HLP, CAD, and others (Table 10.2) [71]. Another meta-analysis of 16 RCTs has demonstrated the positive effect of garlic on the reduction of TC and TG in 952 subjects with HLP and CHD, with effective doses from 600 mg/d to 900 mg/d (Table 10.2) [72].

Adverse effects of garlic, including vomiting, insomnia, dizziness, heartburn, abdominal discomfort, diarrhea, bloating, nausea, headache, and flatulence, were observed. Besides, oral consumption of garlic may increase the risk of bleeding [73]. Human studies have shown that garlic as a food is safe during pregnancy and lactation [74].

10.3.3 Zingiber officinale *Roscoe*

The rhizome of *Zingiber officinale* Roscoe, known as ginger, is a common spice in the world, belonging to the Zingiberaceae family. Its therapeutic effects on the cardiovascular system, HLP, hyperglycemia, obesity, and cancer have been demonstrated [75]. Gingerols, i.e., 6-gingerol, 12-gingerol, 10-gingerol, 8-gingerol, 4-gingerol, and 5-gingerol, are the main constituents of ginger [76]. In a meta-analysis, Asghari-Jafarabadi and Khalili investigated 21 RCTs that showed the significant effects of ginger on decreasing TG, TC, and LDL-C, as well as increasing HDL-C. The effective dose of ginger for improving lipid profile was more than 1500 mg/d for >8 weeks, in the case of weight control in the subgroup analysis of the study (Table 10.2) [67].

FDA considers ginger root as generally safe, in doses of up to 4 grams daily. However, higher consumption can lead to adverse effects such as gastrointestinal discomfort, allergic reactions, bleeding complications, central nervous system depression, and arrhythmias. Ingesting more than 6 grams daily may exacerbate gastrointestinal issues, promote warfarin toxicity, lower blood pressure, and increase the risk of gallstone formation [77].

Ginger is also recognized as a natural remedy for nausea and motion sickness [78] and has been proposed as a galactagogue for breastfeeding mothers. Research indicates that ginger can enhance breast milk production in the postpartum period without adverse effects. Incorporating ginger into the diet during pregnancy and breastfeeding is generally considered safe, with no reported complications. While ginger has been found to alleviate nausea and vomiting during pregnancy, further research is needed to establish its safety and efficacy comprehensively in pregnant and lactating women [79].

Ginger can interact with some medications, affecting their safety and effectiveness. It can modulate the activity of cytochrome P450s and ATP-binding cassette transporters, potentially leading to interaction with cyclosporine, metronidazole, crizotinib, nifedipine, anticoagulants, and phenprocoumon [80]. It is not recommended for use during pregnancy. Besides, patients who are at risk of bleeding or have gallstone disease should not use it. However, it is safe to use during lactation [81].

10.3.4 Trigonella foenumgraecum *L.*

It contains various phytochemicals such as phytosterols, pectin, and sapogenin that may be related significantly to hypolipidemic effects [40]. Fakhr et al. conducted a meta-analysis of 29 RCTs that indicated a significant improvement in TG and HDL-C in patients with HLP, with an effective dose of 15 g/d of powder or seed extract of fenugreek (Table 10.2) [82]. A meta-analysis of 12 RCTs concluded that fenugreek seed in the form of powder or hydroalcoholic extract, compared with placebo, markedly decreased TC, TG, and LDL-C and increased HDL-C by a dose more than 10 g/d for >8 weeks (Table 10.2) [40].

10.3.5 Nigella sativa *L.*

Black seed or black cumin is the seed of *Nigella sativa* L. which belongs to Ranunculaceae family. It exerts various properties, i.e., anti-inflammatory, antibacterial, antioxidant, immune-potentiating, hypoglycemic, antihypertensive, bronchodilatory, cardioprotective, anti-obesity, and antihyperlipidemic [83–85]. Thymoquinone is the main bioactive phytochemical of black seed, which is responsible for its therapeutic effects. Additionally, black seed contains various other constituents, such as thymol, thymohydroquinone, nigellone, dithymoquinone, and its derivatives, alpha-hederin, flavonoids, and several fatty acids, including linoleic acid and oleic acid [84].

In a meta-analysis of 17 RCTs, Sahebkar et al. indicated that powder or oil of black seed significantly decreased TG, TC, and LDL-C in 1185 patients with HTN, MetS, etc., but no significant change was observed in HDL-C (Table 10.2) [86]. However, in another meta-analysis of 50 RCTs, black seed extract or oil in 3679 subjects with T2DM, HTN, and others showed significant improvement in TC, TG, LDL-C, and HDL-C (Table 10.2) [83]. Differences between the results of the two meta-analyses may be due to different sample sizes, the number of RCTs, the range of dosage, and the type of disorders. A meta-analysis of five RCTs showed the significant effects of 1000 mg/d of black seed on reduction in TG and 3000 mg/d of black seed on improvement in LDL-C in patients with obesity and MetS, for duration of 6–8 weeks [68].

Black seed can cause upset stomach, vomiting, and constipation, as well as interactions with sildenafil, carbamazepine, cyclosporine, amoxicillin, theophylline, glibenclamide, and phenytoin. Also, it is recommended to avoid the use of this herb along with anticoagulants, serotonergic drugs, and immunosuppressive agents, and also *N. sativa* might increase phenytoin blood level, so it should be used with caution in patients taking this medication. Black seed should be used with caution during pregnancy and lactation [87].

10.3.6 Crocus sativus *L.*

Saffron, flower of *Crocus sativus* L., belongs to Iridaceae family [88]. The therapeutic effect of saffron on dyslipidemia, obesity, and hyperglycemia has been reported. Crocetin, picrocrocin, safranal, and crocin are the four main constituents of saffron which were associated with hypolipidemic properties [7, 88]. Significant effects of saffron on reducing TG, TC, and LDL-C by a dose of less than 100 mg/d for ≥12 weeks have been shown in a meta-analysis of 32 RCTs (Table 10.2) [7].

Another meta-analysis has reported a significant improvement of saffron in LDL-C, TC, TG, and HDL-C. The effective dose of saffron is 30–100 mg/d for 12 weeks and 1000 mg/d for 8 weeks (Table 10.2) [88].

Saffron may have some side effects such as anxiety, decreased appetite, nausea, increased appetite, hypomania, sedation, and abnormal bleeding. Some medications of saffron include sedative (CNS depressants) and antihypertensive drugs. Pregnant and lactating women should use saffron with caution [89].

10.3.7 Cinnamomum verum *J. Presl*

A meta-analysis that investigated 12 RCTs concluded cinnamon (capsules or extract) significantly reduced TC, TG, and LDL-C, as well as the dose of ≥1.5 g/d cinnamon elevated HDL-C (Table 10.2) [90]. The dose ranges of 1–6 g/d of cinnamon, mainly in the form of powder, are the recommended effective dose [91].

10.3.8 Combined Herbal Medicines

Combination therapy of herbal medicine is one of the common treatments used in various traditional medicine systems. Some clinical trials have been conducted to investigate their safety and efficacy. In traditional Persian medicine (TPM), an herbal remedy consists of *Portulaca oleracea* L., *Rhus coriaria* L., and *Trigonella foenumgraecum.* In an RCT, this TPM remedy showed a significant reduction in TC and LDL-C in patients with DLP [92]. Another TPM remedy, i.e., black seed, garlic, milk thistle, psyllium seed, aloe vera, and fenugreek seed, displays a significant decrease in TC, TG, and LDL-C in patients with T2DM and DLP [93]. The JTTZ formula, a Chinese herbal remedy, includes *Momordica charantia* L., *Coptis chinensis* Franch., *Anemarrhena asphodeloides* Bunge, *Salvia miltiorrhiza* Bunge, *Schisandra chinensis* (Turcz.) Baill., *Monascus purpureus* Went (red yeast rice), aloe vera, and dried ginger. In an RCT, the JTTZ formula significantly reduced TC, TG, and LDL-C [94].

10.4 Medicinal Plants' Evidences in Management of Obesity

Characterized by excessive accumulation of body fat, obesity is a global health crisis affecting individuals of all ages, genders, and socioeconomic backgrounds and posing a multifaceted challenge to public health systems. As of 2022, about 1 billion people worldwide were obese, encompassing 650 million adults, 340 million adolescents, and 39 million children. This multifactorial metabolic disorder is one of the most important risk factors for several chronic diseases, including diabetes, hyperlipidemia, cardiovascular diseases, nonalcoholic fatty liver disease (NAFLD), and some types of cancer [95, 96].

Conventional treatments for obesity include lifestyle modifications (i.e., behavioral therapy, diet, and exercise), oral pharmacological agents, and surgery. However, only a few drugs have been approved, and some are associated with effects, including hypertension, headache, and dry mouth, especially with long-term use. Hence, complementary medicine modalities, such as herbal medicines, are gaining popularity [96]. Extensive research worldwide has been dedicated to investigating the safety and effectiveness of various medicinal plants and herbal products in the treatment of overweight and obesity [97]. Some of the main proposed mechanisms for the effectiveness of medicinal plants in the treatment of obesity include appetite suppression, increased metabolism and thermogenesis, inhibition of pancreatic lipase activity, reduced fat absorption, increasing lipolysis, and decreased lipogenesis. Thymoquinone, thymol, cinnamaldehyde, catechins, and curcumin can be mentioned among the most important herbal ingredients that cause these effects [98].

In this section, we will review some plants that have been evaluated based on new scientific sources and clinical trials regarding their effectiveness on obesity.

10.4.1 Nigella sativa L.

A recent meta-analysis showed that adding *N. sativa* into diet may have potential benefits in lowering body mass index (BMI) and decreasing overall body weight and waist circumference (WC) [84]. The main compound of *N. sativa* is thymoquinone (TQ) which constitutes a significant portion, approximately 30–48%, of the oil derived from *N. sativa* (Fig. 10.2). Its other components such as nigellone and flavonoids may also contribute to its pharmacological properties. *N. sativa* has the potential to activate peroxisome proliferator-activated receptor gamma-2 (PPAR-γ2), a key player in regulating energy balance. Moreover, no significant adverse reactions or toxic effects have been reported in neither animal nor human studies of *N. sativa* [84]. Based on the search results, the exact dose of black seed in the treatment of obesity has not been determined.

10.4.2 Cinnamon

A systematic review/meta-analysis of 12 RCTs which supplemented cinnamon powder for obese individuals [99] has reported a significant reduction in weight, BMI, and WC.

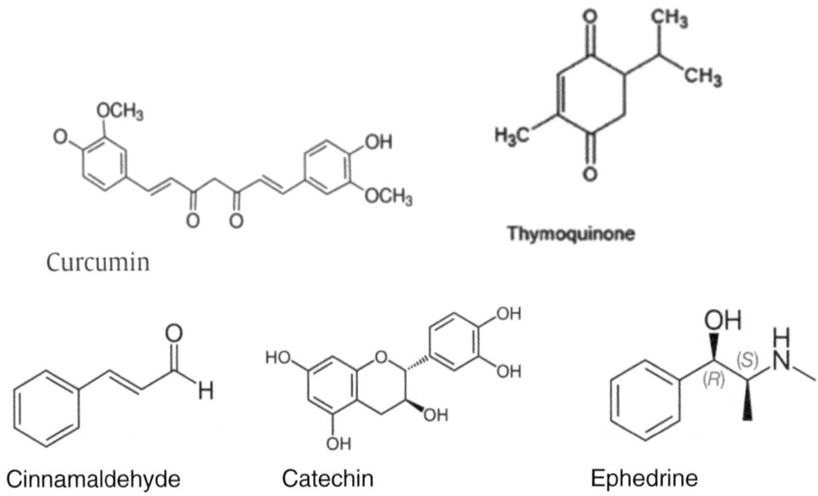

Fig. 10.2 Some of main components of the used herbal medicines to manage obesity

10.4.3 Green Tea

Polyphenols and their primary and secondary metabolites are the main components of green tea, catechins, can promote energy expenditure within fat cells via activation of the sympathetic nervous system. Mechanisms of this activity include inhibiting the enzyme catechol-O-methyltransferase, boosting the process of lipid oxidation, and influencing various metabolic aspects, such as appetite control and thermogenesis. The collective effect of these mechanisms ultimately leads to a reduction in body weight [100].

The National Center for Complementary and Integrative Health (NCCIH) states that green tea as a beverage or dietary supplement is promoted for improving mental alertness, relieving digestive symptoms and headaches, and promoting weight loss.

In numerous meta-analysis studies, the beneficial effects of green tea on reduction of weight, WC, BMI, waist-to-hip ratio, and body fat (BF) were shown (Table 10.3).

10.4.4 Ephedra Sinica

Ephedra sinica, an ancient medicinal plant used for over 5000 years in traditional Chinese medicine, has recently drawn attention for its potential in combating obesity (Fig. 10.2). A key component, ephedrine, is believed to contribute to weight loss and is often combined with caffeine for this purpose. Proposed mechanisms include increased metabolic rate and fat burning via enhancing sympathetic neural activities and increasing heart rate [101].

Table 10.3 Meta-analyses of RCTs evaluating the effects of some common herbal medicines on overweight/obesity

Id	Author, year	Herbal medicine/ control	Meta-analyzed studies (n)/disorders	Participants			Intervention		Significant main outcome	Effective dose
				Sample size (n)	Age (yr)	Sex	Dose/frequency	Duration (w)		
Green tea	Asbaghi et al. [112]	Green tea and green tea extract/placebo	11/type 2 diabetes	687	Mean: 52–64.9	Both	400–10,000 mg/d	8–16	Wt, BMI, WC, BF	NR
	Jurgens et al. [113]	Green tea and green tea extract/placebo	14/obesity, overweight	1562	18–65	Both	140.85–1206.9 mg/d	12–13	Wt, BMI, WC, WHR	NR
	Lin et al. [114]	Green tea and green tea extract/placebo	22/adults	2357	NR	Both	99–20,000 mg/d	2–20	Wt, BMI, WC	NR
Tea	Shen et al. [115]	Green tea, marjoram tea, spearmint herbal tea/ placebo, placebo with metformin	6/women with PCOS	235	20–40	Women	500–540 mg/d	1–12	Wt, BMI, WC, HC, WHR, BF, FBG	NR
Saffron	Tahmasbi et al. [116]	Saffron or crocin/placebo	25/MetS, T2DM, healthy adults, schizophrenic Patients with MetS, MDD, overweight, CAD	1609	NR	Both	15–1000 mg/d	4–12	↓Wt, BMI, WC, HC, WHR	
Garcinia cambogia	Golzarand et al. [117]	Garcinia cambogia/ placebo	8/obese, overweight	530	NR	NR	166–4667 mg/d	8–12	↓Wt, BMI, PFA, and WC	NR

(continued)

Table 10.3 (continued)

Id	Author, year	Herbal medicine/ control	Meta-analyzed studies (n)/disorders	Participants			Intervention		Significant main outcome	Effective dose
				Sample size (n)	Age (yr)	Sex	Dose/frequency	Duration (w)		
Nigella sativa	Namazi et al. [85]	Powder, extract, or oil of *Nigella sativa*/placebo	11/healthy, mild HTN, MetS, overweight, obese, T2DM, AR	839	33–46	Both	100–3000 mg/d	6–12	↓Wt, BMI, WC	NR
Phaseolus vulgaris	Onakpoya et al. [118]	*Phaseolus vulgaris*/ placebo	6/healthy obese, overweight	NR	NR	NR	445–1500 mg/d	4–8	No significant change in Wt, BF	NR
Garlic	Fu et al. [119]	Garlic/placebo	19/hyperlipidemia, NAFLD, MetS	999	NR	NR	188–2400 mg/d	6–16	↓BMI, WC	NR
Almond	Eslampour et al. [120]	Almond/diet, cheese, olive oil, walnuts, placebo	28/adults healthy, hypercholesterolemic, overweight, obese, T2DM, PCOS	1720	24–87	Both	25–100 g/d	3–77.14	↓Wt, BMI, WC, HC, WHR, fat mass, fat-free mass	NR
Cinnamon	Mousavi et al. [99]	Cinnamon powder/ placebo	12/metabolic abnormalities	786	21.8–63.9	Both	1–10 g/d	8–16	↓Wt, BMI, WC	NR

CAD coronary artery disease, *MetS* metabolic syndrome, *NAFLD* nonalcoholic fatty liver disease, *PCOS* polycystic ovary syndrome, *T2DM* type 2 diabetes mellitus, *yr*, year, *NR* not reported, *Wt* weight, *WC* waist circumference, *WHR* waist-to-hip ratio, *BMI* body mass index, *BF* body fat

Anti-obesity effects of *Ephedra sinica* are also attributed to its ability to enhance peroxisome proliferator-activated receptor alpha (PPAR-α) and adiponectin functions while reducing tumor necrosis factor-alpha (TNF-α) activity, addressing both obesity and hyperglycemia. Moreover, it can modulate gut microbiota, resulting in improved glucose tolerance and weight loss.

Recent research has revealed a significant correlation between ephedra and changes in gut microbiota composition. These changes are attributed to reductions in body weight (BW) and body mass index (BMI), underscoring the potential of this herb in gut microbiota modulation [102]. Ephedrine and ephedra have shown a modest short-term weight loss, approximately 0.9 kg/month more than placebo, without any evidence of decreasing weight for long term [103].

Ephedra sinica extract has also shown promise in browning of white adipocytes, representing a practical strategy for management of obesity [104]. Dietary supplementation with *Ephedra sinica* is beneficial in addressing obesity-related concerns, including weight gain, fat accumulation, glucose tolerance, and lipid profiles in high-fat diet-fed mice [102].

The recommended oral dosage of ephedrine for adults is 12.5–25 mg every 4 hours as needed, with a maximum daily dose not exceeding 150 mg [105]. Despite its potential benefits, ephedra is associated with adverse effects, ranging from minor symptoms like tremor and headaches to more severe cardiovascular events. Therefore, a cautious approach is essential, especially for patients prone to adverse reactions [106]. Also, *Ephedra sinica* may interact with antidepressants, amphetamines, aspirin, hypertension medications, and caffeine, potentially causing some side effects [107].

10.4.5 Ginger

A number of studies have investigated the effects of this plant on weight loss and metabolic abnormalities, suggesting it could play an effective role in managing metabolic syndrome. Ginger properties, including hypotensive, anti-obesity, hypoglycemic, and hypolipidemic effects, have garnered attention in this topic [108, 109].

In a meta-analysis of four trials which compared the effect of ginger consumption with placebo, a significant reduction in body weight, WC, WHR, and hip circumference was observed without any significant effect on BMI by ≤1000 mg/d ginger for maximum 12 weeks [110]. Research has shown that ginger extract can mitigate obesity and inflammation by regulating the expression of microRNAs and activating AMPK in white adipose tissue. Ginger supplementation in mice can help alleviate obesity and remodel adipose tissue [108, 111].

The details of the herbal medicines to manage obesity are shown in Table 10.3.

10.5 Herbal Medicines for Management of Metabolic Syndrome

MetS is a health problem that is defined by a cluster of several disorders such as diabetes mellitus, hypertension, obesity, and dyslipidemia. Although its underlying pathophysiology is not clear, numerous researches are conducted to manage it by plant-derived products due to high cost and adverse effects of the synthetic drugs. Some of the suggested natural products are curcumin, resveratrol, *Nigella sativa*, *Hibiscus sabdariffa*, and *Theobroma cacao*. Details of the meta-analysis studies with the herbal medicines and phytochemicals for management of MetS are shown in Table 10.4.

Table 10.4 Meta-analyses of the trials to investigate the effects of the plant-derived products on MetS

Natural products	Author, year	Included meta-analysis studies (n)/ disorders	Intervention		Participants			Significant main outcome	Effective dose
			Dose (mg/d)	Duration (w)	Sample size (n)	Sex	Age (yr)		
Resveratrol	Asgary et al. [121]	10/MetS	100–3000	4–12	396	NR	20–75	↓Glucose, WC	≥ 500 mg/d for >10 w
Curcumin, nano-curcumin, curcuminoid/ placebo	Qiu et al. [122]	13/MetS	20–2400	4–12	785	B	37–67	↓ WC, FBS, DBP ↑ HDL-C	NR
Nigella sativa L.	Payab et al. [68]	5/obesity, MetS	1500–3000	6–8	NR	NR	NR	↓ TG, LDL-C, SBP	*For TG:* 1000 mg/d *For LDL-C*: 3000 mg/d
Trigonella foenumgraecum L./ placebo	Fakhr et al. [82]	29/T2DM, healthy, HLP, NAFLD, PCOS	25–60,000	2–144	1910	B	18–70	↓ TG, FBS,WC, SBP ↑HDL-C	*For FBS, HDL-C and TG:* 15 g/d
Hibiscus sabdariffa L./ placebo	Najafpour Boushehri et al. [123]	7/MetS, HTN, obese with fatty liver, healthy	100–1350	4–12.8	362	B	20–54	↓ FBS, BP, LDL-C	NR

HDL-C high-density lipoprotein cholesterol, *LDL-C* low-density lipoprotein cholesterol, *MetS* metabolic syndrome, *NAFLD* nonalcoholic fatty liver disease, *NR* not reported, *PCOS* polycystic ovary syndrome, *T2DM* type 2 diabetes mellitus, *TC* total cholesterol, *TG* triglyceride, *yr* year, ↓ significant reduction, ↑ significant elevation, *B* both, *HLP* hyperlipidemia, *HTN* hypertension, *SBP* systolic blood pressure, *DBP* diastolic blood pressure

10.6 Herbal Medicines for Management of Osteoporosis

The prevalence of osteoporosis as the most common bone disease is accelerating worldwide. It affected one in three women and one in five men aged >50 years old. The IOF estimated that there are 200 million osteoporotic women in the world. It is prevalent in women especially in postmenopausal condition [124]. There are different pharmacological agents and non-pharmacological approaches to treat osteoporosis [125]. Numerous studies show beneficial effects of some herbal medicines and phytochemicals in the prevention and treatment of osteoporosis, including green tea, quercetin, curcumin, phytoestrogens, and soy isoflavones. Some of these beneficial effects are modulated through inhibition of the transcription factors such as Runx2, stimulation of the molecular signaling pathways such as MAPK, suppression of osteoclast differentiation, influence on calcium absorption/excretion, and osteoblast formation [126]. Some of the meta-analysis studies conducted with the natural products are summarized in Table 10.5.

Table 10.5 Meta-analyses of the trials/observational studies investigating the effects of the plant-derived products on osteoporosis

Natural products	Author, year	Included meta-analysis studies (n)/disorders	Intervention		Participants			Significant main outcome	Effective dose
			Dose (mg/d)	Duration (w)	Sample size (n)	Sex	Age (yr)		
Phytoestrogens	Salari et al. [127]	11 trials/PM women	37.3–126	4–96	1252	F	NR	↓Bone resorption	NR
Isoflavone/placebo, control, calcium	Sansai et al. [128]	63 trials/PM women	10–600	4–144	6427	F	NR	↑BMD	Genistein 54 mg/d, ipriflavone 600 mg/d
Coffee and Tea	Chen et al. [129]	20 observational/men, women, PM women	1500–3000	6–8	508,312	B	NR	Non-sig. effect on fracture or BMD	NR

PM postmenopausal, *NR* not reported, *F* female, *BMD* bone mineral density

10.7 Herbal Medicine in Managing Polycystic Ovary Syndrome

PCOS is a complex endocrine disease that diminishes the quality of life. With a prevalence of 5–21%, PCOS is commonly known for causing infertility in women. Some clinical manifestations of PCOS include hyperandrogenism and associated acne, hair loss of the scalp but hair growth on the body and face, ovarian cysts, anovulation, and, therefore, infertility [130]. PCOS is normally interlinked with metabolic syndrome; hence, women suffering from PCOS are often at a higher risk of insulin resistance and type 2 diabetes, along with high blood pressure (HBP), heart failure, and stroke [131]. Other manifestations are abnormalities in the serum levels of sex hormones and related complications, depression, and anxiety [132]. Common treatments for PCOS are lifestyle modifications as the first and the most efficient step toward the management of PCOS, medications, and surgery [133]. The cardinal intervention of complementary medicine revolves around lifestyle management and herbal therapy for maintaining health and preventing diseases, especially metabolic syndrome and its related complications. The purpose of the present section is to review high-quality meta-analyses concerning phytoconstituents and their effects on the management of PCOS (Table 10.6).

10.7.1 Flaxseed

Linum usitatissimum L. (Linaceae) or flaxseed and its main fatty acid α-linolenic acid (ALA) have been shown to reduce inflammatory factors such as C-reactive protein [133]. ALA could convert to docosahexaenoic acid (DHA) and eicosapentaenoic acid (EPA), later. Flaxseed also contains phytoestrogenic lignans which counters levels of testosterone in patients with PCOS, according to a meta-analysis [134]. Emamat et al. demonstrated that flaxseed can improve menstrual cycle and decrease free testosterone and hirsutism scores in a 2–4-month regular consumption; daily doses include rather 30 mg flaxseed powder or 2 g of the flaxseed oil [134]. Due to high content of fiber and oil, flaxseed may cause various gastrointestinal problems such as nausea, bloating, cramps, and diarrhea. Cautions should be taken while using dose-specific medications such as antiplatelets and antidiabetics [133].

10.7.2 Soy Isoflavones

Isoflavones are another phytoestrogen polyphenols, categorized as flavonoids, that are mostly found in legumes such as soybean. They are normally attached to a glycoside group; however, after fermentation, the isoflavones remain as

Table 10.6 Effects of some herbal medicines on PCOS and hyperprolactinemia

Author, year	Herbal medicine/ control	Meta-analyzed studies (n)/ disorders	Participants			Intervention		Significant main outcome	Effective dose
			Sample size (n)	Age (year)	Sex	Dose/frequency	Duration		
Zilaee et al. [137]	Soy isoflavones/ placebo, controlled diet	4/PCOS	323	25.9 ± 5.3	F	≈50 mg/d	8–12 w	↓TT ↔FSH	NR
Fadlalmola et al. [142]	Resveratrol/placebo	4/PCOS	218	26.3 ± 1.9	F	800–1500 mg/d	6–7 w	↓ TT LH DHEAS	NR
Emamt et al. [134]	Flaxseed/placebo	9/PCOS	293	31.5 ± 13.5	F	30 mg/d	6–20 w	↓TT	30 mg/d
Kilicdag et al. [151, 152]	*Vitex agnus-castus* L./Bromocriptine	1/latent HPL	160	NR	F	Agnucaston®, Biomeks, 40 mg/day	12 w	↓Prolactin ↓Mastalgia	40 mg/d
Man et al. [147]	Peony-glycyrrhiza decoction	1/symptomatic hyperPRL	99	18–45	F	9-g granules equivalent to 22.5-g crude herbal mixture	16 w	↑Menstrual resumption ↓HPL symptoms ↔Prolactin	NR

DHEAS dehydroepiandrosterone sulfate, *FINS* fasting insulin, *HPL* hyperprolactinemia, *LH* luteinizing hormone, *TIS* three times a day, *TT* testosterone

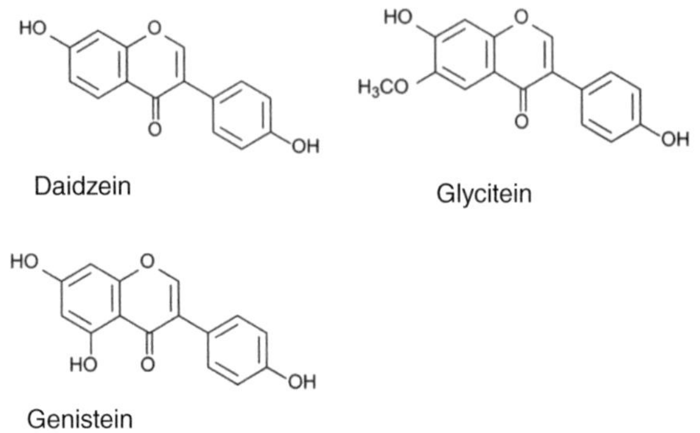

Fig. 10.3 Most common soy isoflavone aglycones

aglycones [135]. Most common soy isoflavone aglycones are glycitein, genistein, and daidzein [136] (Fig. 10.3). Soy isoflavones can interact with estrogen receptors (ER) and are used in estrogen-dependent complications such as osteoporosis, menopause, endometriosis, and ER-positive breast cancers, with precaution [137]. A systematic review and meta-analysis by Zilaee et al. (2023) investigated the data collected from four randomized clinical trials including 162 patients with PCOS, which projected a significant decrease in testosterone levels but no significant one in FSH levels. The administered isoflavones were rather pure isoflavone such as genistein or a mixture of them [137]. Isoflavones should be taken with caution during pregnancy and hypothyroidism . Despite the dosage is not being high while consumed as food and allergic reaction is usually observed in higher amounts, the dose range of the soy isoflavones depend on the source of the plant.

10.7.3 Resveratrol

Resveratrol is a stilbenoid phytoestrogen that is categorized as a polyphenol and is abundant in the peel of red fruits such as different kinds of berries and red grapes [138] (Fig. 10.4). Resveratrol is well known for its high capacity for radical scavenging activities, anti-inflammatory, anticancer, antifungal, and antibacterial properties [139, 140]. As resveratrol is a phytoestrogen, it has shown estrogenic and antiestrogenic effects, in vivo. The level of testosterone has been observed to be lessened by the administration of resveratrol in dehydroepiandrosterone (DHEA)-induced rats [141].

A meta-analysis by Fadlalmola et al. (2023) has presented the effects of resveratrol on 84 patients with PCOS compared to placebo from four clinical trials [142]. The results demonstrated a significant reduction in testosterone, FSH, and LH levels. The results showed no significant effects on pregnancy rate. The dose ranged from 800 to 1500 mg/day [142]. Resveratrol consumption of 1500 mg/day, better be divided into two to three doses, for 3 months is considered to be safe. Higher doses can be associated with stomach upset. It is also considered safe when consumed by pregnant women and children from the fruit and food source. Precaution should be taken with patients who take antiplatelet drugs or expecting surgery [143].

Fig. 10.4 Resveratrol

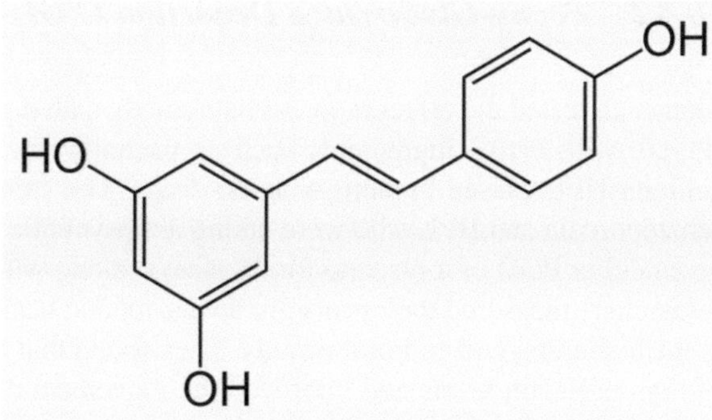

10.8 Herbal Medicine in Managing Hyperprolactinemia

Hyperprolactinemia (HPL) is a condition in which elevated levels of prolactin hormone are detected. Prolactin is a hormone that not only plays part in lactation but also directly affects reproduction by suppressing progesterone secretion during luteal phase. Prolactin normally elevates during breastfeeding; however, other factors can also cause a rise in prolactin level, pathophysiologically [144]. One of the most important neurotransmitters that affects levels of prolactin directly is dopamine. Dopamine prevents prolactin from secretion from pituitary gland; therefore, dopamine antagonist can trigger prolactin release. Other complications that are associated with HPL include menstrual irregularities, sexual dysfunction galactorrhea, and osteoporosis. The most common medication for HPL is dopamine receptor agonists such as bromocriptine and cabergoline, but treatment highly depends on the origin of the disease [145]. Present treatments are often accompanied by adverse effects such as nausea, vomiting, and fatigue. Therefore, patients prefer to try herbal medicine instead, which is commonly associated with less severe side effects. Although there is not sufficient evidence for deciding on the exact herbal treatment for HPL, an attempt was made to cover the exiting well-designed clinical trials in this section (Table 10.6).

10.8.1 Vitex agnus-castus L.

V. agnus-castus (Lamiaceae), commonly known as chasteberry, is often prescribed in various female complications such as menopause and menstrual irregularity. It consists of alkaloids, iridoid glycosides, and essential oils. According to a meta-analysis, vitex can maintain healthy luteal phase in latent HPL by raising progesterone and 17β-estradiol levels in the middle of the cycle. It can also reduce serum prolactin levels and ameliorate mastalgia, comparably to bromocriptine [145, 146]. The recommended daily dose for vitex is 3.2–40 mg orally per day for up to 6 months. Gastrointestinal (GI)-associated side effects are common, and it should be avoided during pregnancy and breastfeeding. As it affects prolactin levels, simultaneous consumption with dopaminergic antagonists should be avoided [147].

10.8.2 Peony-Glycyrrhiza Decoction (PGD)

Man et al. tested the effect of an herbal remedy called peony-glycyrrhiza decoction (PGD), with active ingredients such as paeoniflorin, albiflorin, and glycyrrhizic acid, on HPL caused by antipsychotic drugs. The study involved 99 women with schizophrenia and HPL who were taking antipsychotic drugs. They were randomly given either PGD or a placebo for 16 weeks, along with their usual treatment. The researchers measured their prolactin levels, mental health, and movement disorders at the beginning and end of the study. They found that PGD reduced the symptoms of high prolactin levels and improved the movement disorders more than placebo, without affecting the mental health. Menstruation status was also improved. However, PGD did not lower the serum prolactin levels [148]. This decoction should be avoided during pregnancy, as it may cause uterine contraction, and breastfeeding. As peony may act similar to estrogen, any hormone-sensitive condition should be taken into account while prescribing this decoction [149]. Glycyrrhiza or licorice should be taken with caution in patient with hypertension in long-term use [150].

10.9 Conclusion

This chapter gave a hint about the effects of medicinal plants as traditional medicines on more prevalent metabolic disorders. Herbal medicines such as green tea, garlic, black seed, fenugreek, cinnamon, flaxseed, soy isoflavones, *Vitex agnus-castus L.*, ginger, and saffron can be considered as supplementation with low side effects for the management of the metabolic disorders. However, further studies for determining the effective dose and duration of consumption of these herbs are recommended.

References

1. Tabatabaei-Malazy O, Larijani B, Abdollahi M. Targeting metabolic disorders by natural products. J Diabetes Metab Disord. 2015;14:57. https://doi.org/10.1186/s40200-015-0184-8.
2. Manouchehri A, Abbaszadeh S, Ahmadi M, Nejad FK, Bahmani M, Dastyar N. Polycystic ovaries and herbal remedies: a systematic review. JBRA Assist Reprod. 2023;27(1):85–91.
3. Morvaridi M, Rayyani E, Jaafari M, Khiabani A, Rahimlou M. The effect of green coffee extract supplementation on cardio metabolic risk factors: a systematic review and meta-analysis of randomized controlled trials. J Diabetes Metab Disord. 2020;19(1):645–60.
4. Cui W, Luo K, Xiao Q, Sun Z, Wang Y, Cui C, et al. Effect of mulberry leaf or mulberry leaf extract on glycemic traits: a systematic review and meta-analysis. Food Funct. 2023;14(3):1277–89.
5. Tian J, Feng B, Tian Z. The effect of curcumin on lipid profile and glycemic status of patients with type 2 diabetes mellitus: a systematic review and meta-analysis. Evid Based Complement Alternat Med. 2022;2022:8278744.

6. Abdollahi A, Adelibahram F, Ghassab-Abdollahi N, Araj-Khodaei M, Parsian Z, Mirghafourvand M. The effect of Salvia officinalis on blood glycemic indexes and blood lipid profile in diabetic patients: a systematic review and meta-analysis. J Complement Integr Med. 2023;20(3):521–9.
7. Zamani M, Zarei M, Nikbaf-Shandiz M, Gholami F, Hosseini AM, Nadery M, et al. The effects of saffron supplementation on cardiovascular risk factors in adults: a systematic review and dose-response meta-analysis. Front Nutr. 2022;9:1055517.
8. Asbaghi O, Nazarian B, Reiner Ž, Amirani E, Kolahdooz F, Chamani M, et al. The effects of grape seed extract on glycemic control, serum lipoproteins, inflammation, and body weight: a systematic review and meta-analysis of randomized controlled trials. Phytother Res. 2020;34(2):239–53.
9. Mohammadi-Sartang M, Sohrabi Z, Barati-Boldaji R, Raeisi-Dehkordi H, Mazloom Z. Flaxseed supplementation on glucose control and insulin sensitivity: a systematic review and meta-analysis of 25 randomized, placebo-controlled trials. Nutr Rev. 2018;76(2):125–39.
10. Tabatabaei-Malazy O, Ramezani A, Atlasi R, Larijani B, Abdollahi M. Scientometric study of academic publications on antioxidative herbal medicines in type 2 diabetes mellitus. J Diabetes Metab Disord. 2016;15:48. https://doi.org/10.1186/s40200-016-0273-3.
11. Federation ID. IDF Diabetes Atlas. 10, editor: International Diabetes Federation; 2021.
12. Sohouli MH, Haghshenas N, Hernández-Ruiz Á, Shidfar F. Consumption of sesame seeds and sesame products has favorable effects on blood glucose levels but not on insulin resistance: a systematic review and meta-analysis of controlled clinical trials. Phytother Res. 2022;36(3):1126–34.
13. Bommer C, Heesemann E, Sagalova V, Manne-Goehler J, Atun R, Bärnighausen T, et al. The global economic burden of diabetes in adults aged 20–79 years: a cost-of-illness study. Lancet Diabetes Endocrinol. 2017;5(6):423–30.
14. Sasani N, Kazemi A, Rezaiyan M, Amiri-Ardekani E, Akhlaghi M, Babajafari S, et al. Effect of Artemisia extract on glycemic control: a systematic review and meta-analysis of randomized controlled trial. Int J Clin Pract. 2021;75(11):e14719.
15. Sayed UFSM, Moshawih S, Goh HP, Kifli N, Gupta G, Singh SK, et al. Natural products as novel anti-obesity agents: insights into mechanisms of action and potential for therapeutic management. Front Pharmacol. 2023;14
16. Keramati M, et al. Cinnamon, an effective anti-obesity agent: evidence from an umbrella meta-analysis. J Food Biochem. 2022;46(8):e14166.
17. Jayaprakasha G, Rao LJM. Chemistry, biogenesis, and biological activities of Cinnamomum zeylanicum. Crit Rev Food Sci Nutr. 2011;51(6):547–62.
18. Gothai S, Ganesan P, Park S-Y, Fakurazi S, Choi D-K, Arulselvan P. Natural phyto-bioactive compounds for the treatment of type 2 diabetes: inflammation as a target. Nutrients. 2016;8(8):461.
19. Davis PA, Yokoyama W. Cinnamon intake lowers fasting blood glucose: meta-analysis. J Med Food. 2011;14(9):884–9.
20. Crawford P. Effectiveness of cinnamon for lowering hemoglobin A1C in patients with type 2 diabetes: a randomized, controlled trial. J Am Board Family Med. 2009;22(5):507–12.
21. Kwan HY, Wu J, Su T, Chao X-J, Liu B, Fu X, et al. Cinnamon induces browning in subcutaneous adipocytes. Sci Rep. 2017;7(1):2447.
22. Silva ML, Bernardo MA, Singh J, de Mesquita MF. Cinnamon as a complementary therapeutic approach for dysglycemia and dyslipidemia control in type 2 diabetes mellitus and its molecular mechanism of action: a review. Nutrients. 2022;14(13):2773.
23. Gu D-T, et al. Safety of cinnamon: an umbrella review of meta-analyses and systematic reviews of randomized clinical trials. Front Pharmacol. 2022;12:790901.
24. Vitamins & Supplements. Available from: https://www.webmd.com/ (2023).
25. Espiritu MJ, et al. Mechanisms of herb-drug interactions involving cinnamon and CYP2A6: focus on time-dependent inhibition by Cinnamaldehyde and 2-Methoxycinnamaldehyde. Drug Metab Dispos. 2020;48(10):1028–43.

26. Liu K, Zhou R, Wang B, Chen K, Shi LY, Zhu JD, et al. Effect of green tea on glucose control and insulin sensitivity: a meta-analysis of 17 randomized controlled trials. Am J Clin Nutr. 2013;98(2):340–8.
27. Li Y, Wang C, Huai Q, Guo F, Liu L, Feng R, et al. Effects of tea or tea extract on metabolic profiles in patients with type 2 diabetes mellitus: a meta-analysis of ten randomized controlled trials. Diabetes Metab Res Rev. 2016;32(1):2–10.
28. Hartley L, Flowers N, Holmes J, Clarke A, Stranges S, Hooper L, et al. Green and black tea for the primary prevention of cardiovascular disease. Cochrane Database Syst Rev. 2013;6
29. Khan N, Mukhtar H. Tea polyphenols in promotion of human health. Nutrients. 2018;11(1):39.
30. Zhao T, Li C, Wang S, Song X. Green tea (Camellia sinensis): a review of its phytochemistry, pharmacology, and toxicology. Molecules. 2022;27(12):3909.
31. Zhong J, Xu C, Reece EA, Yang P. The green tea polyphenol EGCG alleviates maternal diabetes–induced neural tube defects by inhibiting DNA hypermethylation. Am J Obstet Gynecol. 2016;215(3):368.
32. (NCCIH), T.N.C.f.C.a.I.H. Green Tea. 2020 October 2020; Available from: https://www.nccih.nih.gov/health/green-tea.
33. Bedrood Z, Rameshrad M, Hosseinzadeh H. Toxicological effects of Camellia sinensis (green tea): a review. Phytother Res. 2018;32(7):1163–80.
34. Cerbin-Koczorowska M, Waszyk-Nowaczyk M, Bakun P, Goslinski T, Koczorowski T. Current view on green tea catechins formulations, their interactions with selected drugs, and prospective applications for various health conditions. Appl Sci. 2021;11(11):4905.
35. Sánchez M, González-Burgos E, Iglesias I, Gómez-Serranillos MP. Pharmacological update properties of aloe Vera and its major active constituents. Molecules. 2020;25(6)
36. Dick WR, Fletcher EA, Shah SA. Reduction of fasting blood glucose and hemoglobin A1c using oral Aloe Vera: a meta-analysis. J Altern Complement Med. 2016;22(6):450–7.
37. Noor A, Gunasekaran S, Vijayalakshmi M. Improvement of insulin secretion and pancreatic β-cell function in streptozotocin-induced diabetic rats treated with Aloe vera extract. Pharm Res. 2017;9(Suppl 1):S99.
38. Deora N, Venkatraman K. Aloe vera in diabetic dyslipidemia: improving blood glucose and lipoprotein levels in pre-clinical and clinical studies. J Ayurveda Integr Med. 2022;13(4):100675.
39. Gong J, Fang K, Dong H, Wang D, Hu M, Lu F. Effect of fenugreek on hyperglycaemia and hyperlipidemia in diabetes and prediabetes: a meta-analysis. J Ethnopharmacol. 2016;194:260–8.
40. Askarpour M, Alami F, Campbell MS, Venkatakrishnan K, Hadi A, Ghaedi E. Effect of fenugreek supplementation on blood lipids and body weight: a systematic review and meta-analysis of randomized controlled trials. J Ethnopharmacol. 2020;253:112538.
41. Nagulapalli Venkata KC, Swaroop A, Bagchi D, Bishayee A. A small plant with big benefits: fenugreek (Trigonella foenum-graecum Linn.) for disease prevention and health promotion. Mol Nutr Food Res. 2017;61(6)
42. Wani SA, Kumar P. Fenugreek: a review on its nutraceutical properties and utilization in various food products. J Saudi Soc Agric Sci. 2018;17(2):97–106.
43. Suksomboon N, Poolsup N, Boonkaew S, Suthisisang CC. Meta-analysis of the effect of herbal supplement on glycemic control in type 2 diabetes. J Ethnopharmacol. 2011;137(3):1328–33.
44. Neelakantan N, Narayanan M, de Souza RJ, van Dam RM. Effect of fenugreek (Trigonella foenum-graecum L.) intake on glycemia: a meta-analysis of clinical trials. Nutr J. 2014;13:7.
45. Patel NB. Khat (Catha edulis Forsk)–and now there are three. Brain Res Bull. 2019;145:92–6.
46. Al-Sharafi BA, Gunaid AA. Effect of habitual khat chewing on glycemic control, body mass index, and age at diagnosis of diabetes in patients with type 2 diabetes mellitus in Yemen. Clin Med Insights Endocrinol Diabetes. 2015;8:S26045.
47. Mengistu Y, Dedefo G, Arkew M, Asefa G, Jebessa G, Atnafu A, et al. Effect of regular Khat chewing on serum fasting sugar level in diabetic patients versus healthy individuals; a comparative study. Nutr Metab Insights. 2021;14:11786388211035220.

48. Alsalahi A, Alshawsh MA, Mohamed R, Alyousefi NA, Alshagga MA, Shwter AN, et al. Conflicting reports on the role of the glycemic effect of Catha edulis (Khat): a systematic review and meta-analysis. J Ethnopharmacol. 2016;186:30–43.
49. Ghorbani A. Clinical and experimental studies on polyherbal formulations for diabetes: current status and future prospective. J Integr Med. 2014;12(4):336–45.
50. Daryabeygi-Khotbehsara R, Golzarand M, Ghaffari MP, Djafarian K. Nigella sativa improves glucose homeostasis and serum lipids in type 2 diabetes: a systematic review and meta-analysis. Complement Ther Med. 2017;35:6–13.
51. Bundgaard Anker CC, Rafiq S, Jeppesen PB. Effect of Steviol glycosides on human health with emphasis on type 2 diabetic biomarkers: a systematic review and meta-analysis of randomized controlled trials. Nutrients. 2019;11(9)
52. Huang FY, Deng T, Meng LX, Ma XL. Dietary ginger as a traditional therapy for blood sugar control in patients with type 2 diabetes mellitus: a systematic review and meta-analysis. Medicine (Baltimore). 2019;98(13):e15054.
53. Huang J, Qin S, Huang L, Tang Y, Ren H, Hu H. Efficacy and safety of Rhizoma curcumea longae with respect to improving the glucose metabolism of patients at risk for cardiovascular disease: a meta-analysis of randomised controlled trials. J Hum Nutr Diet. 2019;32(5):591–606.
54. Ding KX, Gao TL, Xu R, Cai J, Zhang HQ, Sun YY, et al. Quantifying the effect of supplementation with algae and its extracts on glycolipid metabolism: a meta-analysis of randomized controlled trials. Nutrients. 2020;12(6)
55. Jang HH, Lee J, Lee SH, Lee YM. Effects of Capsicum annuum supplementation on the components of metabolic syndrome: a systematic review and meta-analysis. Sci Rep. 2020;10(1):20912.
56. Jamshidi S, Moradi Y, Nameni G, Mohsenpour MA, Vafa M. Effects of cashew nut consumption on body composition and glycemic indices: a meta-analysis and systematic review of randomized controlled trials. Diabetes Metab Syndr. 2021;15(2):605–13.
57. Mohit M, Nouri M, Samadi M, Nouri Y, Heidarzadeh-Esfahani N, Venkatakrishnan K, et al. The effect of sumac (Rhus coriaria L.) supplementation on glycemic indices: a systematic review and meta-analysis of controlled clinical trials. Complement Ther Med. 2021;61:102766.
58. Nchanji EB, Ageyo OC. Do common beans (Phaseolus vulgaris L.) promote good health in humans? A systematic review and meta-analysis of clinical and randomized controlled trials. Nutrients. 2021;13(11)
59. Yargholi A, Najafi MH, Zareian MA, Hawkins J, Shirbeigi L, Ayati MH. The effects of sesame consumption on glycemic control in adults: a systematic review and meta-analysis of randomized clinical trial. Evid Based Complement Alternat Med. 2021;2021:2873534.
60. Kim SJ, Anh NH, Jung CW, Long NP, Park S, Cho YH, et al. Metabolic and cardiovascular benefits of apple and apple-derived products: a systematic review and meta-analysis of randomized controlled trials. Front Nutr. 2022;9:766155.
61. Mirzababaei A, Daneshvar M, Abaj F, Daneshzad E, Hosseininasab D, Clark CCT, et al. The effect of walnut (Juglans regia) leaf extract on glycemic control and lipid profile in patients with type 2 diabetes mellitus: a systematic review and meta-analysis of randomized clinical trials. Clin Nutr Res. 2022;11(2):120–32.
62. Musazadeh V, Golandam F, Faghfouri AH, Abdoli Shadbad M, Keramati M, Moridpour AH, et al. Curcumin supplementation contributes to relieving anthropometric and glycemic indices, as an adjunct therapy: a meta-research review of meta-analyses. J Funct Foods. 2022;99:105357.
63. Shabil M, Bushi G, Bodige PK, Maradi PS, Patra BP, Padhi BK, et al. Effect of fenugreek on hyperglycemia: a systematic review and meta-analysis. Medicina (Kaunas). 2023;59(2)
64. Adel Mehraban MS, Tabatabaei-Malazy O, Rahimi R, Daniali M, Khashayar P, Larijani B. Targeting dyslipidemia by herbal medicines: a systematic review of meta-analyses. J Ethnopharmacol. 2021;280:114407.

65. Pirillo A, Casula M, Olmastroni E, Norata GD, Catapano AL. Global epidemiology of dyslipidaemias. Nat Rev Cardiol. 2021;18(10):689–700.
66. Onakpoya I, Spencer E, Heneghan C, Thompson M. The effect of green tea on blood pressure and lipid profile: a systematic review and meta-analysis of randomized clinical trials. Nutr Metab Cardiovasc Dis. 2014;24(8):823–36.
67. Asghari-Jafarabadi M, Khalili L. The effect of ginger (Zingiber officinale) on improving blood lipids and body weight; a systematic review and multivariate meta-analysis of clinical trials. Curr Pharm Des. 2022;28(35):2920–43.
68. Payab M, Hasani-Ranjbar S, Shahbal N, Qorbani M, Aletaha A, Haghi-Aminjan H, et al. Effect of the herbal medicines in obesity and metabolic syndrome: a systematic review and meta-analysis of clinical trials. Phytother Res. 2020;34(3):526–45.
69. Chan W-JJ, McLachlan AJ, Luca EJ, Harnett JE. Garlic (Allium sativum L.) in the management of hypertension and dyslipidemia–a systematic review. J Herbal Med. 2020;19:100292.
70. Shabani E, Sayemiri K, Mohammadpour M. The effect of garlic on lipid profile and glucose parameters in diabetic patients: a systematic review and meta-analysis. Prim Care Diabetes. 2019;13(1):28–42.
71. Ried K, Toben C, Fakler P. Effect of garlic on serum lipids: an updated meta-analysis. Nutr Rev. 2013;71(5):282–99.
72. Silagy C, Neil A. Garlic as a lipid lowering agent – a meta-analysis. J R Coll Physicians Lond. 1994;28(1):39.
73. El-Saber Batiha G, Magdy Beshbishy A, et al. Chemical constituents and pharmacological activities of garlic (Allium sativum L.): a review. Nutrients. 2020;12(3)
74. Sarecka-Hujar B, Szulc-Musioł B. Herbal medicines – are they effective and safe during pregnancy? Pharmaceutics. 2022;14(1):171.
75. Mao QQ, et al. Bioactive compounds and bioactivities of ginger (Zingiber officinale roscoe). Foods. 2019;8(6)
76. Zhang M, Zhao R, Wang D, Wang L, Zhang Q, Wei S, et al. Ginger (Zingiber officinale Rosc.) and its bioactive components are potential resources for health beneficial agents. Phytother Res. 2021;35(2):711–42.
77. Modi MMK. Ginger Root. 2022 November 28, 2022.; Available from: https://www.ncbi.nlm.nih.gov/books/NBK565886/.
78. Lien HC, et al. Effects of ginger on motion sickness and gastric slow-wave dysrhythmias induced by circular vection. Am J Physiol Gastrointest Liver Physiol. 2003;284(3):G481–9.
79. Paritakul P, et al. The effect of ginger on breast milk volume in the early postpartum period: a randomized. Double-Blind Controlled Trial Breastfeed Med. 2016;11:361–5.
80. Qiu J-X, Zhou Z-W, He Z-X, Zhang X, Zhou S-F, Zhu S. Estimation of the binding modes with important human cytochrome P450 enzymes, drug interaction potential, pharmacokinetics, and hepatotoxicity of ginger components using molecular docking, computational, and pharmacokinetic modeling studies. Drug Des Devel Ther. 2015:841–66.
81. Crichton M, Davidson AR, Innerarity C, Marx W, Lohning A, Isenring E, et al. Orally consumed ginger and human health: an umbrella review. Am J Clin Nutr. 2022;115(6):1511–27.
82. Fakhr L, Chehregosha F, Zarezadeh M, Chaboksafar M, Tarighat-Esfanjani A. Effects of fenugreek supplementation on the components of metabolic syndrome: a systematic review and dose-response meta-analysis of randomized clinical trials. Pharmacol Res. 2023;187:106594.
83. Hallajzadeh J, Milajerdi A, Mobini M, Amirani E, Azizi S, Nikkhah E, et al. Effects of Nigella sativa on glycemic control, lipid profiles, and biomarkers of inflammatory and oxidative stress: a systematic review and meta-analysis of randomized controlled clinical trials. Phytother Res. 2020;34(10):2586–608.
84. Ahmad MF, et al. An updated knowledge of black seed (Nigella sativa Linn.): review of phytochemical constituents and pharmacological properties. J Herbal Med. 2021;25:100404.
85. Namazi N, et al. The effects of Nigella sativa L. on obesity: a systematic review and meta-analysis. J Ethnopharmacol. 2018;219:173–81.

86. Sahebkar A, Beccuti G, Simental-Mendía LE, Nobili V, Bo S. Nigella sativa (black seed) effects on plasma lipid concentrations in humans: a systematic review and meta-analysis of randomized placebo-controlled trials. Pharmacol Res. 2016;106:37–50.
87. Hannan MA, Rahman MA, Sohag AAM, Uddin MJ, Dash R, Sikder MH, et al. Black cumin (Nigella sativa L.): a comprehensive review on Phytochemistry, health benefits, molecular pharmacology, and safety. Nutrients. 2021;13(6):1784.
88. Roshanravan B, Samarghandian S, Ashrafizadeh M, Amirabadizadeh A, Saeedi F, Farkhondeh T. Metabolic impact of saffron and crocin: an updated systematic and meta-analysis of randomised clinical trials. Arch Physiol Biochem. 2022;128(3):666–78.
89. Ayati Z, Yang G, Ayati MH, Emami SA, Chang D. Saffron for mild cognitive impairment and dementia: a systematic review and meta-analysis of randomised clinical trials. BMC Complement Med Ther. 2020;20:1–10.
90. Wu T, Huang W, He M, Yue R. Effects of cinnamon supplementation on lipid profiles among patients with metabolic syndrome and related disorders: a systematic review and meta-analysis. Complement Ther Clin Pract. 2022;49:101625.
91. Santos HO, da Silva GA. To what extent does cinnamon administration improve the glycemic and lipid profiles? Clinical nutrition ESPEN. 2018;27:1–9.
92. Niknafs A, Rezvanfar M, Kamalinejad M, Latifi SA, Almasi-Hashiani A, Salehi M. The effect of a Persian herbal medicine compound on the lipid profiles of patients with dyslipidemia: a randomized double-blind placebo-controlled clinical trial. Evid Based Complement Alternat Med. 2021;2021:6631963.
93. Ghorbani A, Zarvandi M, Rakhshandeh H. A randomized controlled trial of a herbal compound for improving metabolic parameters in diabetic patients with uncontrolled dyslipidemia. Endocrine, metabolic & immune disorders – drug targets (formerly current drug targets – immune). Endocr Metab Disorders. 2019;19(7):1075–82.
94. Yu X, Xu L, Zhou Q, Wu S, Tian J, Piao C, et al. The efficacy and safety of the Chinese herbal formula, JTTZ, for the treatment of type 2 diabetes with obesity and hyperlipidemia: a multicenter randomized, positive-controlled, open-label clinical trial. Int J Endocrinol. 2018;2018:1.
95. Tiwari A, Balasundaram P. Public health considerations regarding obesity; 2021.
96. Organization, W.H. World Obesity Day 2022 – Accelerating action to stop obesity. 2022.; Available from: https://www.who.int/news/item/04-03-2022-world-obesity-day-2022-accelerating-action-to-stop-obesity.
97. Aghabeiglooei Z, et al. Effects of Komouni formulation (herbal product of Persian medicine) with a low-calorie diet on Cardiometabolic risk factors in overweight and obese women: a triple-blinded randomized clinical trial. Iran J Pharm Res. 2023;22(1):e136114.
98. Hasani-Ranjbar S, Jouyandeh Z, Abdollahi M. A systematic review of anti-obesity medicinal plants-an update. J Diabetes Metab Disord. 2013;12:1–10.
99. Mousavi SM, et al. Cinnamon supplementation positively affects obesity: a systematic review and dose-response meta-analysis of randomized controlled trials. Clin Nutr. 2020;39(1):123–33.
100. Rondanelli M, et al. Effect of acute and chronic dietary supplementation with green tea Catechins on resting metabolic rate, energy expenditure and respiratory quotient: a systematic review. Nutrients. 2021;13(2)
101. Kim BS, Song MY, Kim H. The anti-obesity effect of Ephedra sinica through modulation of gut microbiota in obese Korean women. J Ethnopharmacol. 2014;152(3):532–9.
102. Song MK, et al. Beneficial effect of dietary Ephedra sinica on obesity and glucose intolerance in high-fat diet-fed mice. Exp Ther Med. 2012;3(4):707–12.
103. Shekelle PG, Hardy ML, Morton SC, Maglione M, Mojica WA, Suttorp MJ, Rhodes SL, Jungvig L, Gagné J. Efficacy and safety of ephedra and ephedrine for weight loss and athletic performance: a meta-analysis. JAMA. 2003;289(12):1537–45.
104. Park SJ, et al. Extract of Ephedra sinica Stapf induces browning of mouse and human white adipocytes. Foods. 2022;11(7)

105. UpToDate. Ephedrine (systemic): Drug information. 2023; Available from: https://medilib.ir/uptodate/show/9114.
106. Bahramsoltani R, Tabatabaei-Malazy O. Ephedra. In: Wexler P, editor. Encyclopedia of toxicology. 4th ed. Academic Press; 2024. p. 305–12. https://doi.org/10.1016/B978-0-12-824315-2.01010-1.
107. Haller CA, Benowitz NL. Adverse cardiovascular and central nervous system events associated with dietary supplements containing ephedra alkaloids. N Engl J Med. 2000;343(25):1833–8.
108. Salaramoli S, et al. The effects of ginger and its constituents in the prevention of metabolic syndrome: a review. Iran J Basic Med Sci. 2022;25(6):664–74.
109. Cheng Z, et al. 6-gingerol ameliorates metabolic disorders by inhibiting hypertrophy and hyperplasia of adipocytes in high-fat-diet induced obese mice. Biomed Pharmacother. 2022;146:112491.
110. Maharlouei N, Tabrizi R, Lankarani KB, Rezaianzadeh A, Akbari M, Kolahdooz F, Rahimi M, Keneshlou F, Asemi Z. The effects of ginger intake on weight loss and metabolic profiles among overweight and obese subjects: a systematic review and meta-analysis of randomized controlled trials. Crit Rev Food Sci Nutr. 2019;59(11):1753–66.
111. Kim S, et al. Ginger extract ameliorates obesity and inflammation via regulating MicroRNA-21/132 expression and AMPK activation in white adipose tissue. Nutrients. 2018;10(11)
112. Asbaghi O, et al. Effect of green tea on anthropometric indices and body composition in patients with type 2 diabetes mellitus: a systematic review and meta-analysis. Complement Med Res. 2021;28(3):244–51.
113. Jurgens TM, et al. Green tea for weight loss and weight maintenance in overweight or obese adults. Cochrane Database Syst Rev. 2012;12
114. Lin Y, et al. The effect of green tea supplementation on obesity: a systematic review and dose–response meta-analysis of randomized controlled trials. Phytother Res. 2020;34(10):2459–70.
115. Shen W, et al. Effects of tea consumption on anthropometric parameters, metabolic indexes and hormone levels of women with polycystic ovarian syndrome: a systematic review and meta-analysis of randomized controlled trials. Front Endocrinol. 2021;12:736867.
116. Tahmasbi F, et al. Effects of saffron (Crocus sativus L.) on anthropometric and cardiometabolic indices in overweight and obese patients: a systematic review and meta-analysis of randomized controlled trials. Phytother Res. 2022;36(9):3394–414.
117. Golzarand M, Omidian M, Toolabi K. Effect of Garcinia cambogia supplement on obesity indices: a systematic review and dose-response meta-analysis. Complement Ther Med. 2020;52:102451.
118. Onakpoya I, et al. The efficacy of Phaseolus vulgaris as a weight-loss supplement: a systematic review and meta-analysis of randomised clinical trials. Br J Nutr. 2011;106(2):196–202.
119. Fu Z, et al. Effects of garlic supplementation on components of metabolic syndrome: a systematic review, meta-analysis, and meta-regression of randomized controlled trials. BMC Complement Med Ther. 2023;23(1):260.
120. Eslampour E, et al. The effect of almond intake on anthropometric indices: a systematic review and meta-analysis. Food Funct. 2020;11(9):7340–55.
121. Asgary S, Karimi R, Momtaz S, Naseri R, Farzaei MH. Effect of resveratrol on metabolic syndrome components: a systematic review and meta-analysis. Rev Endocr Metab Disorders. 2019;20:173–86.
122. Qiu L, Gao C, Wang H, Ren Y, Li J, Li M, et al. Effects of dietary polyphenol curcumin supplementation on metabolic, inflammatory, and oxidative stress indices in patients with metabolic syndrome: a systematic review and meta-analysis of randomized controlled trials. Front Endocrinol (Lausanne). 2023;14:1216708. https://doi.org/10.3389/fendo.2023.1216708.
123. Najafpour Boushehri S, Karimbeiki R, Ghasempour S, Ghalishourani SS, Pourmasoumi M, Hadi A, et al. The efficacy of sour tea (Hibiscus sabdariffa L.) on selected cardiovascular disease risk factors: a systematic review and meta-analysis of randomized clinical trials. Phytother Res. 2020;34(2):329–39.

124. Epidemiology. Available at: http://www.osteoporosis.foundation/health-professionals/about-osteoporosis/epidemiology (2023).
125. Sohi YH, Golestani A, Panahi G, Tabatabaei-Malazy O, Khalagi K, Fahimfar N, Ostovar A, Sanjari M, Larijani B, Nabipour I. The association between anti-diabetic agents and osteoporosis, sarcopenia, and osteosarcopenia among Iranian older adults; Bushehr elderly health (BEH) program. Daru. 2023; https://doi.org/10.1007/s40199-023-00497-5.
126. Tabatabaei-Malazy O, Salari P, Khashayar P, Larijani B. New horizons in treatment of osteoporosis. Daru. 2017;25(1):2. https://doi.org/10.1186/s40199-017-0167-z.
127. Salari Sharif P, Nikfar S, Abdollahi M. Prevention of bone resorption by intake of phytoestrogens in postmenopausal women: a meta-analysis. Age (Dordr). 2011;33:421–31.
128. Sansai K, Na Takuathung M, Khatsri R, Teekachunhatean S, Hanprasertpong N, Koonrungsesomboon N. Effects of isoflavone interventions on bone mineral density in postmenopausal women: a systematic review and meta-analysis of randomized controlled trials. Osteoporos Int. 2020;31(10):1853–64. https://doi.org/10.1007/s00198-020-05476-z.
129. Chen CC, Shen YM, Li SB, Huang SW, Kuo YJ, Chen YP. Association of Coffee and Tea intake with bone mineral density and hip fracture: a meta-analysis. Medicina (Kaunas). 2023;59(6):1177. https://doi.org/10.3390/medicina59061177.
130. CDC. PCOS (Polycystic Ovary Syndrome) and Diabetes 2022 Available from: https://www.cdc.gov/diabetes/basics/pcos.html
131. Meyer C, McGrath BP, Teede HJ. Overweight women with polycystic ovary syndrome have evidence of subclinical cardiovascular disease. J Clin Endocrinol Metabol. 2005;90(10):5711–6.
132. Barry JA, Kuczmierczyk AR, Hardiman PJ. Anxiety and depression in polycystic ovary syndrome: a systematic review and meta-analysis. Hum Reprod. 2011;26(9):2442–51.
133. Griffin RM. Flaxseed 2023. Available from: https://www.webmd.com/a-to-z-guides/supplement-guide-flaxseed-oil
134. Aly JM, Decherney AH. Lifestyle modifications in PCOS. Clin Obstet Gynecol. 2021;64(1):83–9.
135. Emamat H, Najafpour Boushehri S, Eslami MA, Saneei Totmaj A, Ghalandari H. The effects of flaxseed or its oil supplementations on polycystic ovary syndrome: a systematic review of clinical trials. Phytother Res. 2023;37(3):1082–91.
136. Lampe JW. Isoflavonoid and lignan phytoestrogens as dietary biomarkers. J Nutr. 2003;133(Suppl 3):956s–64s.
137. Kim I-S. Current perspectives on the beneficial effects of soybean isoflavones and their metabolites for humans. Antioxidants. 2021;10(7):1064.
138. Zılaee M, Mansoori A, Ahmad HS, Mohaghegh SM, Asadi M, Hormoznejad R. The effects of soy isoflavones on total testosterone and follicle-stimulating hormone levels in women with polycystic ovary syndrome: a systematic review and meta-analysis. Eur J Contracept Reprod Health Care. 2020;25(4):305–10.
139. Kalantari H, Das DK. Physiological effects of resveratrol. Biofactors. 2010;36(5):401–6.
140. Malhotra A, Bath S, Elbarbry F. An organ system approach to explore the Antioxidative, anti-inflammatory, and Cytoprotective actions of resveratrol. Oxidative Med Cell Longev. 2015;2015:803971.
141. Weber K, Schulz B, Ruhnke M. Resveratrol and its antifungal activity against Candida species. Mycoses. 2011;54(1):30–3.
142. Furat Rencber S, Kurnaz Ozbek S, Eraldemır C, Sezer Z, Kum T, Ceylan S, Guzel E. Effect of resveratrol and metformin on ovarian reserve and ultrastructure in PCOS: an experimental study. J Ovarian Res. 2018;11:1–16.
143. Fadlalmola HA, Elhusein AM, Al-Sayaghi KM, Albadrani MS, Swamy DV, Mamanao DM, et al. Efficacy of resveratrol in women with polycystic ovary syndrome: a systematic review and meta-analysis of randomized clinical trials. Pan Afr Med J. 2023:44.
144. WebMD. Resveratrol – uses, side effects, and more. Available from: https://www.webmd.com/vitamins/ai/ingredientmono-307/resveratrol

145. Majumdar A, Mangal NS. Hyperprolactinemia. J Hum Reprod Sci. 2013;6(3):168–75.
146. van Die MD, Burger HG, Teede HJ, Bone KM. Vitex agnus-castus extracts for female reproductive disorders: a systematic review of clinical trials. Planta Med. 2013;79(07):562–75.
147. Daniele C, Thompson Coon J, Pittler MH, Ernst E. Vitex agnus castus: a systematic review of adverse events. Drug Saf. 2005;28(4):319–32.
148. Man SC, Li XB, Wang HH, Yuan HN, Wang HN, Zhang RG, et al. Peony-Glycyrrhiza decoction for antipsychotic-related hyperprolactinemia in women with schizophrenia: a randomized controlled trial. J Clin Psychopharmacol. 2016;36(6):572–9.
149. Feng Z-t, Xu J, He G-c, Cai S-j, Li J, Mei Z-g. A systemic review and meta-analysis of the clinical efficacy and safety of total glucosides of peony combined with methotrexate in rheumatoid arthritis. Clin Rheumatol. 2018;37:35–42.
150. Nazari S, Rameshrad M, Hosseinzadeh H. Toxicological effects of Glycyrrhiza glabra (licorice): a review. Phytother Res. 2017;31(11):1635–50.
151. Puglia LT, Lowry J, Tamagno G. Vitex agnus castus effects on hyperprolactinaemia. Front Endocrinol. 2023;14:1269781. https://doi.org/10.3389/fendo.2023.1269781.
152. Kilicdag EB, Tarim E, Bagisa T, Erkanli S, Aslan E, Ozsahin K, et al. Fructus agni casti and bromocriptine for treatment of hyperprolactinemia and mastalgia. Int J Gynaecol Obstet. 2004;85:292–3. https://doi.org/10.1016/j.ijgo.2004.01.001.

Chapter 11
Gender Identity and Endocrinology

Maryam Mirahmad, Mahnaz Pejman Sani, Seyed Reza Yahyazadeh, Amirahmad Shojaei, and Sayed Mahmoud Sajjadi-Jazi

11.1 Introduction to Gender Identity

As early as the twentieth century, the term "transsexual" was first used by sexologist Hirschfeld to describe people who desired a life congruent with their experienced gender, in place of their assigned gender [1]. It was the time when social awareness emerged for women and men, who believed that they were "trapped in the wrong body" [2]. The terminology in this field is evolving persistently. Gender identity refers to each person's deep and internal sense of being a female, male, neither, or some combination of both [3]. Transgender is a term used to refer to a broad spectrum of persons whose gender identity is not conforming to their assigned sex at birth [3].

M. Mirahmad
Endocrinology and Metabolism Research Center, Endocrinology and Metabolism Clinical Sciences Institute, Tehran University of Medical Sciences, Tehran, Iran

M. Pejman Sani · S. M. Sajjadi-Jazi (✉)
Endocrinology and Metabolism Research Center, Endocrinology and Metabolism Clinical Sciences Institute, Tehran University of Medical Sciences, Tehran, Iran

Department of Endocrinology, Shariati Hospital, School of Medicine, Tehran University of Medical Sciences, Tehran, Iran
e-mail: mpsani@sina.tums.ac.ir; m_sajadi@tums.ac.ir

S. R. Yahyazadeh
Department of Urology, Shariati Hospital, Tehran University of Medical Sciences, Tehran, Iran

Urology Research Center, Tehran University of Medical Sciences, Tehran, Iran

A. Shojaei
Medical Ethics and History of Medicine Research Center, Tehran University of Medical Sciences, Tehran, Iran

H. Gharib et al. (eds.), *Interdisciplinary Advances in Endocrinology*,
https://doi.org/10.1007/978-981-95-2286-6_11

The size of transgender population is difficult to accurately estimate and is probably underestimated because of the attached stigma. However, over the past decades, social awareness has improved, and people feel more comfortable expressing their gender identity [4]. Population-based studies estimate that gender incongruence ranges from 0.4% to 1.2% for birth-assigned females and from 0.5% to 1.3% for birth-assigned males, leading to an estimate of about 25 million people worldwide [5, 6]. It has been widely observed that there are a growing number of transgender people who may seek medical and/or surgical care worldwide [7].

Transgender individuals can experience varying degrees of distress related to their biological sex, primary and secondary sexual characteristics, and social gender roles [8]. Therefore, they may go through a social transition. Social transition can include changing the individual's name, physical appearance, and pronouns and taking social roles in alignment with their gender identity [9]. A more radical approach is medical transition comprising puberty suppression, hormone therapy, and surgical interventions. Mounting evidence supports the use of medical and surgical approaches in individuals seeking care for gender dysphoria [10–12]. This chapter provides a discussion of gender dysphoria definition, hormonal and surgical intervention for gender affirmation, mental healthcare, and ethical considerations for transgender care.

11.2 Gender Dysphoria

The terminology used to describe transgender and gender-diverse individuals has undergone significant evolution within psychiatric and medical disciplines. Diagnostic manuals such as the International Classification of Diseases (ICD) and the Diagnostic and Statistical Manual of Mental Disorders, Fifth Edition (DSM-5), have progressively updated their diagnostic criteria and terminology for transgender people. Earlier terms like "gender identity disorder" and "transsexualism" have been replaced in ICD-11 by "gender incongruence" and in DSM-5 by "gender dysphoria" to better reflect present understanding and reduce stigma [13]. The term "dysphoria" by itself refers to a general state of distress and dissatisfaction; in this context, gender dysphoria specifically describes an individual's discomfort or discontent with their assigned gender. The DSM-5 defines gender dysphoria as a strong and persistent incongruence between expressed or experienced gender and assigned gender, lasting at least 6 months [14]. The DSM-5 provides distinct diagnostic criteria for children and for adolescents and adults.

11.2.1 Diagnostic Criteria for Children

Diagnosis of gender dysphoria in children can be made when there is clinically significant impairment or distress in school, social, or everyday functions, accompanied by a pronounced incongruence between the assigned gender and the child's expressed or experienced gender. This incongruence must be present for at least 6 months and be manifested by at least six of the following: (1) a marked desire to be, or an insistence that one is, another gender; (2) a marked preference for cross-gender clothing; (3) a marked preference for adopting cross-gender roles during fantasy or make-believe play; (4) a marked preference for activities, games, or toys stereotypically associated with the other gender; (5) a marked preference for play-mates of the other gender; (6) a marked rejection of activities, games, or toys typical of one's assigned gender; (7) a marked dislike of one's own sexual anatomy; (8) and a marked desire for the primary and/or secondary sex characteristics that align with one's experienced gender [11, 15].

11.2.2 Diagnostic Criteria for Adolescents and Adults

Diagnosis requires a strong incongruence between assigned and experienced gender lasting at least 6 months, accompanied by clinically significant impairment or distress in daily functioning. At least two of the following criteria must be met: (1) a strong incongruence between one's expressed or experienced gender and primary and/or secondary sex characteristics or, in the case of younger adolescents, the expected development of secondary sex characteristics; (2) a marked desire to be rid of one's primary and/or secondary sex characteristics or, in the case of younger adolescents, a desire to stop the development of expected secondary sex characteristics; (3) a marked desire to possess the primary and/or secondary sex characteristics of the other gender; (4) a marked desire to be another gender; (5) a marked desire to be treated as another gender; and (6) a firm conviction of having the typical feelings and reactions of a gender other than one's assigned gender [11, 15].

11.3 Hormonal Gender Reassignment Treatment

Since 1979, evidence-based guidelines have developed focusing on the care of transgender individuals. Endocrine Society [11] and the World Professional Association for Transgender Health (WPATH) [16] provide clinical practice guidelines concerning transgender health. Transgender persons may need puberty blockers and/or gender-affirming hormone therapy (GAHT).

11.3.1 Puberty Suppression and GAHT in Adolescent

Gender-dysphoric/gender-incongruent adolescents may be eligible for treatment by puberty blockers as soon as they reach Tanner stage II of puberty [11]. Puberty blockers suppress the development of secondary sexual characteristics allowing adolescents and their families more time to explore gender identity and investigate the possible outcomes of available treatments. Pubertal development can be suppressed via gonadotropin-releasing hormone agonists (GnRHa). Constant administration of GnRHa suppresses gonadotropin secretion from the pituitary gland. This response is followed by decreased gonadal activity, reduced secretion of endogenous sex hormones to prepubertal levels, halted pubertal progression, and partial regression of secondary sexual characteristics if already developed [17, 18]. The most frequently used GnRH formulation is an intramuscular injection given every 3 months. However, longer-acting forms and surgically implanted antagonists are also available [19].

In case of persistent gender dysphoria, transgender adolescents may seek sex hormone treatment to induce sexual characteristics consistent with the affirmed gender. Based on the timing of GnRHa treatment, sex steroid treatment consists of two main regimens [16].

In those who received GnRHa treatment at early Tanner stages of pubertal development, sex hormones in line with affirmed gender can be used. In this context, the desired sexual characteristics are induced with sex hormones at doses comparable to those of peripubertal hypogonadal adolescents [16, 19]. Then, the dose of steroid hormones is gradually increased over a period of about 2 years in order to achieve levels of adult sex hormones [20].

When GnRHa treatment is started in postpubertal or late pubertal stages, sex hormones can be started in higher doses and more rapidly increased, similar to treatment regimens used in transgender adults [11, 19].

Adolescents are eligible for treatment by puberty blockers if [11]:

1. A qualified mental health professional confirmed the following: (a) diagnosis of long-lasting gender incongruence or gender dysphoria; (b) began or worsened gender dysphoria by the start of puberty; (c) any coexisting social, psychological, or medical problems that may interfere with treatment have been addressed and controlled; and (d) the adolescent is competent to give informed consent to the (reversible) treatment.
2. And the adolescent: (a) is informed about the potential effects and side effects of the treatment, including loss of fertility and fertility preservation options; and (b) gives informed consent for the treatment, while the parents, guardians, or caretakers also consent to the treatment and support the adolescent during treatment.
3. And an experienced clinician or a pediatric endocrinologist: (a) agrees with the indication of treatment, (b) confirmed that there are no contraindications to the GnRHa, and (c) confirmed puberty has started (Tanner stage II or greater).

11.3.2 GAHT in Adults

GAHT allows transgender adults to maintain their gender identity or cross-gender sexual characteristics [16]. A growing body of evidence has shown the safety and efficacy of GAHT in short- and mid-term follow-up studies [21–23]. The Endocrine

Society Clinical Guideline recommends adults seeking GAHT should meet particular criteria: well-documented and persistent gender dysphoria, capacity to make an informed consent for treatment, controlled mental health concerns, if exist, and have reached the age of maturity [11].

GAHT is used for two main goals: The first is to decrease levels of endogenous sex hormones resulting in decreased sexual characteristics of one's assigned gender at birth. The second is to substitute endogenous sex hormones consistent with one's gender identity by using the principles of hormone replacement therapy for hypogonadism [11]. Based on the goals of treatment, GAHT can be divided into feminizing hormone therapy and masculinizing hormone therapy.

11.3.2.1 Masculinizing Hormone Therapy

Various androgen preparations have been reported to be effective in masculinizing transgender men. Transdermal or parenteral preparations can be used to reach testosterone levels within the normal male range (typically 320–1000 ng/dL) [24, 25].

With testosterone, clitoromegaly, body virilization, deepening of the voice, facial and body hair growth, increased muscle mass, and usually menstrual suppression may occur [26]. Typically, within a few months of testosterone alone, cessation of menses may occur. In some cases, menstrual cessation may not be driven by testosterone alone, and progestational agents or endometrial ablation should be recommended [11]. There are various regimens for GAHT in transgender people. Suggested doses and types of hormones based on present guidelines are presented in the following. GAHT available for transgender men is presented in Table 11.1 [11, 27, 28].

Table 11.1 Gender-affirming hormone treatment in transgender men

Drug class	Route of administration	Drug	Dose
Testosterone	Intramuscular	Testosterone enanthate or cypionate	50–100 mg weekly or 100–200 mg every 2 weeks
		Testosterone undecanoate	1000 mg every 10–12 weeks
	Subcutaneous	Testosterone enanthate or cypionate	50–100 mg weekly
	Oral	Testosterone undecanoate	160 mg/day
	Transdermal	Testosterone gel	50–100 mg/day
		Testosterone patch	2.5–7.5 mg/day
Progestational agents	Oral	Medroxyprogesterone	5–10 mg/day
		Lynestrenol	5–10 mg/day
	Intramuscular	Medroxyprogesterone	150 mg every 3 months

11.3.2.2 Feminizing Hormone Therapy

GAHT for transgender women is more complex than for transgender men. Estrogen therapy within physiologic doses can reduce testosterone levels, but estrogen alone is not sufficient to suppress testosterone to the reference ranges seen in cisgender women [29]. Thus, adjunctive agents, such as GnRHa and progestins, with antiandrogen activity help additional reduction of testosterone levels [11]. Cyproterone acetate has antiandrogenic properties and is also a potent progesterone receptor agonist that causes suppression of the hypothalamic-pituitary-gonadal axis [30]. Spironolactone inhibits androgens by blocking androgen receptors and may have estrogenic activity [30]. 5-Alpha reductase inhibitors reduce the conversion of testosterone into 5-alpha dihydrotestosterone, which is a more potent androgen [30]. Suggested doses and hormones available for transgender women are presented in Table 11.2 [11, 27, 28].

11.4 Surgical Gender Reassignment Treatment

Parallel to the increasing number of transgender people, there are a growing number of transgender individuals who are seeking surgical care worldwide [31, 32]. This increasing surgical trend is owing to social, institutional, and patient-related factors; for instance, insurance policies and laws are changing dynamically; social awareness is increasing; and the availability and capacity of surgical techniques are improving [31]. Gender-affirming surgery is generally irreversible and often the

Table 11.2 Gender-affirming hormone treatment in transgender women

Drug class	Route of administration	Drug	Dose
Estrogen	Oral	Estradiol (17-beta-estradiol valerate)	2–6 mg/day
	Intramuscular	Estradiol cypionate	2–10 mg weekly
		Estradiol valerate	5–30 mg every 1–2 weeks
	Transdermal	Estradiol gel	1.5 mg/day
		Estradiol patch	0.025–0.2 mg/day, new patch placed once or twice weekly based on preparation type
Antiandrogens	Oral	Cyproterone acetate	25–50 mg/day
		Spironolactone	100–300 mg/day
Gonadotropin-releasing hormone agonists	Intramuscular	Leuprolide acetate	3.75 mg monthly or 11.25 mg every 3 months
		Triptorelin	3.75 mg monthly or 11.25 mg every 3 months
	Subcutaneous	Goserelin	3.6 mg monthly or 10.8 mg every 3 months

final step in the medical transition. Patients and clinicians should contribute to a multidisciplinary medical decision-making process that includes a discussion on available surgical approaches, benefits and possible complications, and patient's personal values and expectations [16]. In the following, we will review present trends in male-to-female and female-to-male gender-affirming surgery.

11.4.1 Male-to-Female Sex Reassignment Surgery

Male-to-female gender reassignment surgery can include facial feminization procedures, breast augmentation, and genital surgeries.

11.4.1.1 Facial Feminization

In recent years, facial gender-affirming surgery has received increased attention, and present evidence supports its benefits [33]. There is a substantial difference between female and male craniofacial skeleton and soft tissue, which are mainly evident at the forehead, mandible, nose, and chin. Facial feminization surgery is a group of procedures on bone and soft tissue aimed to change masculine anatomic features to that of feminine features. More commonly utilized procedures include forehead contouring, mandible angle reduction, genioplasty, chondrolaryngoplasty, rhinoplasty, and lip lift [34]. A profound understanding of differences in facial characteristics that convey femininity and masculinity is required for surgeons who perform facial feminization procedures. When comparing females with males, females have softer, rounder, and smaller facial features, while males have more angular and larger facial characteristics [35]. Female hairline tends to be more O-shaped, in contrast to the M-shaped male hairline [34]. The female forehead has little or no brow ridge. Procedures in the forehead involve hairline advancement, brow lift, lateral supraorbital recontouring, and anterior frontal sinus wall setback [36]. The female nose tends to be smaller and shorter, with a more projected tip, and a more obtuse nasofrontal angle. Standard operative rhinoplasty approaches may be sufficient to affect the desired changes [24]. Females have wider zygomatic bones with prominent malar eminences and narrow chin, making a more heart-shaped and rounder face compared to square male face. To achieve these feminine characteristics, mandibular angle reduction and genioplasty narrowing may be performed [37]. The lips are typically fuller, with a lesser distance from the nasal base to the vermillion border in females than in males. Lip feminization approaches include lip augmentation using fat, fillers, or fascia and removing a piece of skin below the nose [37]. More prominent thyroid cartilage in males can be modified by tracheal shave or chondrolaryngoplasty. During these procedures, a superior V-shaped portion of the thyroid cartilage is excised, and, if necessary, submental adipose tissue can also be removed while dissecting [34, 37].

11.4.1.2 Breast Augmentation

Breast augmentation is a common procedure, which is desired in transfeminine individuals. Previous studies demonstrated a direct and consistent enhancement in general satisfaction and body image satisfaction following this procedure [16]. The most commonly used approach is to modify breast size and shape by breast implant. Fat transfer could be an adjunct or alternative surgical procedure [38]. Estrogen is often administered in conjugation with androgen blockers such as spironolactone, which have breast-enhancing effects, for about 6–12 months before surgical breast augmentation [39].

11.4.1.3 Male-to-Female Sex Reassignment

Genital sex reassignment surgery in transgender women may involve bilateral orchiectomy, gender-confirming vulvoplasty, and vaginoplasty. The most frequently performed surgical procedure and the gold standard of vaginoplasty in feminizing genital surgery is penile-inversion vaginoplasty [40, 41]. In this procedure, pedicled inverted penile skin flap will form a neovaginal cavity. Neovaginal cavity is created between the urethra and rectum [40]. In some cases, the penile skin flap is insufficient to cover the whole canal. Accordingly, the scrotal skin graft is augmented to form the distal and/or posterior wall of the neovagina [42]. Another novel technique for vaginoplasty is cultured autologous oral epithelial cells [43]. In addition to forming and lining a neovaginal canal, vaginoplasty may comprise urethral shortening, penectomy, clitoroplasty, and labiaplasty [31]. There are various subtypes of vaginoplasty, based on the way the neovaginal canal is lined. Other choices are intestinal vaginoplasty, skin graft vaginoplasty, or peritoneal vaginoplasty [41, 44]. The labia majora and minora are created from the scrotum. Clitoroplasty is performed using the glans penis while preserving its neurosensory supply [45]. In order to avoid urological complications like urethral stricture and urinary incontinence, the prostate is not removed as a part of genital sex reassignment surgery [46].

11.4.2 Female-to-Male Gender Reassignment Surgery

Female-to-male gender reassignment surgeries comprised facial masculinization, chest reconstruction, and genital surgeries.

11.4.2.1 Facial Masculinization

Compared with facial feminization, present data on facial masculinization approaches are minimal [10]. The available techniques commonly use cadaveric or autologous costal cartilages, fat grafts, or exogenous implants and are augmentative in nature [47]. Although some transgender individuals may achieve the desired facial appearance using hormonal therapy alone, in many individuals the resulting changes do not provide the desired degree of masculinization. A few examples of frontal cranioplasty approaches involve forehead augmentation with methyl methacrylate or polyethylene orbitofrontal implant to increase frontal bossing [48, 49]. Another facial masculinization surgical approach is rhinoplasty. To achieve a masculine nose, some procedures like tip counter rotation and techniques for greater tip projection, dorsal augmentation, and increasing tip and dorsal width can be applied. During midface contouring, the buccal fat pad is removed, and autologous fat is transplanted over the zygoma for superolateral cheek augmentation [47]. Mandibular angle implants can be placed to create a square jaw [50], and laryngeal prominence can be augmented to create a modestly sized and visible Adam's apple using rib cartilage [51]. Favorable masculine facial norms can be reached using these procedures. Nevertheless, further research is required on surgical techniques and long-term outcomes of masculinizing craniofacial surgeries in transgender individuals.

11.4.2.2 Chest Reconstruction

One of the most common transmasculine surgeries is masculinizing chest surgery, with the goals of forming an aesthetic male nipple areolar complex and creating smooth masculine chest contours [34]. Findings from recent literature demonstrated improved quality of life, satisfaction with appearance and body, and decrease in gender dysphoria in those who have undergone mastectomy [52, 53]. Present guidelines recommend assessment of risk factors related to breast cancer, prior to chest surgeries [11, 16]. Surgical techniques involve transareolar or semicircular incisions to free nipple grafting following mastectomy [54]. Corrective follow-up surgery is occasionally required to manage complications, ptosis, scar alterations, and repositioning of nipple-areolar complex [10].

11.4.2.3 Female-to-Male Sex Reassignment

The aims of female-to-male genital surgery are highly variable and may comprise providing the ability to micturate in the standing position, forming a male-like genitalia, and enabling sexual function with good cosmetic outcomes [55]. Preferably, these goals should be reached with the preservation of sufficient erogenous sensation [56]. Two main options for reconstructive surgical procedures are metoidioplasty and total phalloplasty [57].

Due to concerns about endometrial carcinoma or reproductive tract cancer after exposure to exogenous hormones, healthcare providers should determine the necessity of bilateral salpingo-oophorectomy and hysterectomy [11, 58].

11.4.2.3.1 Metoidioplasty

Metoidioplasty is a demanding surgical procedure that can be performed separately or combined, as a part of single-stage procedure that comprises hysterectomy, salpingo-oophorectomy and vaginectomy, urethroplasty, scrotoplasty with/without insertion of testicular implants, and reconstruction of the neophallus [59]. In this type of procedure, neophallus is created from clitoris, which is hypertrophied by androgen hormone intake prior to surgery. Additionally, the urethra is lengthened to the tip of neophallus, and the scrotum can be made from labia [59]. Techniques of metoidioplasty have been modified multiple times. Some techniques may use genital flaps (e.g., vaginal epithelium flap) or buccal mucosal grafts in order to lengthen the urethra [55, 60]. Metoidioplasty is an alternative to phalloplasty and has the advantage of blood flow conservation and engorgement, as well as intrinsic tactile and erogenous sensation, with no risk of donor site scarring or morbidity [10]. The main limitation of metoidioplasty is that the length of the neophallus is usually short, making it incapable of sexual penetration, and does not produce bulk under clothes [60]. Urethrocutaneous fistula, postvoid dribbling, flap necrosis, and buccal complications have been reported following metoidioplasty [12].

11.4.2.3.2 Phalloplasty

Phalloplasty uses distant flaps to construct phallus. Various types of free flaps have been used in female-to-male phalloplasty, such as radial forearm flap, anterolateral thigh flap, latissimus dorsi flap, different abdominal wall flaps, scapular free flap, free deltoid flap, tensor fasciae latae, free sensate osteocutaneous fibula flap, dorsalis pedis flap, and deep epigastric artery perforator flap [59]. Presently, radial forearm free-flap phalloplasty has been proposed as the gold standard phalloplasty surgical procedure [57]. Radial forearm has a consistent anatomy with relatively thin and supple tissue enabling the flap to be easily shaped and tubed to form neourethra and phallus. Forearm is relatively hairless and has various nerves available for coaptation [61]. An erectile device is usually implanted within neophallus following phalloplasty, for sufficient rigidity during penetrative intercourse [62]. Complications include urethral fistula, urethral stricture, partial or total flap loss, and donor site morbidity [12, 63].

11.5 Mental Health Considerations in Transgender Individuals

Transgender and nonbinary individuals are disproportionately affected by outcomes related to poor mental health as a result of increased discrimination and stigma in addition to decreased social support [64]. Transgender youth are at higher risk of life-threatening behaviors and internalizing disorders [65]. Several studies on transgender youth have demonstrated an increased prevalence of psychological distress, major depressive episodes, anxiety disorder, self-harm, suicidal ideation, and suicide attempts [66–71]. Transgender youth experience both internal and external stressors, which can impair their mental health [72].

11.5.1 External Stressors

Members of many minority groups face external stressors, such as discrimination, peer victimization, rejection, and non-affirmation. Family satisfaction and resilience can have an important influence on the mental health of transgender and binary individuals, particularly for youths. High rates of family rejection place transgender youth at greater risk for disparate mental health outcomes [73]. In other words, family support is associated with a lower risk of psychological distress, self-harm, depression, and anxiety and higher levels of self-esteem, life satisfaction, and resilience among youths and young adults [74]. Another important source of stress for transgender youth is peer and school-based relationships. High rates of verbal harassment, cyberbullying perpetrated, and physical victimization against transgender youth have been reported by studies [75]. Higher rates of discrimination and more difficulties with peers strongly predict impaired psychological functioning in transgender children and adolescents [73, 76, 77]. Non-affirmation of gender is another external stressor facing transgender youth that can result in a particular psychological distress, known as social dysphoria or interpersonal gender dysphoria [78, 79].

11.5.2 Internal Stressors

In addition to external stressors, internal stressors can also negatively affect the mental health of transgender youth. Internal stressors include negative expectations, body dysphoria, identity confusion, internalized transphobia, and identity concealment [80]. Cultural, social, and community stigma influence their beliefs about themselves and their future expectations [72, 79]. They report concerns about future expectations of victimization, discrimination, and rejection [72]. The physical dysphoria as a result of incongruence between their identity and their appearance and/or body also affects mental health of transgender individuals [81].

11.5.3 Interventions

Due to inadequate high-quality data specific to transgender individuals, there is presently no evidence-based intervention for mental health outcomes in transgender individuals. However, present interventions aim to target factors related to mental health function including internal and external stressors, universal risks for psychopathology, and protective factors [82].

Social Support: Social support interventions such as coping skills training, psychoeducation, family support, and promoting positive identity construction improve mental health outcomes [74, 83]. Given the crucial role of family acceptance in positive mental health for transgender youth, family-based interventions are effective in preventing or reducing poor psychological outcomes. Clinical family-based interventions include providing psychoeducation to families, emphasizing the protective role of family support, connecting families to community services and resources, and facilitating access to advocacy [80].

Medical Treatment: Studies reported short-term and long-term benefits of gender-affirming medical care in mental health outcomes [64]. Gender-affirming care is associated with improvement in multiple measures of mental health and psychological functioning. Receipt of gender-affirming hormones, puberty blockers, and gender-affirming surgeries is associated with decreased rates of emotional and behavioral problems, anxiety, depression, and gender dysphoria, in addition to improvement in body satisfaction and general functioning [84–87]. Surgeries such as facial, genital, chest/breast surgeries, voice therapy, and/or hair removal reduce gender dysphoria and improve psychological well-being, quality of life, and self-esteem [74].

Treatment Onset: Among gender-incongruent youth who received medical care, older age and late pubertal stage are associated with poorer mental health, pointing to possible benefits of earlier access to gender-affirming medical interventions [88, 89].

Access to Treatment: Recent studies suggest that access to gender-affirming care is associated with improved mental health among transgender youths [64, 90]. Over a short period, access to pharmacological interventions was shown to be linked to the mitigation of mental health disparities and lower odds of depression, self-harm, and suicide among transgender youths [64]. Similar results were also reported among adults. Access to pubertal suppression intervention during adolescence was associated with favorable mental health outcomes and decreased lifetime suicidal ideation among adults [90].

11.6 Ethical Issues in Gender-Affirming Care

There are several restrictions and issues that influence the treatment of transgender persons. Optimal gender-affirming care includes particular attention to legal and ethical aspects of practice. The main ethical principles are justice, beneficence, non-maleficence, and autonomy [91]. All persons must have the ultimate right to make judgments and independent informed decisions for their treatment [92]. The patient's autonomy can be compromised by exaggerating the benefits of medical interventions and de-emphasizing doubts and risks. Healthcare providers need to detect when the individual has the maturational capacity to consent to irreversible interventions [93]. To ensure non-maleficence and beneficence, healthcare providers should do only good and ensure that the treatment is in the patient's best interest and does not cause physical, psychological, and social sequelae [8]. Presently, there is significant disagreement on how to support transgender children and adolescents. Some public health authorities assert that the risks of youth gender-affirming care and puberty suppression outweigh the benefits and consequently have restricted gender affirmation of adolescents and prioritized psychological interventions as the first line of treatment [94]. One of the main challenges in the medical management of individuals during their transition age is due to the possibility of regret and the risk of infertility after irreversible medical interventions [8]. Limited evidence is available on the long-term consequences of GAHT on future fertility. Accordingly, guidelines recommend highlighting probable infertility and discussing fertility preservation options prior to hormone therapy [11, 16].

11.6.1 Informed Consent

In ethical considerations for transgender individuals, the core principle of patient autonomy is becoming the dominant principle of medical ethics instead of "non-maleficence."

In transgender health, the "informed consent model" is an alternative to the "standard model of care." The standard model of care provided by the WPATH Standards of Care (SoC) emphasizes the importance of gender dysphoria diagnosis by mental health professionals. By contrast, the informed consent model, as a more patient-centered approach, is designed to support autonomy and the patient's capability for understanding and weighing potential treatments, without the necessity of external evaluations by mental health professionals. Rather, this approach facilitates a collaborative choice of the best available treatment through a discussion of benefits and risks by the patient and clinician [95–97]. The concepts of shared decision-making and informed consent are crucial to the healthcare practice, highlighting the importance of the active contribution of patients in their medical care treatments and open and complete disclosure of relevant data by clinicians [97, 98]. For active participation of patients, the ability of decision-making competence is required, which can be translated as the ability to comprehend the pertinent data, perceive the situation and its impacts, communicate a choice, and weigh treatment choices [99].

11.6.1.1 Minimum Age for Treatment

The age at which children and adolescents have the capacity to appropriately give informed consent to such treatments is still in question [100, 101]. The World Health Organization considers adolescents as the second decade of life, from ages 10 to 19 years. The age limit for decision-making rights is recognized as 18 years of age, in most countries. However, the age limit for children and younger adolescents differs greatly across the governments and countries [100]. The most recent version of WPATH SoC (eighth version) removed age-based recommendations, instead, suggesting a more personalized approach and evaluation of the patient's best interest [16]. Generally, pubertal suppression is not recommended earlier than Tanner stage II. Hormone therapy could be initiated during older adolescence, considering long-term outcomes and consequences on fertility within a shared decision-making approach between the patient, physician, and family [102].

11.6.1.2 Fertility

The Endocrine Society recommends gender-affirming surgeries that affect fertility (e.g., hysterectomy or gonadectomy) should be delayed until the patient is at least at the legal age of majority in his/her country. Gender-affirming surgeries that do not affect fertility like breast surgery can be considered on a case-by-case basis [16]. The previous version of the WPATH standard of care (SoC7) also recommended performing genital surgery, at least when the patient reached the legal age of adulthood [103].

11.7 Knowledge Gaps and Future Directions

In the past decades, notable advancement has been achieved regarding our knowledge of transgender and nonbinary individuals, but rigorous investigation remains limited.

Puberty suppression and cross-sex hormone therapy are relatively new and require long-term longitudinal follow-up studies investigating long-term outcomes of pubertal blockers and GnRHas on bone health, neurocognition, and fertility [65].

Well-designed randomized controlled trials would investigate the superiority of available therapies. For instance, they would assess the efficacy of sublingual or intramuscular estrogens, with or without progestogens, as feminizing treatment and its impact on psychological and physical health [4].

Similar to hormonal therapies, there is a knowledge gap regarding standardized surgical approaches. Male-to-female surgery has been partly standardized, but additional refinements are required to improve outcomes. On the other hand, in female-to-male surgery, the optimal technique of surgery has not yet been achieved, and complications are more frequent [55]. Moreover, surgeons might be challenged by varying expectations of transgender individuals. The collaboration of medical professionals in making proper diagnoses, selecting appropriate candidates, and determining the optimal timing and type of surgery can effectively reduce surgical complications, fulfill patient expectations, and minimize dissatisfaction and regret [55]. Since revision surgery is commonly required, long-term follow-up studies investigating outcomes and satisfaction rates are severely lacking, particularly in female-to-male gender-affirming surgeries [10, 44].

Another notable challenge in this field is fertility preservation, specifically for those who undergo puberty suppression. Although promising novel findings reported that in vivo maturation of oocytes can be achieved in the clinical setting, further investigation is required for both transgender women and transgender men [65, 104]. In addition to fertility, gender-affirming medical care can influence sexual function. One major gap in the present literature is regarding sexual health and satisfaction. Most studies only focus on sexual functioning and ignore sexual satisfaction [105]. Future research ideally should address the mentioned knowledge gaps, including multicenter standardized prospective design, with sufficient sample size.

References

1. Hirschfeld M. Was muss das Volk vom Dritten Geschlecht wissen. Leipzig: Verlag Max Spohr; 1901.
2. Bullough VL. Transsexualism in history. Arch Sex Behav. 1975;4(5):561–71. https://doi.org/10.1007/bf01542134.
3. Gary B, Nastasja De G, Bernadette W, Polly C. Assessment and support of children and adolescents with gender dysphoria. Arch Dis Child. 2018;103(7):631. https://doi.org/10.1136/archdischild-2018-314992.
4. D'Hoore L, T'Sjoen G. Gender-affirming hormone therapy: an updated literature review with an eye on the future. J Intern Med. 2022;291(5):574–92. https://doi.org/10.1111/joim.13441.
5. Winter S, Diamond M, Green J, Karasic D, Reed T, Whittle S, et al. Transgender people: health at the margins of society. Lancet. 2016;388(10042):390–400. https://doi.org/10.1016/s0140-6736(16)00683-8.
6. Goodman M, Adams N, Corneil T, Kreukels B, Motmans J, Coleman E. Size and distribution of transgender and gender nonconforming populations: a narrative review. Endocrinol Metab Clin N Am. 2019;48(2):303–21. https://doi.org/10.1016/j.ecl.2019.01.001.
7. Wiepjes CM, Nota NM, de Blok CJM, Klaver M, de Vries ALC, Wensing-Kruger SA, et al. The Amsterdam cohort of gender dysphoria study (1972–2015): trends in prevalence, treatment, and regrets. J Sex Med. 2018;15(4):582–90. https://doi.org/10.1016/j.jsxm.2018.01.016.
8. Bizic MR, Jeftovic M, Pusica S, Stojanovic B, Duisin D, Vujovic S, et al. Gender dysphoria: bioethical aspects of medical treatment. Biomed Res Int. 2018;2018:1.
9. de Castro Peraza ME, Lorenzo Rocha N-D, García Acosta JM, Díez Fernández O, Rodríguez Novo N, Pérez Ramos A, et al. Benefits of early social transition in transgender minors. Family perspectives: qualitative study. Rev Esp Salud Publica. 2023;97:e202301007.
10. Morrison SD, Chen ML, Crane CN. An overview of female-to-male gender-confirming surgery. Nat Rev Urol. 2017;14(8):486–500. https://doi.org/10.1038/nrurol.2017.64.
11. Hembree WC, Cohen-Kettenis PT, Gooren L, Hannema SE, Meyer WJ, Murad MH, et al. Endocrine treatment of gender-dysphoric/gender-incongruent persons: an Endocrine Society* clinical practice guideline. J Clin Endocrinol Metabol. 2017;102(11):3869–903. https://doi.org/10.1210/jc.2017-01658.
12. Hadj-Moussa M, Agarwal S, Ohl DA, Kuzon WM. Masculinizing genital gender confirmation surgery. Sexual Medicine Reviews. 2019;7(1):141–55. https://doi.org/10.1016/j.sxmr.2018.06.004.
13. Amengual T, Kunstman K, Lloyd RB, Janssen A, Wescott AB. Readiness assessments for gender-affirming surgical treatments: a systematic scoping review of historical practices and changing ethical considerations. Front Psych. 2022:13. https://doi.org/10.3389/fpsyt.2022.1006024.
14. Butler G, Graaf ND, Wren B, Carmichael P. Assessment and support of children and adolescents with gender dysphoria. Arch Dis Child. 2018;103(7):631–6. https://doi.org/10.1136/archdischild-2018-314992.

15. American Psychiatric Association D, Association AP. Diagnostic and statistical manual of mental disorders: DSM-5: American psychiatric association Washington, DC; 2013.
16. Coleman E, Radix AE, Bouman WP, Brown GR, de Vries ALC, Deutsch MB, et al. Standards of Care for the Health of transgender and gender diverse people, version 8. Int J Transgend Health. 2022;23(Suppl 1):S1–s259. https://doi.org/10.1080/26895269.2022.2100644.
17. Schagen SEE, Cohen-Kettenis PT, Delemarre-van de Waal HA, Hannema SE. Efficacy and safety of gonadotropin-releasing hormone agonist treatment to suppress puberty in gender dysphoric adolescents. J Sex Med. 2016;13(7):1125–32. https://doi.org/10.1016/j.jsxm.2016.05.004.
18. Bangalore Krishna K, Fuqua JS, Rogol AD, Klein KO, Popovic J, Houk CP, et al. Use of gonadotropin-releasing hormone analogs in children: update by an international consortium. Horm Res Paediatr. 2019;91(6):357–72.
19. Claahsen-van der Grinten H, Verhaak C, Steensma T, Middelberg T, Roeffen J, Klink D. Gender incongruence and gender dysphoria in childhood and adolescence – current insights in diagnostics, management, and follow-up. Eur J Pediatr. 2021;180(5):1349–57. https://doi.org/10.1007/s00431-020-03906-y.
20. Chantrapanichkul P, Stevenson MO, Suppakitjanusant P, Goodman M, Tangpricha V. Serum hormone concentrations in transgender individuals receiving gender-affirming hormone therapy: a longitudinal retrospective cohort study. Endocr Pract. 2021;27(1):27–33. https://doi.org/10.4158/ep-2020-0414.
21. Spratt DI, Stewart II, Savage C, Craig W, Spack NP, Chandler DW, et al. Subcutaneous injection of testosterone is an effective and preferred alternative to intramuscular injection: demonstration in female-to-male transgender patients. J Clin Endocrinol Metab. 2017;102(7):2349–55. https://doi.org/10.1210/jc.2017-00359.
22. Cunha FS, Domenice S, Sircili MHP, Mendonca BB, Costa EMF. Low estrogen doses normalize testosterone and estradiol levels to the female range in transgender women. Clinics. 2018;73:73.
23. Meyer G, Mayer M, Mondorf A, Flügel AK, Herrmann E, Bojunga J. Safety and rapid efficacy of guideline-based gender-affirming hormone therapy: an analysis of 388 individuals diagnosed with gender dysphoria. Eur J Endocrinol. 2020;182(2):149–56. https://doi.org/10.1530/eje-19-0463.
24. Moore E, Wisniewski A, Dobs A. Endocrine treatment of transsexual people: a review of treatment regimens, outcomes, and adverse effects. J Clin Endocrinol Metab. 2003;88(8):3467–73. https://doi.org/10.1210/jc.2002-021967.
25. Pelusi C, Costantino A, Martelli V, Lambertini M, Bazzocchi A, Ponti F, et al. Effects of three different testosterone formulations in female-to-male transsexual persons. J Sex Med. 2014;11(12):3002–11. https://doi.org/10.1111/jsm.12698.
26. Vaccaro CJ, Karageuzian SA, McFadden E. The importance of safely prescribing hormones in the transgender community. Cureus. 2023;15(9):e44639. https://doi.org/10.7759/cureus.44639.
27. T'Sjoen G, Arcelus J, De Vries ALC, Fisher AD, Nieder TO, Özer M, et al. European Society for Sexual Medicine position statement "assessment and hormonal Management in Adolescent and Adult Trans People, with attention for sexual function and satisfaction". J Sex Med. 2020;17(4):570–84. https://doi.org/10.1016/j.jsxm.2020.01.012.
28. Iuliano S, Izzo G, Zagari MC, Vergine M, Brunetti FS, Brunetti A, et al. Endocrine management of transgender adults: a clinical approach. Sexes. 2021;2(1):104–18.
29. Gooren LJ, Giltay EJ, Bunck MC. Long-term treatment of transsexuals with cross-sex hormones: extensive personal experience. J Clin Endocrinol Metab. 2008;93(1):19–25. https://doi.org/10.1210/jc.2007-1809.
30. Maheshwari A, Nippoldt T, Davidge-Pitts C. An approach to nonsuppressed testosterone in transgender women receiving gender-affirming feminizing hormonal therapy. J Endocr Soc. 2021;5(9):bvab068. https://doi.org/10.1210/jendso/bvab068.

31. Nolan IT, Kuhner CJ, Dy GW. Demographic and temporal trends in transgender identities and gender confirming surgery. Transl Androl Urol. 2019;8(3):184.
32. Arcelus J, Bouman WP, Van Den Noortgate W, Claes L, Witcomb G, Fernandez-Aranda F. Systematic review and meta-analysis of prevalence studies in transsexualism. Eur Psychiatry. 2015;30(6):807–15.
33. Morrison SD, Capitán-Cañadas F, Sánchez-García A, Ludwig DC, Massie JP, Nolan IT, et al. Prospective quality-of-life outcomes after facial feminization surgery: an international multicenter study. Plast Reconstr Surg. 2020;145(6):1499–509. https://doi.org/10.1097/prs.0000000000006837.
34. Van Boerum MS, Salibian AA, Bluebond-Langner R, Agarwal C. Chest and facial surgery for the transgender patient. Transl Androl Urol. 2019;8(3):219–27.
35. Fisher M, Lu SM, Chen K, Zhang B, Di Maggio M, Bradley JP. Facial feminization surgery changes perception of patient gender. Aesthet Surg J. 2020;40(7):703–9. https://doi.org/10.1093/asj/sjz303.
36. Pansritum K. Forehead and hairline surgery for gender affirmation. Plast Reconstr Surg Glob Open. 2021;9(3)
37. Barnett SL, Choe J, Aiello C, Bradley JP. Facial feminization surgery: anatomical differences, preoperative planning, techniques, and ethical considerations. Medicina. 2023;59(12):2070.
38. Bekeny JC, Zolper EG, Fan KL, Del Corral G. Breast augmentation for transfeminine patients: methods, complications, and outcomes. Gland Surg. 2020;9(3):788–96. https://doi.org/10.21037/gs.2020.03.18.
39. Maycock LB, Kennedy HP. Breast care in the transgender individual. J Midwifery Womens Health. 2014;59(1):74–81. https://doi.org/10.1111/jmwh.12066.
40. Buncamper ME, van der Sluis WB, van der Pas RS, Özer M, Smit JM, Witte BI, et al. Surgical outcome after penile inversion vaginoplasty: a retrospective study of 475 transgender women. Plast Reconstr Surg. 2016;138(5):999–1007.
41. van der Sluis WB, de Nie I, Steensma TD, van Mello NM, Lissenberg-Witte BI, Bouman MB. Surgical and demographic trends in genital gender-affirming surgery in transgender women: 40 years of experience in Amsterdam. Br J Surg. 2022;109(1):8–11. https://doi.org/10.1093/bjs/znab213.
42. Safa B, Lin WC, Salim AM, Deschamps-Braly JC, Poh MM. Current concepts in feminizing gender surgery. Plast Reconstr Surg. 2019;143(5):1081e–91e.
43. Dessy LA, Mazzocchi M, Corrias F, Ceccarelli S, Marchese C, Scuderi N. The use of cultured autologous oral epithelial cells for vaginoplasty in male-to-female transsexuals: a feasibility, safety, and advantageousness clinical pilot study. Plast Reconstr Surg. 2014;133(1):158–61.
44. Morrison SD, Satterwhite T, Grant DW, Kirby J, Laub DR Sr, VanMaasdam J. Long-term outcomes of Rectosigmoid Neocolporrhaphy in male-to-female gender reassignment surgery. Plast Reconstr Surg. 2015;136(2):386–94. https://doi.org/10.1097/prs.0000000000001459.
45. Kanhai RC. Sensate vagina pedicled-spot for male-to-female transsexuals: the experience in the first 50 patients. Aesth Plast Surg. 2016;40:284–7.
46. Trum HW, Hoebeke P, Gooren LJ. Sex reassignment of transsexual people from a gynecologist's and urologist's perspective. Acta Obstet Gynecol Scand. 2015;94(6):563–7.
47. Patel NN, Gulati A, Knott PD, Seth R. Facial masculinization surgery. Oper Tech Otolaryngol Head Neck Surg. 2023;34(1):69–73. https://doi.org/10.1016/j.otot.2023.01.011.
48. Ousterhout DK. Paul Tessier and facial skeletal masculinization. Ann Plast Surg. 2011;67(6):S10–S5.
49. Afshari A, Nguyen L, Winocour JS. Transgender facial aesthetics and regenerative techniques. In: Plastic and aesthetic regenerative surgery and fat grafting: clinical application and operative techniques. Springer; 2022. p. 799–812.
50. Massenburg BB, Ettinger RE, Morrison SD. Gender-affirming surgery of the mandible: lower jaw feminization and masculinization. Facial Plastic Surg Clin. 2023;31(3):381–92.

51. Deschamps-Braly JC. Approach to feminization surgery and facial masculinization surgery: aesthetic goals and principles of management. J Craniofac Surg. 2019;30(5):1352–8. https://doi.org/10.1097/scs.0000000000005391.
52. van de Grift TC, Elaut E, Cerwenka SC, Cohen-Kettenis PT, Kreukels BP. Surgical satisfaction, quality of life, and their association after gender-affirming surgery: a follow-up study. J Sex Marital Ther. 2018;44(2):138–48.
53. Agarwal CA, Scheefer MF, Wright LN, Walzer NK, Rivera A. Quality of life improvement after chest wall masculinization in female-to-male transgender patients: a prospective study using the BREAST-Q and body uneasiness test. J Plast Reconstr Aesthet Surg. 2018;71(5):651–7. https://doi.org/10.1016/j.bjps.2018.01.003.
54. Monstrey S, Selvaggi G, Ceulemans P, Van Landuyt K, Bowman C, Blondeel P, et al. Chest-wall contouring surgery in female-to-male transsexuals: a new algorithm. Plast Reconstr Surg. 2008;121(3):849–59.
55. Selvaggi G, Bellringer J. Gender reassignment surgery: an overview. Nat Rev Urol. 2011;8(5):274–82.
56. Kocjancic E, Acar O, Talamini S, Schechter L. Masculinizing genital gender-affirming surgery: metoidioplasty and urethral lengthening. Int J Impot Res. 2022;34(2):120–7. https://doi.org/10.1038/s41443-020-0259-z.
57. Spennato S, Ederer IA, Borisov K, Kueenzlen L, Rothenberger J, Kühn S, et al. Radial forearm free flap Phalloplasty in female-to-male transsexuals – a comparison between Gottlieb and Levine's and Chang and Hwang's technique. J Sex Med. 2022;19(4):661–8. https://doi.org/10.1016/j.jsxm.2022.01.004.
58. Mueller A, Gooren L. Hormone-related tumors in transsexuals receiving treatment with cross-sex hormones. Eur J Endocrinol. 2008;159(3):197–202. https://doi.org/10.1530/eje-08-0289.
59. Djordjevic ML. Novel surgical techniques in female to male gender confirming surgery. Transl Androl Urol. 2018;7(4):628–38. https://doi.org/10.21037/tau.2018.03.17.
60. Djordjevic ML, Stojanovic B, Bizic M. Metoidioplasty: techniques and outcomes. Transl Androl Urol. 2019;8(3):248–53. https://doi.org/10.21037/tau.2019.06.12.
61. Akhavan AA, Sandhu S, Ndem I, Ogunleye AA. A review of gender affirmation surgery: what we know, and what we need to know. Surgery. 2021;170(1):336–40. https://doi.org/10.1016/j.surg.2021.02.013.
62. Chiriaco G, Looney A, Christopher AN, Ralph D, Lee WG. Erectile device insertion following phalloplasty in transgender and non-binary individuals assigned female at birth: a narrative review. Int J Impot Res. 2023;35(7):664–71. https://doi.org/10.1038/s41443-023-00764-8.
63. Heston AL, Esmonde NO, Dugi DD III, Berli JU. Phalloplasty: techniques and outcomes. Transl Androl Urol. 2019;8(3):254–65.
64. Tordoff DM, Wanta JW, Collin A, Stepney C, Inwards-Breland DJ, Ahrens K. Mental health outcomes in transgender and nonbinary youths receiving gender-affirming care. JAMA Netw Open. 2022;5(2):e220978. https://doi.org/10.1001/jamanetworkopen.2022.0978.
65. Rosenthal SM. Challenges in the care of transgender and gender-diverse youth: an endocrinologist's view. Nat Rev Endocrinol. 2021;17(10):581–91.
66. Reisner SL, Vetters R, Leclerc M, Zaslow S, Wolfrum S, Shumer D, et al. Mental health of transgender youth in care at an adolescent urban community health center: a matched retrospective cohort study. J Adolesc Health. 2015;56(3):274–9.
67. Kuper LE, Mathews S, Lau M. Baseline mental health and psychosocial functioning of transgender adolescents seeking gender-affirming hormone therapy. J Dev Behav Pediatr. 2019;40(8):589–96.
68. Spack NP, Edwards-Leeper L, Feldman HA, Leibowitz S, Mandel F, Diamond DA, et al. Children and adolescents with gender identity disorder referred to a pediatric medical center. Pediatrics. 2012;129(3):418–25.
69. Olson J, Schrager SM, Belzer M, Simons LK, Clark LF. Baseline physiologic and psychosocial characteristics of transgender youth seeking care for gender dysphoria. J Adolesc Health. 2015;57(4):374–80.

70. Davey A, Arcelus J, Meyer C, Bouman WP. Self-injury among trans individuals and matched controls: prevalence and associated factors. Health Soc Care Community. 2016;24(4):485–94.
71. Veale JF, Watson RJ, Peter T, Saewyc EM. Mental health disparities among Canadian transgender youth. J Adolesc Health. 2017;60(1):44–9.
72. Wittlin NM, Kuper LE, Olson KR. Mental health of transgender and gender diverse youth. Annu Rev Clin Psychol. 2023;19(1):207–32. https://doi.org/10.1146/annurev-clinpsy-072220-020326.
73. Price-Feeney M, Green AE, Dorison S. Understanding the mental health of transgender and nonbinary youth. J Adolesc Health. 2020;66(6):684–90.
74. Tebbe EA, Budge SL. Factors that drive mental health disparities and promote well-being in transgender and nonbinary people. Nat Rev Psychol. 2022;1(12):694–707. https://doi.org/10.1038/s44159-022-00109-0.
75. Greytak EA, Kosciw JG, Diaz EM. Harsh realities: the experiences of transgender youth in Our Nation's Schools: ERIC; 2009.
76. Sievert ED, Schweizer K, Barkmann C, Fahrenkrug S, Becker-Hebly I. Not social transition status, but peer relations and family functioning predict psychological functioning in a German clinical sample of children with gender dysphoria. Clin Child Psychol Psychiatry. 2021;26(1):79–95.
77. Van Cauwenberg G, Dhondt K, Motmans J. Ten years of experience in counseling gender diverse youth in Flanders, Belgium. A clinical overview. Int J Impot Res. 2021;33(7):671–8.
78. Price-Feeney M, Green AE, Dorison SH. Impact of bathroom discrimination on mental health among transgender and nonbinary youth. J Adolesc Health. 2021;68(6):1142–7.
79. Toomey RB. Advancing research on minority stress and resilience in trans children and adolescents in the 21st century. Child Dev Perspect. 2021;15(2):96–102.
80. Malpas J, Pellicane MJ, Glaeser E. Family-based interventions with transgender and gender expansive youth: systematic review and best practice recommendations. Transgend Health. 2022;7(1):7–29. https://doi.org/10.1089/trgh.2020.0165.
81. Kozee HB, Tylka TL, Bauerband LA. Measuring transgender individuals' comfort with gender identity and appearance: development and validation of the transgender congruence scale. Psychol Women Q. 2012;36(2):179–96. https://doi.org/10.1177/0361684312442161.
82. Coyne CA, Poquiz JL, Janssen A, Chen D. Evidence-based psychological practice for transgender and non-binary youth: defining the need, framework for treatment adaptation, and future directions. Evid-Based Pract Child Adolesc Mental Health. 2020;5(3):340–53. https://doi.org/10.1080/23794925.2020.1765433.
83. Matsuno E, Israel T. The parent support program: development and acceptability of an online intervention aimed at increasing supportive behaviors among parents of trans youth. J GLBT Fam Stud. 2021;17(5):413–31.
84. Chew D, Anderson J, Williams K, May T, Pang K. Hormonal treatment in young people with gender dysphoria: a systematic review. Pediatrics. 2018;141(4)
85. Mahfouda S, Moore JK, Siafarikas A, Hewitt T, Ganti U, Lin A, et al. Gender-affirming hormones and surgery in transgender children and adolescents. Lancet Diabetes Endocrinol. 2019;7(6):484–98.
86. De Vries AL, McGuire JK, Steensma TD, Wagenaar EC, Doreleijers TA, Cohen-Kettenis PT. Young adult psychological outcome after puberty suppression and gender reassignment. Pediatrics. 2014;134(4):696–704.
87. de Vries ALC, Steensma TD, Doreleijers TAH, Cohen-Kettenis PT. Puberty suppression in adolescents with gender identity disorder: a prospective follow-up study. J Sex Med. 2011;8(8):2276–83. https://doi.org/10.1111/j.1743-6109.2010.01943.x.
88. Sorbara JC, Chiniara LN, Thompson S, Palmert MR. Mental health and timing of gender-affirming care. Pediatrics. 2020;146(4)
89. Chen D, Abrams M, Clark L, Ehrensaft D, Tishelman AC, Chan Y-M, et al. Psychosocial characteristics of transgender youth seeking gender-affirming medical treatment: baseline findings from the trans youth care study. J Adolesc Health. 2021;68(6):1104–11.

90. Turban JL, King D, Carswell JM, Keuroghlian AS. Pubertal suppression for transgender youth and risk of suicidal ideation. Pediatrics. 2020;145(2)
91. Varkey B. Principles of clinical ethics and their application to practice. Med Princ Pract. 2021;30(1):17–28. https://doi.org/10.1159/000509119.
92. Guyer P. Kant on the theory and practice of autonomy. Soc Philos Policy. 2003;20(2):70–98.
93. McNamara M, Lepore C, Alstott A, Kamody R, Kuper L, Szilagyi N, et al. Scientific misinformation and gender affirming care: tools for providers on the front lines. J Adolesc Health. 2022;71(3):251–3.
94. Cohn J. Some limitations of "challenges in the Care of Transgender and Gender-Diverse Youth: an endocrinologist's view". J Sex Marital Ther. 2023;49(6):599–615. https://doi.org/10.1080/0092623x.2022.2160396.
95. Cavanaugh T, Hopwood R, Lambert C. Informed consent in the medical care of transgender and gender-nonconforming patients. AMA J Ethics. 2016;18(11):1147–55.
96. Gerritse K, Hartman LA, Bremmer MA, Kreukels BPC, Molewijk BC. Decision-making approaches in transgender healthcare: conceptual analysis and ethical implications. Med Health Care Philos. 2021;24(4):687–99. https://doi.org/10.1007/s11019-021-10023-6.
97. Tomson A. Gender-affirming care in the context of medical ethics–gatekeeping v. informed consent. South Afr J Bioethics Law. 2018;11(1):24–8.
98. Barry MJ, Edgman-Levitan S. Shared decision making – pinnacle of patient-centered care. N Engl J Med. 2012;366(9):780–1. https://doi.org/10.1056/NEJMp1109283.
99. Appelbaum PS. Assessment of patients' competence to consent to treatment. N Engl J Med. 2007;357(18):1834–40.
100. Hein IM, Troost PW, Broersma A, de Vries MC, Daams JG, Lindauer RJL. Why is it hard to make progress in assessing children's decision-making competence? BMC Med Ethics. 2015;16(1):1. https://doi.org/10.1186/1472-6939-16-1.
101. Kimberly LL, Folkers KM, Friesen P, Sultan D, Quinn GP, Bateman-House A, et al. Ethical issues in gender-affirming Care for Youth. Pediatrics. 2018;142(6) https://doi.org/10.1542/peds.2018-1537.
102. Giordano S, Horowicz E. Gender-affirming surgery for transgender adolescents: ethical and legal considerations. Best Pract Res Clin Obstet Gynaecol. 2023;86:102295. https://doi.org/10.1016/j.bpobgyn.2022.102295.
103. Coleman E, Bockting W, Botzer M, Cohen-Kettenis P, DeCuypere G, Feldman J, et al. Standards of Care for the Health of transsexual, transgender, and gender-nonconforming people, version 7. Int J Trans. 2012;13(4):165–232. https://doi.org/10.1080/15532739.2011.700873.
104. Rothenberg SS, Witchel SF, Menke MN. Oocyte cryopreservation in a transgender male adolescent. N Engl J Med. 2019;380(9):886–7. https://doi.org/10.1056/NEJMc1813275.
105. Stephenson R, Riley E, Rogers E, Suarez N, Metheny N, Senda J, et al. The sexual health of transgender men: a scoping review. J Sex Res. 2017;54(4–5):424–45. https://doi.org/10.1080/00224499.2016.1271863.

Chapter 12
Exercise and Endocrine Diseases

Maryam Selk-Ghaffari, Mohammad Hosein Pourgharib Shahi, and Ramin Kordi

12.1 Introduction

Physical activity is defined as any type of bodily movement that is a result of the skeletal muscles' contraction and leads to energy consumption [1]. Exercise is a structured, repetitive, and planned physical activity that results in improvement in physical fitness [1].

Performing regular exercise and physical activity reduces the risk of noncommunicable diseases, including diabetes, cardiovascular disease, cerebrovascular disease, hypertension, breast cancer, and colon cancer [2]. Moreover, performing exercise and physical activity leads to improved mental health, reduces the risk of depression, and postpones the onset of dementia [2]. The American College of Sports Medicine (ACSM) with the main purpose of prescribing exercise as a mandated step in disease prevention and treatment announced Exercise is Medicine (EIM) initiative in 2007 [3].

Long-term benefits of exercise in the cardiovascular system and anti-inflammatory impact of exercise propose exercise as a treatment for inflammatory rheumatic diseases [4]. Skeletal muscles interact with other organs by producing myokine proteins with each exercise session [4]. The anti-inflammatory effect of exercise is related to the released myokines [4]. Additionally, exercise improves tissue regeneration including cardiac regeneration, muscle regeneration, and neural regeneration [5].

The physiologic effect of endocrine hormones consists of a variety of actions including regulation of metabolism, growth and development, hydration status, cardiovascular modifications, reproduction, and immune system function [6]. The role

M. Selk-Ghaffari (✉) · M. H. Pourgharib Shahi · R. Kordi
Sports Medicine Research Center, Neuroscience Institute, Tehran University of Medical Sciences, Tehran, Iran
e-mail: mselkghaffari@sina.tums.ac.ir

H. Gharib et al. (eds.), *Interdisciplinary Advances in Endocrinology*,
https://doi.org/10.1007/978-981-95-2286-6_12

of exercise in the process of production of endocrine hormones and related functions has been demonstrated [6]. Performing a well-structured individualized health-enhancing exercise program will improve the function of endocrine hormones. However, an improper exercise program may have harmful consequences on the health status [6].

Based on the World Health Organization (WHO) 2020 guidelines, children and adolescents are recommended to perform moderate- to vigorous-intensity aerobic exercise lasting at least 60 min per day, during the week [7]. Resistance exercise, bone-strengthening exercise, and vigorous-intensity exercise are recommended for at least 3 days a week [7]. Individuals aged between 18 and 64 years are recommended to perform aerobic exercise with moderate intensity for at least 150–300 min during the week or aerobic exercise with vigorous intensity for at least 75–150 min during the week [7]. Resistance exercises with moderate intensity or higher intensities involving all major muscle groups are recommended for 2 days per week or more [7]. Aerobic exercise recommendations for older individuals aged ≥65 years are similar to recommendation for individuals aged between 18 and 64 years, and resistance exercise and balance training are recommended for 3 or more days per week [7].

In this chapter, we will discuss the evidence regarding exercise prescription in diabetes and special consideration in the general population and professional athletes with diabetes. Also, we will review the existing evidence on exercise and growth hormone levels and thyroid functions.

12.2 Exercise and Diabetes

Engaging in physical activity and exercise has been proven to be beneficial for managing blood glucose levels and general health in the patients with diabetes and prediabetes [8]. The benefits of engaging in physical activity and exercise in individuals with diabetes consist of enhanced glycemic control, reduced insulin resistance, improved cardiorespiratory fitness, better lipid profile, decreased blood pressure, improved vigor, and weight loss maintenance [9]. Engaging in regular exercise has been proposed as a protective factor against the development of type 2 diabetes and also delays its onset [8].

Systematic reviews and meta-analysis evaluating randomized controlled trials have indicated that exercise-based interventions reduced glycated hemoglobin (HbA1C) [10–12] in individuals with type 2 diabetes in comparison to no exercise control groups [10].

Outcomes of aerobic exercise consist of an increase in oxidative enzymes and increase in mitochondrial density and also improved cardiac output and lung function, as well as improved insulin sensitivity and enhanced immune function [8, 13]. Engaging in aerobic exercise results in reduced insulin resistance, improved endothelial function, improved lipid profiles, and enhanced cardiorespiratory fitness in patients with type 1 diabetes [14]. Engaging in aerobic exercise results in reduced triglycerides, blood pressure, HbA1C, and insulin resistance in patients with type 2 diabetes [15]. A higher level of exercise training in individuals with type 1 and type 2 diabetes is associated with reduced overall and cardiovascular mortality [8, 16].

High-intensity interval training (HIIT) is defined as alternating exercise cycles between short-duration episodes of higher and lower exercise intensities [8, 9]. Engaging in HIIT exercise in patients with type 2 diabetes leads to improvement in the oxidative capacity of skeletal muscles, enhanced glycemic control, and insulin sensitivity [8, 17, 18]. HIIT results in higher improvement in cardiorespiratory fitness in individuals with or without diabetes [9, 17, 19].

HIIT exercise is associated with a lower risk of hypoglycemia during the exercise compared to continuous aerobic exercise [9, 20–22].

Engaging in resistance exercise results in improved body composition, improved physical performance, enhanced muscle mass and strength, increased bone mineral density, decreased blood pressure, better mental health, improved lipid levels, and insulin sensitivity in healthy individuals [13]. Individuals with diabetes are at higher risk for decreased muscle strength [23, 24]. Individuals with type 2 diabetes engaging in resistance exercises have indicated improved insulin resistance, better glycemic control, reduced fat mass, increased lean body mass, improved muscular strength, and lower blood pressure [25].

Exercise plays a crucial role in the management and prevention of diabetes. In general, exercise is a powerful tool for individuals with diabetes to manage their condition, reduce diabetes-related complications, improve their overall health, and enhance their quality of life [26]. By incorporating regular physical activity into their daily routine, individuals with diabetes can reap the numerous benefits that exercise has offered. However, exercise and physical activity in individuals with diabetes should be undertaken with special considerations regarding controlling blood glucose level and hydration status. It is important to note that individuals with diabetes should monitor their blood glucose levels before, during, and after exercise to ensure they remain within a safe range. They should also stay hydrated by drinking a sufficient amount of water before, during, and after exercise.

12.3 Exercise Prescription in Diabetes

Exercise training and physical activity is one of the suggested methods in the diabetes prevention and management approaches [27]. The main objective in the management of diabetes is glycemic control which could be achieved via medications, lifestyle modifications including correction of diet, and engaging in exercise and physical activity. Accurate and precise blood glucose control reduces the probability of the development and progression of diabetes complications.

Exercise testing is not needed in patients with diabetes who are asymptomatic for cardiovascular diseases and plan to start a light- to moderate-intensity exercise program. The American College of Sports Medicine (ACSM) recommends that sedentary individuals with diabetes should obtain a medical clearance prior to starting any intensity of exercise program. However, the *American* Diabetes Association (ADA) states that no medical clearance is required for patients with diabetes who are asymptomatic for cardiovascular diseases and are planning to start a light- to moderate-intensity exercise program [28].

It is recommended that individuals with type 1 and type 2 diabetes perform a combination of aerobic and resistance exercise [28]. Moderate- to vigorous-intensity aerobic exercise for 3–7 days per week including rhythmic, prolonged physical activities using large muscle groups (e.g., cycling, walking, swimming) as continuous physical activity or high-intensity interval training is recommended. The recommended duration of moderate- to vigorous-intensity aerobic exercise is 150 min per week [28]. Moderate- to vigorous-intensity resistance exercise is recommended for at least 2 nonconsecutive days per week. Resistance exercise is advised to consist of a minimum of eight to ten exercises with one to three sets of 10–15 repetitions to near fatigue per set using free weights, resistance machines, resistance bands, and/or body weight [28]. Balance and flexibility exercises are recommended for at least 2–3 days per week. Light- to moderate-intensity balance training with any duration is recommended. Static or dynamic flexibility exercises are advised. Static stretches are recommended to be held for 10–30 s as two to four repetitions for each exercise [28].

Occurrence of hypoglycemic episodes during exercise (blood glucose level < 70 mg • dL − 1) is the main concern in individuals with diabetes using insulin or oral hypoglycemic medications which enhance the secretion of insulin [8]. Common hypoglycemia symptoms consist of weakness, shakiness, abnormal sweating, anxiety, nervousness, tingling of the fingers, headache, mental dullness, visual disturbances, confusion, seizures, amnesia, and coma [28]. Fast reduction in blood glucose levels in exercise and physical activity might induce the symptoms even in blood glucose >70 mg • dL − 1. On the other hand, a decrease in blood glucose levels might not produce the obvious hypoglycemia symptoms defined as hypoglycemic unawareness which should be considered [28]. Patients with diabetes using insulin or insulin-related medications should measure blood glucose levels prior to, during (if required), and following the training session. Recommended pre-exercise blood glucose levels are between 90 and 250 mg • dL − 1 (5.0 and 13.9 mmol • L − 1). Consuming carbohydrate snacks and adjustment of the medication is required in hypo- and hyperglycemia [28]. Urine ketones should be evaluated in the blood glucose levels above 250 mg • dL − 1, and the detection of ketones in the urine is the indication of cancelling the training [8, 28]. If blood sugar levels are above 350 mg • dL − 1 (≥19.4 mmol • L − 1), termination of the training session is mandated [28].

12.4 Exercise and Professional Athletes with Diabetes

Overall, individuals with type 1 diabetes have the ability to engage in any types of sports, including high-intensity sports or competitive sports [29]. Nevertheless, sports that enhance the probability of impaired consciousness or damaged judgment as a result of hypoglycemia including extreme climbing, diving, high-altitude ski touring, parachuting, hang gliding, and water canoeing are not recommended [29]. Engaging in the mentioned sports needs particularly cautious behavior, numerous years of personal experience, individualized preparation programs, and working out [29].

Long-standing diabetes-related complications must be evaluated prior to starting a sport [30]. According to the existing complications, exercise modification is mandated. Delayed or immediate exercise-induced hypoglycemia is the main challenge in athletes with diabetes consuming oral insulin secretagogues medication or insulin [30]. It has been proposed that doing strengthening exercises prior to aerobic exercise results in a reduced risk of exercise-induced hypoglycemia [31]. Individuals with insulin-dependent diabetes are recommended to consume carbohydrates prior to and following exercise. In exercise sessions with a duration longer than 60 minutes, athletes should consume carbohydrate snacks during the exercise session. Another solution to prevent exercise-induced hypoglycemia in athletes using insulin is the adjustment of insulin dose. Athletes using insulin are recommended to measure their blood sugar prior, during, and following exercise sessions [30]. Recommended blood glucose levels before exercise are between 90 and 250 mg • dL − 1 (5.0 and 13.9 mmol • L − 1). Using carbohydrate snacks and modification of the medication should be considered if needed [28], since the exercise-induced stress might aggravate the hyperglycemia and result in ketoacidosis [30]. If blood glucose levels are ≥250 mg • dL − 1 (13.9 mmol • L − 1) prior to the exercise session, assessment of urine ketones is mandated. If the ketones in urine are detected and the blood glucose levels are ≥250 mg • dL − 1, the exercise session should be postponed [8, 28].

If blood sugar levels are ≥350 mg • dL − 1 (≥19.4 mmol • L − 1), the exercise session should be postponed, and insulin therapy is mandated prior to exercise. Athletes should be aware and educated regarding the symptoms of hypoglycemia and consume rapidly absorbable glucose if any symptoms are detected. Exercise and physical activity is a vital component of diabetes management. Recreational and elite athletes receiving proper education regarding precautions can safely contribute to sports [30].

12.5 Exercise and Growth Hormone

Growth hormone (GH) secretion has a pulsatile style according to a circadian rhythm. Exercise and sleep are the main physiologic determinants of GH secretion [32]. Exercise and physical activity stimulate GH secretion in both children and adults [33]. The mechanisms suggested for exercise-related GH release consist of direct stimulation by catecholamines, lactate, and nitric oxide, neural input, decreased production of somatostatin, increased production of growth hormone-releasing hormone (GHRH), and alterations in acid–base balance [32]. The amount of GH released in response to exercise depends on a number of factors, including the intensity of exercise, duration, and type of exercise [33]. Moderate- to vigorous-intensity aerobic exercises and resistance exercises both lead to a substantial, acute rise in GH secretion [33]. Exercise intensity and the amount of the amplified GH secretion have indicated a linear association. The GH response to exercise can be blunted by several factors including older age, obesity, diabetes, and medications such as corticosteroids which can suppress GH secretion. Young female individuals indicate a higher increase in GH secretion in comparison to young male individuals in response to exercise. Older individuals' GH secretion in response to exercise is lower at four- to sevenfold in comparison to younger individuals. Individuals with diabetes and obesity and who consume corticosteroids indicate lower increases in exercise-induced GH release [33]. Following a single bout of aerobic exercise, GH secretion transiently decreases. Consequently, GH concentrations in 24 hours are not usually raised with a single episode of training. Nevertheless, repeated episodes of aerobic training during 24 hours lead to augmented GH release [33]. Resistance training has indicated significant exercise-induced GH release. Intensity and frequency are the main determinants of the amount of GH secretion [32]. Several studies have shown that high-intensity interval training (HIIT) can effectively increase GH levels, particularly when performed at intensities close to maximal effort [34, 35].

12.6 Exercise and Thyroid Function

The existing data on the effect of exercise on thyroid functions are inconsistent. In some studies, it has been demonstrated that exercise with short duration at intensity exceeding lactate threshold or 60% maximal oxygen uptake (VO2max) leads to an increase in TSH levels [36, 37]. As a result of this increase in TSH, total and free T4 levels increase. Also, a reduction in total and free T3 is detected [36]. The suggested mechanism is exercise-related hemoconcentration including thyroid-binding globulin concentration in vascular space [37]. Exercise-related reduction detected in total and free T3 might be due to increased uptake of target tissues or reduced production

[37]. The inconsistency in various studies' results might be due to the required delay to have the effect of the exercise on the secretion of thyroid hormones [37].

Studies assessing the effect of submaximal exercises longer than 60 min on thyroid function have indicated inconsistent results. Some studies have indicated no effect on TSH level [38]. However, some studies have indicated progressive increase in TSH or free T3 levels by nearly 40 minutes of exercise. Some studies have reported reaching a steady-state plateau in T3 or TSH levels by nearly 40 min of exercise [37].

Exercise has various effects on the peripheral metabolism of the thyroid hormones and the pituitary–thyroid axis [39]. Parameters affecting the variability in exercise effect on thyroid function consist of age, nutritional status, present fitness level, altitude, and ambient temperature [39]. Simultaneously, the duration, type, intensity, and frequency of the exercise affect the exercise-induced results [39]. The most constant impact of the exercise on the pituitary–thyroid axis consists of an increase in reverse T3 [39].

In a systematic review by Duñabeitia et al., the effect of exercise on patients with hypothyroidism was investigated [40]. The majority of the participants in the studies consisted of female individuals with subclinical hypothyroidism. The studies which were evaluated indicated low to moderate methodological quality. Physical and mental health of the individuals with hypothyroidism performing aerobic and resistance exercises indicated improvement [40]. Results of the meta-analysis indicated no significant effect of exercise on TSH, free T3, and free T4 levels in individuals with hypothyroidism [40]. In individuals with hyperthyroidism consuming medication, resistance exercises improve the skeletal muscle performance recovery and support weight gain via lean body mass improvement [41].

12.7 Conclusion

Exercise has indicated benefits in controlling blood glucose and improving general health in individuals with diabetes and prediabetes. The benefits of performing exercise in individuals with diabetes consist of reduced insulin resistance, improved glycemic control, improved cardiorespiratory fitness, better lipid profile, decreased blood pressure, improved vigor, and weight loss maintenance. Engaging in aerobic, resistance, and balance exercises in general population and athletes with diabetes is recommended. However, exercise requires special consideration regarding blood glucose level control prior to, during, and following exercise sessions.

Exercise and physical activity have been proposed as one of the main physiologic stimulators of growth hormone secretion in both children and adults. The studies regarding exercise's effect on thyroid function have indicated controversy. However, improved physical and mental health of individuals with hypothyroidism has been demonstrated by exercise.

References

1. Norton K, Norton L, Sadgrove D. Position statement on physical activity and exercise intensity terminology. J Sci Med Sport. 2010;13(5):496–502.
2. Guthold R, Stevens GA, Riley LM, Bull FC. Worldwide trends in insufficient physical activity from 2001 to 2016: a pooled analysis of 358 population-based surveys with 1·9 million participants. Lancet Glob Health. 2018;6(10):e1077–e86.
3. Thompson WR, Sallis R, Joy E, Jaworski CA, Stuhr RM, Trilk JL. Exercise is medicine. Am J Lifestyle Med. 2020;14(5):511–23.
4. Benatti FB, Pedersen BK. Exercise as an anti-inflammatory therapy for rheumatic diseases – myokine regulation. Nat Rev Rheumatol. 2015;11(2):86–97.
5. Liu C, Wu X, Vulugundam G, Gokulnath P, Li G, Xiao J. Exercise promotes tissue regeneration: mechanisms involved and therapeutic scope. Sports Med Open. 2023;9(1):27.
6. Hackney AC, Lane AR. Exercise and the regulation of endocrine hormones. In: Progress in molecular biology and translational science, vol. 135; 2015. p. 293–311.
7. Bull FC, Al-Ansari SS, Biddle S, Borodulin K, Buman MP, Cardon G, et al. World Health Organization 2020 guidelines on physical activity and sedentary behaviour. Br J Sports Med. 2020;54(24):1451–62.
8. Colberg SR, Sigal RJ, Yardley JE, Riddell MC, Dunstan DW, Dempsey PC, et al. Physical activity/exercise and diabetes: a position statement of the American Diabetes Association. Diabetes Care. 2016;39(11):2065.
9. Sigal RJ, Armstrong MJ, Bacon SL, Boule NG, Dasgupta K, Kenny GP, et al. Physical activity and diabetes. Can J Diabetes. 2018;42:S54–63.
10. Umpierre D, Ribeiro PA, Kramer CK, Leitao CB, Zucatti AT, Azevedo MJ, et al. Physical activity advice only or structured exercise training and association with HbA1c levels in type 2 diabetes: a systematic review and meta-analysis. JAMA. 2011;305(17):1790–9.
11. Umpierre D, Ribeiro P, Schaan B, Ribeiro J. Volume of supervised exercise training impacts glycaemic control in patients with type 2 diabetes: a systematic review with meta-regression analysis. Diabetologia. 2013;56:242–51.
12. Liubaoerjijin Y, Terada T, Fletcher K, Boulé NG. Effect of aerobic exercise intensity on glycemic control in type 2 diabetes: a meta-analysis of head-to-head randomized trials. Acta Diabetol. 2016;53:769–81.
13. Garber CE, Blissmer B, Deschenes MR, Franklin BA, Lamonte MJ, et al. Quantity and quality of exercise for developing and maintaining cardiorespiratory, musculoskeletal, and neuromotor fitness in apparently healthy adults: guidance for prescribing exercise. Med Sci Sports Exerc. 2011;43:1334–59.
14. Chimen M, Kennedy A, Nirantharakumar K, Pang T, Andrews R, Narendran P. What are the health benefits of physical activity in type 1 diabetes mellitus? A literature review. Diabetologia. 2012;55:542–51.
15. Snowling NJ, Hopkins WG. Effects of different modes of exercise training on glucose control and risk factors for complications in type 2 diabetic patients: a meta-analysis. Diabetes Care. 2006;29(11):2518–27.
16. Sluik D, Buijsse B, Muckelbauer R, Kaaks R, Teucher B, Tj A, et al. Physical activity and mortality in individuals with diabetes mellitus: a prospective study and meta-analysis. Arch Intern Med. 2012;172(17):1285–95.
17. Jelleyman C, Yates T, O'Donovan G, Gray LJ, King JA, Khunti K, et al. The effects of high-intensity interval training on glucose regulation and insulin resistance: a meta-analysis. Obes Rev. 2015;16(11):942–61.
18. Little JP, Gillen JB, Percival ME, Safdar A, Tarnopolsky MA, Punthakee Z, et al. Low-volume high-intensity interval training reduces hyperglycemia and increases muscle mitochondrial capacity in patients with type 2 diabetes. J Appl Physiol. 2011;111(6):1554–60.

19. Weston KS, Wisløff U, Coombes JS. High-intensity interval training in patients with lifestyle-induced cardiometabolic disease: a systematic review and meta-analysis. Br J Sports Med. 2014;48:1227–34.
20. Bally L, Zueger T, Buehler T, Dokumaci AS, Speck C, Pasi N, et al. Metabolic and hormonal response to intermittent high-intensity and continuous moderate intensity exercise in individuals with type 1 diabetes: a randomised crossover study. Diabetologia. 2016;59:776–84.
21. Moser O, Tschakert G, Mueller A, Groeschl W, Pieber TR, Obermayer-Pietsch B, et al. Effects of high-intensity interval exercise versus moderate continuous exercise on glucose homeostasis and hormone response in patients with type 1 diabetes mellitus using novel ultra-long-acting insulin. PLoS One. 2015;10(8):e0136489.
22. Iscoe K, Riddell M. Continuous moderate-intensity exercise with or without intermittent high-intensity work: effects on acute and late glycaemia in athletes with type 1 diabetes mellitus. Diabet Med. 2011;28(7):824–32.
23. Nishitani M, Shimada K, Sunayama S, Masaki Y, Kume A, Fukao K, et al. Impact of diabetes on muscle mass, muscle strength, and exercise tolerance in patients after coronary artery bypass grafting. J Cardiol. 2011;58(2):173–80.
24. Anton SD, Karabetian C, Naugle K, Buford TW. Obesity and diabetes as accelerators of functional decline: can lifestyle interventions maintain functional status in high risk older adults? Exp Gerontol. 2013;48(9):888–97.
25. Gordon B, Benson A, Bird S, Fraser S. Resistance training improves metabolic health in type 2 diabetes: a systematic review. Diabetes Res Clin Pract. 2009;83(2):157–75.
26. Kirwan JP, Sacks J, Nieuwoudt S. The essential role of exercise in the management of type 2 diabetes. Cleve Clin J Med. 2017;84(7 Suppl 1):S15.
27. Hassabi M, Esteghamati A, Halabchi F, Abedi-Yekta AH, Mahdaviani B, Hassanmirzaie B, et al. Iranian National Clinical Practice Guideline for exercise in patients with diabetes. Int J Endocrinol Metab. 2021;19(3)
28. Liguori G. ACSM'S guidelines for exercise testing and prescription. Lippincott Williams & Wilkins; 2020.
29. Esefeld K, Kress S, Behrens M, Zimmer P, Stumvoll M, Thurm U, et al. Diabetes, sports and exercise. Exp Clin Endocrinol Diabetes. 2021;129(01):S52–S9.
30. Shugart C, Jackson J, Fields KB. Diabetes in sports. Sports Health. 2010;2(1):29–38.
31. Yardley JE, Kenny GP, Perkins BA, Riddell MC, Malcolm J, Boulay P, et al. Effects of performing resistance exercise before versus after aerobic exercise on glycemia in type 1 diabetes. Diabetes Care. 2012;35(4):669–75.
32. Godfrey RJ, Madgwick Z, Whyte GP. The exercise-induced growth hormone response in athletes. Sports Med. 2003;33:599–613.
33. Wideman L, Weltman JY, Hartman ML, Veldhuis JD, Weltman A. Growth hormone release during acute and chronic aerobic and resistance exercise: recent findings. Sports Med. 2002;32:987–1004.
34. Avazpour S, Kalkhoran JF, Avazpour K, Mohseni F. The effect of two types of high-intensity interval training on serum value of GH and IGF-1 in overweight nurses. Asian J Sports Med. 2020;11(4)
35. Wahl P, Zinner C, Achtzehn S, Bloch W, Mester J. Effect of high-and low-intensity exercise and metabolic acidosis on levels of GH, IGF-I, IGFBP-3 and cortisol. Growth Hormon IGF Res. 2010;20(5):380–5.
36. Ciloglu F, Peker I, Pehlivan A, Karacabey K, İlhan N, Saygin O, et al. Exercise intensity and its effects on thyroid hormones. Neuroendocrinol Lett. 2005;26(6):830–4.
37. Hackney AC, Saeidi A. The thyroid axis, prolactin, and exercise in humans. Curr Opin Endocr Metab Res. 2019;9:45–50.
38. Berchtold P, Berger M, Cüppers H, Herrmann J, Nieschlag E, Rudorff K, et al. Non-glucoregulatory hormones (T4, T3, rT3, TSH, testosterone) during physical exercise in juvenile-type diabetics. Horm Metab Res. 1978;10(04):269–73.

39. Klubo-Gwiezdzinska J, Bernet VJ, Wartofsky L. Exercise and thyroid function. In: Endocrinology of physical activity and sport. 2nd ed; 2013. p. 85–119.
40. Duñabeitia I, González-Devesa D, Varela-Martínez S, Diz-Gómez JC, Ayán-Pérez C. Effect of physical exercise in people with hypothyroidism: systematic review and meta-analysis. Scand J Clin Lab Invest. 2023:1–10.
41. Bousquet-Santos K, Vaisman M, Barreto ND, Cruz-Filho RA, Salvador BA, Frontera WR, et al. Resistance training improves muscle function and body composition in patients with hyperthyroidism. Arch Phys Med Rehabil. 2006;87(8):1123–30.

MIX
Papier aus verantwortungsvollen Quellen
Paper from responsible sources
FSC® C105338
FSC
www.fsc.org

If you have any concerns about our products,
you can contact us on
ProductSafety@springernature.com

In case Publisher is established outside the EU,
the EU authorized representative is:
Springer Nature Customer Service Center GmbH
Europaplatz 3, 69115 Heidelberg, Germany

Printed by Libri Plureos GmbH
in Hamburg, Germany